MANUAL

— OF —

FIRST AID

Professional English

MANUAL

— OF —

FIRST AID

Professional English

Part 3—Case Studies

IRENA BAUMRUKOVÁ

To order additional copies of this book, contact:
Xlibris
800-056-3182
www.Xlibrispublishing.co.uk
Orders@Xlibrispublishing.co.uk
750239

Contents

The second volume (revision lessons) is divided into 24 units, each of which contains about 20 casuistics on different topics.

Bibliography

Cambridge English Pronouncing Dictionary. 17th ed. Cambridge University Press. 2006. 559p

Marchetta Mark: Barron's Paramedic Exam. Baron's Educational Series 2008, 2nd ed. 275 p.

Paramedic Certification Exam. Learning Express. New York 2009. 4th ed. 210 p.

Preface

The book is the third (practical) part of the Manual of First Aid. All texts are short, understandable and always contain the right answer (marked with ◀), which makes them suitable for self-study and testing the paramedics' professional knowledge as well.

In the first volume the cases concern the following topics: airway and breathing assessment, proper interventions for patients with respiratory compromise, oxygen delivery systems, ventilatory support, respiratory anatomy and physiology, basic airway management, basic cardiopulmonary resuscitation, advanced interventions, cardiology, medical emergencies, traumatic injuries, gynaecology, obstetrics and paediatrics. The last chapter deals with legal considerations, communication, scene safety and scene management, vehicle operations, hazardous materials and mass casualty incidents.

VOLUME 1
Part 1
Airway and breathing

Airway and breathing assessment; proper interventions for patients with respiratory compromise; oxygen delivery systems; ventilatory support; respiratory anatomy and physiology; basic airway management; basic cardiopulmonary resuscitation; advanced interventions

Unit 1
Case study 1

The absence of carbon dioxide in 1_____ ___ indicates the endotracheal tube has been: placed in the oesophagus. ◄

The 2_____ ___ carbon dioxide likely indicates that the 3_____ _____ has been placed in the oesophagus. 4

4_____ correct endotracheal tube placement is absolutely essential.

• Your next action is: remove the endotracheal tube and provide several ventilations prior to attempting intubation again. ◄

The endotracheal tube is likely placed in the 5_____.
Your next action is to 6_____ the endotracheal tube and provide 7_____ _____ with supplemental oxygen 8_____ __ attempting another intubation.

a. remove; b. prior to; c. several ventilations; d. oesophagus; e. Verifying; f. absence of; g. endotracheal tube; h. exhaled air

Case study 2

The 1_____ used to describe normal breath sounds heard over most of the 2_____ _____ is:

• 3_____
• 4_____
• vesicular ◄
• bronchovesicular

a. chest wall; b. term; c. bronchial; d. adventitious

Case study 3

Breath sounds such as 1_____ ___ _____ that are not normally heard are 2_____ __:

• bronchial
• adventitious ◄
• vesicular
• bronchovesicular

a. crackles and rhonchi; b. defined as

Case study 4

The following correctly describes the flow of air from outside the body into the trachea: - Nose, 1_____ _____, nasopharynx, oropharynx, 2_____, larynx,3 _____. ◄

```
a. nasal cavities; b. trachea;
c. laryngopharynx
```

Case study 5

You are called for an unresponsive 29-year-old man. Bystanders report he has been drinking heavily all day. Assessment reveals the patient to be responsive only to painful stimuli. His breathing is shallow at a rate of four times per minute.

- How would you manage this patient? – Bag-valve device with a reservoir at 10-15 LPM ◄

Breathing must be supported with a 1___-_____ _____ with 2_____ high-flow oxygen. This patient's breathing is too 3_____ and too 4_____ to receive enough oxygen for proper 5___ _____ to take place.

```
a. slow; b. gas exchange; c. bag-valve device;
d. shallow; e. supplemental
```

Case study 6

The area where the trachea 1_____ into the right and left mainstem 2_____ is known as the:
- pleura
- xiphoid process

- carina ◄
- 3_____ angle

```
a. divides; b. bronchi; c. sternal
```

Case study 7

The administration of which of the following may result in a decrease in the respiratory rate? – Morphine sulphate. ◄

1_____ is an opiate that can cause 2_____ _____ _____ depression. Administration may result in a 3_____ in the respiratory rate. Patients receiving morphine must be monitored closely for 4_____ _____.

```
a. respiratory depression; b. central nervous
system; c. Morphine; d. decrease
```

Case study 8

The 1_____ _____ between the base of the 2_____ and the 3_____ into which the tip of the curved blade (Macintosh blade) is placed during 4_____ intubation is the:

- carina
- vallecula ◄
- glottis
- oesophagus

```
a. tongue; b. orotracheal; c. anatomical
structure; d. epiglottis
```

Case study 9

When blood levels of carbon dioxide or hydrogen ions 1_____ above normal, the respiratory centre of the brain responds by: increasing the rate and depth of respiration. ◄

2____ ___ _____ of respiration are increased to 3_____ excess CO_2 and therefore decreasing hydrogen ion concentrations. This is a normal 4_____ _____ of the body.

> a. compensatory mechanism; b. increase; c. Rate and depth; e. eliminate

Case study 10

The blood component 1_____ for transporting oxygen from the 2_____ to the 3____ _____ and transporting 4_____ _____ from the body tissues to the lungs is the:

- plasma
- platelets
- leukocytes
- erythrocytes ◄

> a. responsible; b. carbon dioxide; c. lungs; d. body tissues

Case study 11

Which is the 1_____ of the laryngeal mask airway (2___)? – It is blindly inserted. ◄

LMA insertion does not require 3_____.

> a. LMA; b. laryngoscopy; b. advantage

Case study 12

What is often a 1____ _____ in patients with respiratory distress? – Cyanosis ◄

2_____ is a late finding and may not 3__ _____ even when the patient is severely 4_____.

> a. Cyanosis; b. hypoxic; c. be present; d. late finding

Case study 13

You have a female patient with a long history of COPD who complains of worsening shortness of breath. She is on continuous 2 LMP of home oxygen.

- You are concerned that increasing the oxygen flow may eliminate the hypoxic drive to breathe because the hypoxic rate is regulated by: low PaO2. ◄

1_____ _____ to breathe is common in patients with COPD or other 2_____ respiratory disorders. Hypoxic drive is regulated by a low PaO2. (3_____ _____ __ _____). Delivering an 4_____ _____ of oxygen may increase the PaO2. and therefore eliminate the drive to breathe.

> a. increased concentration; b. degenerative; c. Hypoxic drive; d. partial pressure of oxygen

Case study 14

You arrive on the scene of a patient who is receiving bag-valve-mask ventilation. The abdomen is extremely distended. After intubation, you have resistance while 1_____ the patient. Lung sounds are diminished 2_____ and the trachea is midline.

- What should you do? – Insert a naso/oral gastric tube. ◄

When 3_____ _____ interferes with 4_____, insertion of a naso/oral gastric tube into the stomach 5__ _____.

> a. ventilations; b. is indicated; c. gastric distension; d. bagging; e. bilaterally

Case study 15

The simplest airway management 1_____ in a patient without suspected 2_____ _____ injury is: head-tilt/chin-lift 3_____.

> a. manoeuvre;◄ b. cervical spine; c. technique

Case study 16

The proper size 1_____ airway is determined 2__ _____: from the corner of the mouth to the tip of the earlobe at the angle of the jaw. ◄

It is essential that the OPA be sized appropriately because improper sizing can lead to 3_____ _____.

> a. airway obstruction; b. by measuring; c. oropharyngeal

Case study 17

The maximum water pressure recommended for 1_____ _____ ventilation should not exceed: 30 cm. ◄

The valve opening at the cardiac sphincter (opening into the 2_____) is approximately 30 cm/H_2O. Not exceeding 30 cm/H_2O will

reduce (not eliminate) the occurrence of 3_____ _____.

> a. positive pressure; b. stomach; c. gastric distension

Case study 18

Manual manoeuvres used 1__ _____ a patient's airway: include head tilt/chin lift and jaw-thrust. ◄

The 2_____ ____/____ ____ and 3____-_____ manoeuvre are both very effective in initial management of the airway.

> a. head tilt/chin lift; b. jaw-thrust; c. to open

Case study 19

Advantages of the Oesophageal Tracheal Combi/Tube include all of the following:

- 1_____ is rapid and easy. ◄
- It can be used on 2_____ patients. ◄
- It can provide ventilation when 3_____ in the oesophagus. ◄

It is not indicated for 4_____ patients due to its large diameter and the risk of 5_____ of the oesophagus.

> a. insertion; b. paediatric; c. perforation; d. trauma; e. placed

Case study 20

Causes for decreased ETC 0_2 readings include:

- nonperfusing patient ◄

4

- presence of severe
  1_____ ◄
- presence of 2_____
  emboli ◄

All the conditions listed
will result in a decreased ETC0$_2$
reading. Other 3_____ include
shock, bronchospasm, and
incomplete airway obstruction
(such as 4_____ plugging).

a. causes; b. mucus; c. acidosis; d. pulmonary

Case study 21

You are caring for a male patient
in ventricular tachycardia. He is
lethargic, diaphoretic, pale, and has
vomited once. His vital signs are: BP
74/P, pulse 184, respirations 14. You
are assigned to manage the airway.

1_____ _____
should include: 2_____
the airway for vomitus. ◄

Remember the basics!
You must first open the airway
and suction it 3_____ any
other airway management.

- Your patient becomes
  unresponsive and apnoeic.
  Further airway management
  should include: endotracheal
  4_____. ◄

a. intubation; b. Initial management;
c. before; d. suctioning

Case study 22

Succinylcholine is
contraindicated in patients
with crush injures because of:
risk of hyperkalemia. ◄

Succinylcholine should
not be used in 1_____ trauma,
2_____, or 3_____ injuries
because these conditions can
result in 4_____.

a. crush; b. hyperkalemia; c. blunt; d. burns

Vocabulary 1

abdomen /ˈæb.də.mən/
acidosis /ˌæs.ɪˈdəʊ.sɪs/
administration /ədˌmɪn.ɪˈstreɪ.ʃən/
advanced /ədˈvɑːnt st/
advantage /ədˈvɑːn.tɪdʒ/
adventitious /ˌæd.vənˈtɪʃ.əs/
airway /ˈeə.weɪ/
angle /ˈæŋgəl/
apnoeic /æpˈniː.ɪk/
appropriately /əˈprəʊ.pri.ət.li/
assessment /əˈses.mənt/
assign /əˈsaɪn/
attempt /əˈtemp t/
bag /bæg/
bag /bæg/ **valve** /vælv/
bag-valve mask /mɑːsk/
base /beɪs/
basic /ˈbeɪ.sɪk/
bilaterally /ˌbaɪˈlæt.ər.ə.li/
blade /bleɪd/
blindly /ˈblaɪnd.li/
blunt / blʌnt/
brain /breɪn/
bronchospasm /ˌbrɒŋ.kəʊ.ˈspæz.əm/
bronchus /ˈbrɒŋ.kəs/ pl **bronchi** /-kaɪ/
burn /bɜːn/
bystander /ˈbaɪˌstæn.dər/
carbon /ˈkɑː.bən/ **dioxide** /
daɪˈɒk.saɪd/
care / keə/ **for** / fɔː/
carina /kəˈraɪn.ə/
cavity /ˈkæv.ɪ.ti/
chest /tʃest/ **wall** /wɔːl/
chin-lift /tʃɪn/, /lɪft/
Combi tube /komˈbi.tjuːb/

common /ˈkɒmən/
compensatory /ˌkɒm.pənˈseɪt.ə ri/
complain /kəmˈpleɪn/
component /kəmˈpəʊnənt/
compromise /ˈkɒmprəˌmaɪz/
concern /kənˈsɜːn/
continuous /kənˈtɪn.ju.əs/
contraindicate /ˌkɒn.trəˈɪn.dɪ.keɪt/
corner /ˈkɔː.nər/
correct /kəˈrekt/
crackle /ˈkræk.l/
crush /krʌʃ/
curved /kɜːvd/
cyanosis /ˌsaɪəˈnəʊ.sɪs/
decrease /dɪˈkriːs/
degenerative /dɪˈdʒen.ər.ə.tɪv/
delivery /dɪˈlɪv.ər.i/
depression /dɪˈpreʃ.ən/
depth /depθ/
device /dɪˈvaɪs/
diameter /daɪˈæm.ɪ.tər/
diaphoretic /ˌdaɪ.ə.fəˈret.ɪk/
diminish /dɪˈmɪnɪʃ/
disorder /dɪˈsɔː.dər/
distend /dɪˈstend/
distension /dɪˈsten.t ʃən/
divide /dɪˈvaɪd/
drive /draɪv/
due /djuː/ to /tʊ/
earlobe /ˈɪə.ləʊb/
eliminate /ɪˈlɪm.ɪ.neɪt/
endotracheal /en.dɒ.trəˈkiː.əl/ tube /tjuːb/ (ET tube)
epiglottis /ˌep.ɪˈglɒt.ɪs/
erythrocyte /ɪˈrɪθ.rəʊ.saɪt/
essential /ɪˈsen.t ʃəl/
excess /ekˈses/
exchange /ɪksˈtʃeɪndʒ/
extremely /ɪkˈstriːm.li/
flow /fləʊ/
gastric /ˈɡæs.trɪk/
gastric /ˈɡæs.trɪk/ tube /tjuːb/
glottis /ˈɡlɒt.ɪs/ pl glotides
hydrogen /ˈhaɪ.drɪ.dʒən/
hyperkalaemia /ˌhaɪ.pə.kæˈliː.mi.ə/

hypoxic /haɪˈpɒk.sɪk/ drive /draɪv/
improper /ɪmˈprɒp.ər/
incomplete /ˌɪn.kəmˈpliːt/
initial /ɪˈnɪʃəl/
insert /ɪnˈsɜːt/
insertion /ɪnˈsɜː.ʃən/
interfere /ˌɪn.təˈfɪər/
intervention /ˌɪn.təˈven.ʃən/
intubation /ˌɪn.tjuːˈbeɪ.ʃən/
ion /ˈaɪ.ɒn/
jaw /dʒɔː/
jaw /dʒɔː/ thrust /θrʌst/
laryngeal /ləˈrɪn.dʒi.əl/
laryngoscopy /ˌlærɪŋˈɡɒ.skə.pi/
larynx /ˈlær.ɪŋks/ (pl. larynges)
lead /liːd/
lethargic /ləˈθɑː.dʒɪk/
leukocyte /ˈljuː.kə.saɪt/
likely /ˈlaɪklɪ/
LPM, Liter /ˈliːtə/ Per / pə/ Minute /ˈmɪnɪt/
lung /lʌŋ/
mainstem /meɪn.stəm/
bronchus /ˈbrɒŋ.kəs/
manage /ˈmæn.ɪdʒ/
management /ˈmænɪdʒmənt/
manoeuvre /məˈnuː.və/
manual /ˈmæn.ju.əl/
measure /ˈmeʒ.ər/
midline /ˈmɪd.laɪn/
morphine /ˈmɔː.fiːn/
sulphate /ˈsʌl.feɪt/
mouth /maʊθ/
mucus /ˈmjuː.kəs/
nasal /ˈneɪ.zəl/
nasopharynx /ˌneɪ.zəˈfær.ɪŋks/
obstruction /əbˈstrʌk.ʃən/
occurrence /əˈkʌr.ənt s/
oesophagus /ɪˈsɒf.ə.ɡəs/
OPA, Oropharyngeal /ˈɔː.rə.fəˈrɪn.dʒi.əl/ airway /ˈeə.weɪ/
reveal /rɪˈviːl/
rhonchus /rongˈkəs/ pl. -chi
shallow /ˈʃæl.əʊ/
shortness /ˈʃɔːt.nəs/

shortness /ˈʃɔːt.nəs/ **of breath** /breθ/
size /saɪz/
sound /saʊnd/
sphincter /ˈsfɪŋk.tər/
sternal /ˈstɔː.nəl/
stimulus /ˈstɪm.jʊ.ləs/ pl **stimuli**
suction /ˈsʌk.ʃən/
supplemental /ˌsʌp.lɪˈmen.təl/
support /ˈsəˌpɔːt/
tachycardia /ˌtæk.ɪˈkɑː.di.ə/
therefore /ˈðeə.fɔːr/
tilt /tɪlt/
tip /tɪp/
tissue /ˈtɪʃ.uː/, /ˈtɪs.juː/
tongue /tʌŋ/
trachea /trəˈkiː.ə/
trauma /ˈtrɔː.mə/
unresponsive /ˌʌn.rɪˈspɒnt.sɪv/
vallecula /vəˈlek.jʊl.ə/
ventilation /ˌven.tɪˈleɪ.ʃən/
ventilatory /ˈventɪˌleɪtə.rɪ/
ventricular /venˈtrɪk.jə.lər/
verify /ˈver.ɪ.faɪ/
vomitus /ˈvɒm.ɪ.təs/
xiphoid /zi.foid/ **process** /ˈproʊ.ses/

Unit 2

Case study 1

What effects does hyperventilation have on cerebral circulation and intracranial pressure? – More pronounced decrease in circulation than decrease in intracranial pressure. ◄

A CO_2 is a very potent 1_____. When a patient is hyperventilated, CO_2 is removed and the 2_____ will become constricted. This vasoconstriction leads to decreased 3_____ _____ by 4_____ cerebral blood flow.

> a. decreasing; b. vessels; c. vasodilator; d. cerebral pressure

Case study 2

A respiratory pattern characterized by an 1_____ _____, rate, and volume with 2_____ periods of apnoea is: Biot's (ataxic). ◄

This pattern is seen in patients with increased 3_____ _____.

> a. intermittent; b. intracranial pressure, c. irregular pattern

Case study 3

A 1_____ _____ characterized by deep, rapid 2_____ is: central neurogenic hyperventilation. ◄

This breathing pattern is usually seen in a loss of normal 3_____ of ventilatory control.

> a. regulation; b. respiratory pattern; c. respirations

Case study 4

A respiratory pattern characterized by 1_____, shallow, irregular respirations is: bradypnoea.◄

This breathing pattern can be associated with 2_____ or several other 3_____ _____ disorders.

> a. nervous system; b. stroke; c. slow

Case study 5

All of the following can affect the accuracy reading of a pulse oximeter:

- hypoperfusion ◄
- anaemia ◄
- carbon monoxide poisoning ◄

Other circumstances that can affect the 1_____ include exposure to nail polish or acrylic nails, dark pigmentation or 2_____, high bilirubin concentration. Hyperthermia (fever) should not affect the accuracy of a pulse oximeter 3_____.

a. bruising; b. reading; c. accuracy

Case study 6

Complications of endotracheal intubation include all of the following:

- 1_____ to the teeth ◄
- oesophageal intubation ◄
- laryngospasm ◄

Gastric distension usually occurs with bag-valve mask ventilations 2_____ __ intubation. A correctly placed endotracheal tube should not contribute to 3_____ _____.

a. gastric distension; b. prior to; c. trauma

Case study 7

Confirmation of 1_____ ____ placement should be evaluated:

- 2_____ after insertion, ◄
- each time the patient is moved, ◄
- by 3 __ ____ two methods. ◄

a. immediately; b. at least; c. endotracheal tube

Case study 8

You are using an end-tidal carbon dioxide detector as a tool to assist for proper endotracheal intubation placement. The absence of carbon dioxide in exhaled air indicates that the endotracheal tube has been:

- placed in the right mainstem bronchus
- correctly placed in the trachea
- placed in the oesophagus ◄
- placed in the left mainstem bronchus

The use of end-tidal 1_____ _____ detection (ETCO$_2$) is one tool to assess for proper 2_____ ____ placement. The 3_____ of carbon dioxide likely indicates that the endotracheal tube has been placed in the 4_____. Verifying correct endotracheal tube placement is absolutely 5_____. ETCO$_2$ is only one method to assist in verification of proper placement.

a. endotracheal tube; b. absence, c. essential; d. carbon dioxide; e. oesophagus

Case study 9

The minimum size bag-valve mask device used for neonates, infants, and children should be: 450 ml. ◄

Although it is likely that the 1___-_____ _____ will not deliver 450 ml of volume, it is important to have a device 2_____ __ delivering excessive volumes because, as the bag 3__ _____, there is dead space, from which air cannot be 4_____ expelled.

> a. is compressed; b. fully; c. bag-valve mask; d. capable of

Case study 10

A high-pitched noise associated with upper airway 1_____ is known as:

- wheezing
- rhonchi
- stridor ◄
- rales

This can be 2__ _____ of pending complete airway obstruction when associated with 3_____ such as anaphylactic shock.

> a. conditions; b. an indication; c. constriction

Case study 11

The next 5 questions are basic life support questions

- Before providing 1_____ _____ to an unresponsive victim, you must 2_____ ___ breathing. You do this by: looking, listening, and feeling 3_____ through the victim's nose or mouth. ◄

- You are performing rescue breathing on an adult. How many 4_____ do you give? – One breath every 5 seconds. ◄

- Where would you place your hands on the chest of an adult victim when you are performing 5_____ _____? – On the lower half of the sternum, at the nipple line ◄

- What is the ratio of compressions to 6_____ when performing one-person CPR on an adult? – 30 compressions to 2 ventilations. ◄

- What is the correct rate you should use to perform chest compressions for an adult victim of 7_____ _____? – 100 times per minute. ◄

> a. airflow; b. check for; c. ventilations; d. chest compressions; e. rescue breathing; f. breaths; g. cardiac arrest

Case study 12

You are 1_____ rescue breathing with a 2___-_____ device for an apnoeic child. How often should you provide rescue breaths? – 3____ _____ 3 seconds.◄

> a. performing; b. once every; c. bag-mask

Case study 13

In a patient in 1_____
_____, the development of which
sign/symptom would lead you 2___
_____ the patient is significantly
3_____? - Cyanosis ◄

a. decompensating; b. respiratory distress;
c. to believe

Case study 14

You respond to a cafeteria
for a 16-year-old patient who is
choking. Your patient is conscious
and coughing forcefully. She
appears anxious and is difficult
to communicate with due to the
coughing but is able to 1_____
_____. Assessment reveals a
respiratory rate of 28, 2_____,
diminished breath sounds on the
right side, and a SpO_2 reading of
96%. Based on the history and
3_____ _____, you
suspect: aspiration of food into
the right mainstem bronchus
causing obstruction. ◄

Based on the history of the
patient 4_____, a constant
cough (from broncho spasm),
and diminished breath sounds
(obstruction) on the right should lead
you to suspect 5_____ of food.

a. shallow; b. choking; c. assessment findings;
d. follow commands; e. aspiration

Case study 15

Nasotracheal intubation
is 1_____ in
a patient with: a suspected
basilar skull fracture. ◄

A suspected basilar 2_____
_____ is a contraindication for
nasotracheal intubation because the
3_____ ____ of the endotracheal
tube could enter the 4_____
_____ through the fracture site.

a. skull fracture; b. cranial cavity;
c. contraindicated; d. distal tip

Case study 16

Blind nasotracheal intubation:
should be attempted on a patient
with spontaneous respirations.◄

1_____ nasotracheal
intubation requires the patient to
have 2_____ respirations
because the endotracheal tube 3___
_____ as the patient inhales.

a. spontaneous; b. is inserted; c. Blind

Case study 17

You arrive on the scene of a
40-year-old male with a 1_____
__ palpitations and dizziness.
2_____ are BP 102/78, pulse 128
slightly irregular, and respirations
of 26. A pulse oximeter reading
of 86% is obtained. He has 3___
_____ medical problems. With
this information you suspect:

- hyperventilation syndrome
- hypoxemia ◄
- congestive heart failure
- pending respiratory arrest

A patient with a pulse oximeter
reading of 86% with no significant
past medical history of 4_____
_____ is considered hypoxic.

> a. no past; b. pulmonary disorders;
> c. complaint of; d. Vitals

Case study 18

The presence of rhonchi in a patient 1_____ _____ pneumonia indicates:

- narrowing of the airways
- normal finding in a pneumonia patient
- onset of bronchitis
- mucus in the airways ◄

Rhonchi are abnormal 2_____ _____ heard on auscultation of airway that is obstructed by thick 3_____.

> a. lung sounds; b. secretions; c. diagnosed with

Case study 19

When using a bulb syringe device to assist in verification of proper endotracheal tube placement, all of the following are true:

- If the 1_____ _____ easily inflates, the endotracheal tube is correctly placed in the trachea. ◄
- If the bulb syringe does not 2_____, the endotracheal tube is placed in the oesophagus. ◄
- The 3_____ on the endotracheal tube should not be inflated prior to using a bulb syringe device. ◄

If the endotracheal tube has been placed in the 4_____,

inflating the cuff on the endotracheal tube will hold the oesophagus 5_____ and allow the bulb syringe to inflate. It is important to not inflate the endotracheal tube cuff prior to using any bulb syringe device.

> a. inflate; b. bulb syringe; c. oesophagus; d. cuff; e. open

Case study 20

You respond to a 17-year old male because his father was unable to wake him. The father states that his son was at a party last night and has a history of 1_____ _____ ___. He is unconscious and unresponsive. BP is not obtainable, pulse 42 and weak, and respirations of 4. You have orally intubated the patient. Auscultation of lung sounds post intubation 2_____ breath sounds heard over the right chest and an absence of breath sounds over the left chest. Your 3_____ _____ would be to: deflate the endotracheal tube cuff, withdraw the tube 2 cm and reevaluate breath sounds, and reinflate the cuff. ◄

This patient was 4_____ _____ intubated in the right mainstem bronchus. Deflating the endotracheal tube cuff, withdrawing the tube slightly, 5_____ the cuff, and 6_____ breath sounds is the proper procedure when a right mainstem bronchus intubation is suspected.

> a. reveal; b. most likely; c. recreational drug use; d. reinflating; e. next action; f. reevaluating

Case study 21

All of the following are reasons for a pulse oximeter to read "Error":

- low capillary blood 1_____ ◄
- 2_____
  vasoconstriction ◄
- extremity 3_____ ◄

---
a. flow; b. movement; c. peripheral

Case study 22

Field extubation is indicated if the patient: is awake and able to maintain his or her own airway. ◄

Field extubation is 1___ _____.
If it must be 2_____, the patient must clearly be able to
3_____ ___ _____
his or her own airway and have
4_____ spontaneous respirations.

---
a. maintain and protect; b. adequate;
c. performed; d. not common

Vocabulary 2

accuracy /ˈæk.jʊ.rə.si/
acrylic /əˈkrɪl.ɪk/
adequate /ˈæd.ə.kwət/
adult /ˈæd.ʌlt/,/əˈdʌlt/
affect /əˈfekt/
airflow /ˈeə.fləʊ/
anaemia /əˈniːmɪə/
anxious /ˈæŋk.ʃəs/
apnoea /ˈæp.ni.ə/
apnoeic /æpˈniː.ɪk/
appear /əˈpɪər/
arrest /əˈrest/
aspiration /ˌæspɪˈreɪʃən/
associated /əˈsəʊ.si.eɪ.tɪd/
at /ət/ **least** /liːst/
ataxic /əˈtæk.sɪk/
attempt /əˈtempt/

auscultation /ˌɔː.skəlˈteɪ.ʃən/
awake /əˈweɪk/
based /beɪst/
basilar /ˈbæz.ɪ.lər/
bilirubin /ˌbɪl.ɪˈruː.bɪn/
blind /blaɪnd/
bradypnoea /ˌbræd.ɪˈpni.ə/
breath /breθ/
bronchitis /brɒŋˈkaɪ.tɪs/
bruising /ˈbruː.zɪŋ/
bulb /bʌlb/
cafeteria /ˌkæf.əˈtɪə.ri.ə/
capillary /kəˈpɪl.ər.i/
carbon monoxide /ˌkɑː.bən.məˈnɒk.saɪd/
cardiac arrest /ˈkɑr.di.æk əˈrest/
central /ˈsen.trəl/
cerebral /ˈser.ɪ.brəl/
check /tʃek/
choke /tʃəʊk/
circulation /ˌsɜː.kjʊˈleɪ.ʃən/
circumstance /ˈsɜː.kəm.stɑːnts/
command /kəˈmɑːnd/
communicate /kəˈmjuː.nɪ.keɪt/
complaint /kəmˈpleɪnt/
complete /kəmˈpliːt/
compression /kəmˈpreʃən/
condition /kənˈdɪʃ.ən/
confirmation /ˌkɒn.fəˈmeɪ.ʃən/
congestive /kənˈdʒes.tɪv/ **heart** /hɑːt/ **failure** /ˈfeɪ.ljər/
conscious /ˈkɒn.tʃəs/
constant /ˈkɒn.stənt/
constricted /kənˈstrɪkt.ɪd/
constriction /kənˈstrɪk.ʃən/
contraindication /ˌkɒn.trə.ɪn.dɪˈkeɪ.ʃən/
contribute /kənˈtrɪb.juːt/
cough /kɒf/
cranial /ˈkreɪ.ni.əl/
cuff /kʌf/
decompensation /diːˌkɒm.pen.senˈseɪ.ʃən/
deflate /dɪˈfleɪt/
detector /dɪˈtek.tər/
device /dɪˈvaɪs/

12

diagnose /ˈdaɪəɡˌnəʊz/
distal /dɪ.stəl/
dizziness /ˈdɪz.ɪ.nəs/
effect /ɪˈfekt/
error /ˈer.ər /
exposure /ɪkˈspəʊ.ʒə/
extremity /ɪkˈstrem.ɪ.ti/
extubation /ˌeks.tjʊˈbeɪ.ʃən/
feeling /ˈfiː.lɪŋ/
fever /ˈfiː.vər/
field /fiːld/
finding /ˈfaɪndɪŋ/
fracture /ˈfræk.tʃə/
high-pitched /ˌhaɪˈpɪtʃt/
history /ˈhɪs.tər.i/
hyperthermia /ˌhaɪ.pəˈθɜː.mɪ.ə/
hyperventilation /ˌhaɪ.pəˌven.tɪˈleɪ.ʃən/
hypoperfusion /ˌhaɪ.pəʊ.pəˈfjuː.ʒən/
hypoxaemia /ˌhai.pɒkˈsiː.mi.ə/
immediately /ɪˈmiː.di.ət.li/
indication /ˌɪn.dɪˈkeɪ.ʃən/
inflate /ɪnˈfleɪt/
inhale /ɪnˈheɪl/
intermittent /ˌɪn.təˈmɪt.ənt/
intracranial /ɪn.trəˈkreɪ.ni.əl/
irregular /ɪˈreg.jə.lər/
laryngospasm /læˈrɪŋ.gə.spæz.əm/
life support /ˈlaɪf.səˌpɔːt/
listening /ˈlɪs.ən.ɪŋ /
looking /lʊk.ɪŋ/
loss /lɒs/
maintain /meɪnˈteɪn/
move /muːv/
movement /ˈmuːv.mənt/
nail /neɪl/ polish /ˈpɒl.ɪʃ/
narrow /ˈnær.əʊ/
nasotracheal /ˌneɪ.zə.trəˈkiː.əl/
neurogenic /ˌnjʊə.rəˈdʒen.ɪk/
niple /ˈnɪp.l̩/
noise /nɔɪz/
obstruct /əbˈstrʌkt/
onset /ˈɒnˌset/
palpitations /ˌpæl.pɪˈteɪ.ʃənz/
pattern /ˈpæt.ən/

pending /ˈpen.dɪŋ/
perform /pəˈfɔːm/
period /ˈpɪə.ri.əd/
pigmentation /ˌpɪg.mənˈteɪ.ʃən/
pneumonia /njuːˈməʊ.ni.ə/
poisoning /ˈpɔɪ.zən.ɪŋ/
potent /ˈpəʊ.tənt/
procedure /prəˈsiː.dʒə/
pronounced /prəˈnaʊnst/
pulse /pʌls/ oximetry /ˈɒk.sɪ.m.ə.tri/
rale /raːl/
ratio /ˈreɪ.ʃi.əʊ/
reading /ˈriː.dɪŋ/
reevaluate /ˌriː.ɪˈvæljueɪt/
regulation /ˌreg.jʊˈleɪ.ʃən/
reinflate /ˌriː.ɪnˈfleɪt/
rescue /ˈreskjuː/
secretion /sɪˈkriː.ʃən/
shallow /ˈʃæl.əʊ/
significant /sɪgˈnɪf.ɪ.kənt/
skull /skʌl/
slightly /ˈslaɪt.li/
spontaneous /spɒnˈteɪ.ni.əs/
sternum /ˈstɜː.nəm/
stridor /straɪd.ər/
stroke /strəʊk/
suspect /səˈspekt/
syringe /sɪˈrɪndʒ/
thick /θɪk/
times /taɪmz/
tool /tuːl/
upper /ˈʌp.ər/
vasoconstriction /ˌveɪ.zə.kənˈstrɪk.ʃən/
vasodilator /ˌveɪ.zə.daɪˈleɪ.tər/
verification /ˌver.ɪ.fɪˈkeɪ.ʃən/
vessel /ˈves.əl/
victim /ˈvɪk.tɪm/
vitals /ˈvaɪ.təlz/
volume /ˈvɒl.juːm/
wheeze /wiːz/
withdraw /wɪðˈdrɔː/

Unit 3

Case study 1

You have successfully resuscitated a patient who suffered a cardiac arrest. You are 1_____ to the hospital when the patient wakes up and is not tolerating the endotracheal tube. The medical director at the 2_____ _____ has ordered you to extubate the patient. All of the following should be done:

- removing the endotracheal tube on a cough or respiration ◄
- deflating the endotracheal tube cuff 3_____ ◄
- providing 4_____ oxygen once the tube is removed ◄

The endotracheal tube must be removed swiftly on a 5_____ __ _____.

a. en route; b. supplemental; c. cough or expiration; d. receiving hospital; e. completely

Case study 2

You have orally intubated a patient. While your partner ventilates the patient with a bag-valve device, you assess for proper placement. Auscultation reveals sounds heard over the right chest and an absence of breath sounds over the left chest.

Your best course of action would be to: deflate the endotracheal tube cuff, withdraw the tube 2 cm and reevaluate breath sounds, and reinflate the cuff. ◄

This patient was most likely intubated in the right 1_____ _____.

2_____ the endotracheal tube cuff, 3_____ the tube slightly, reinflating the cuff and 4_____ breath sounds is the proper procedure.

a. Deflating; b. reevaluating; c. mainstem bronchus; d. withdrawing

Case study 3

The Sellick manoeuvre: may be used to minimize gastric distention and facilitate placement of an endotracheal tube into the glottic opening. ◄

Posterior pressure exerted on the 1_____ _____ (The Sellick manoeuvre) will effectively 2_____ the oesophagus, minimizing the potential for gastric 3_____. This manoeuvre will also reposition the 4_____ _____ for clearer 5_____ of anatomic structures.

a. compress; b. visualization; c. distention; d. cricoid cartilage; e. vocal cords

Case study 4

You arrive at the scene of an accident in which a car 1___ _____ a telephone pole. You find a 17-year-old female 2_____ from her vehicle, lying 25 feet from the point of impact.

- Which is an 3_____ method of opening the airway? – Jaw thrust. ◄

This is a trauma victim and should be managed utilizing c-spine 4_____.

> a. Ejected; b. precautions; c. has struck; d. acceptable

Case study 5

Which is NOT considered a 1____ __ _____ indicating a tension pneumothorax?

- dyspnoea
- hyperresonance to percussion
- distended jugular veins
- clear lung sounds ◄

2_____ lung sounds do not indicate the presence of a 3_____ pneumothorax.

> a. Clear; b. tension; c. sign or symptom

Case study 6

When confirming endotracheal tube placement, it is imperative to auscultate:

- at the midaxillary line ◄
- over the trachea ◄
- over the epigastrium ◄

1_____ individual lung fields is of great benefit because they help to 2_____ tube placement. Auscultation of the epigastrium is beneficial because it will help to verify 3_____ tube placement or problems with the 4____ _____ of the tube.

> a. improper; b. cuff seal; c. Auscultating; d. confirm

Case study 7

A respiratory pattern characterized by a gradually increasing rate, and tidal volume followed by a gradual 1_____ with intermittent periods of 2_____ is:

- Cheyne-Stokes ◄
- Biot's (ataxic)
- central neurogenic hyperventilation
- agonal

This breathing pattern is usually seen in patients with 3_____ _____ or elderly patients with terminal illness.

> a. brain injury; b. decrease; c. apnoea

Case study 8

You observe a COPD patient utilizing the pursed-lip breathing technique. – It helps maintain pressure within the airways. ◄
1_____-___ breathing technique helps 2_____ _____ within the airways (even during exhalation) to 3_____ bronchial walls that have been damaged as a result of 4_____.

> a. support; b. maintain pressure; c. Pursed-lip; d. disease

Case study 9

When intubating an adult patient with a 1_____ _____ (Macintosh blade), the tip of the blade should 2__ _____: in the vallecula, 3__ ___ _____ of the tongue.◄

a. at the base; b. curved blade; c. be placed

Case study 10

After 1_____ the chest of the victim with a tension pneumothorax, you determine your 2_____ was successful by observing for: an improvement in the patient's ventilatory and circulatory status. ◄

In a tension pneumothorax, the patient is dealing with 3_____ _____ and circulation problems. This tension pneumothorax creates an intrathoracic shift, impending 4_____ ____ return to the heart.

a. venous blood; b. intervention; c. oxygenation problems; d. decompressing

Case study 11

During needle decompression, 1___ _____ is inserted on the top of the rib for what purpose? – To ensure that the vein, artery, and 2_____ _____ under each rib are not damaged.◄

Each 3_____ _____ contains a vein, artery, and nerve, which lie underneath each rib.

a. the needle; b. intercostal space; c. nerve bundle

Case study 12

You have intubated a patient with a long history of chronic bronchitis. During transport you notice that 1_____ are becoming increasingly difficult. You 2_____ the chest, and hear faint equal breath sounds.

What intervention is most likely indicated for this patient? – Tracheobronchial suctioning.◄

In this scenario, suctioning is indicated. A patient with 3_____ _____ produces copious amounts of 4_____, which is capable of plugging the larger airways of an 5__ _____. This would result in difficult ventilation.

a. ET tube; b. mucus; c. chronic bronchitis; d. ventilations; e. auscultate

Case study 13

A drop in systolic 1_____ _____ of 10 mmHg or more or the absence of a 2_____ _____ during inspiration is known as:

- pericardial tamponade
- pulsus paradoxus ◄
- orthostatic 3_____
- pulse pressure change

a. radial pulse; b. change; c. blood pressure

Case study 14

Suctioning (application of 1_____ _____) should be activated: upon extraction of the suction catheter. ◄

Prolonged suctioning has been found 2__ _____ hypoxia, therefore, suctioning should 3__ _____ to extraction only

a. be limited; b. to cause; c. negative pressure

Case study 15

When using a 1_____ _____ (Miller blade) to 2_____

an adult patient, the tip of the blade should be placed:

- directly 3__ __ _____ the epiglottis. ◄
- above the epiglottis
- in the vellecula
- past the epiglottis at the vocal cord

a. intubate; b. on or under; c. straight blade

Case study 16

Digital intubation may be helpful when:

- there is suspected spinal cord injury. ◄
- the tongue is swollen
- the respiratory rate is 4/minute
- upper airway obstruction is suspected

The sniffing position is not required to perform 1_____ _____. The head can remain in a 2_____ _____, therefore digital intubation may be helpful with 3_____ spinal cord injury.

a. Suspected; b. digital intubation; c. neutral position

Case study 17

An infant should not be 1_____ for more than: 5 seconds. ◄

Suctioning should not 2_____ 10 seconds in a child, and 15 seconds in an 3_____.

a. exceed; b. adult; c. suctioned

Case study 18

A child in respiratory distress may grunt as the child breathes. This is a result of: creating pressure to help maintain open airways. ◄

1_____ involves exhaling against a partially closed glottis. This creates pressure to help maintain open 2_____ _____ similar to pursed-lip breathing in adults with COPD. This short low-pitched sound is often 3_____ ___ whimpering and suggests 4_____ _____.

a. mistaken for; b. severe hypoxia; c. Grunting; d. lower airways

Case study 19

You are caring for a 77-year-old male patient who is short of breath and has a history of 1____. He is alert and oriented to person, place, and time but able to speak only in two-to-three-word sentences. What does the patient's ability to speak in two-to-three-word sentences indicate? – Inadequate tidal volume is present.◄

A patient not being able to speak in full sentences due to 2_____ _____ indicates that the patient does not have an adequate tidal volume. This assessment finding can be a significant 3_____ _____ of pending respiratory failure.

a. breathing difficulty; b. warning sign; c. COPD

Case study 20

One reason the respiratory system of a geriatric patient becomes less effective is that: there is decreased chest wall compliance. ◄

There is no escaping the fact that the body becomes 1___ _____ with age. Decreased chest wall compliance, loss of lung elasticity, 2___ _____, decreased 3_____ of gases, and 4_____ of the respiratory muscles can all contribute to a less active respiratory system in a 5_____ _____.

> a. air trapping; b. geriatric patient; c. hypertrophy; d. less efficient; e. diffusion

Case study 21

You respond to a 72-year-old man with syncope. He is sitting in the kitchen when you arrive. He is alert and oriented to 1_____, _____, and ____. He complains of dizziness. Current vitals are BP 108/60, pulse 96 slightly irregular, and respirations of 28. Pulse oximeter reading is 97%. ECG shows a sinus rhythm with occasional PVC's. This patient should receive oxygen: by nonrebreather mask.◄

This patient needs oxygen by 2_____ ____. He has an increased respiratory rate and PVCs on the monitor that may indicate hypoxia. A normal pulse oximeter of 97% is an excellent 3_____ but oxygen should not be withheld based on this reading. Always remember 4__ _____ your patient and not the pulse oximeter.

> a. nonrebreather mask; b. to treat; c. finding; c. person; place, time

Case study 22

Respiratory acidosis is caused by:

- an excess of 1_____
- excess carbon dioxide ◄
- 2_ _____ __ bicarbonate
- 3_____ carbon dioxide excretion

> a. excess; b. bicarbonate; c. a loss of

Case study 23

The nasopharyngeal airway should be measured:

- from the 1_____ of the mouth to the earlobe
- from the tip of the nose to the earlobe ◄
- from the 2___ __ ___ ____ to the corner of the mouth
- from the tip of the nose to the 3____

> a. corner; b. chin; c. tip of the nose

Vocabulary 3

above /əˈbʌv/
acceptable /əkˈsept.ə.bl̩/
accident /ˈæksɪdənt/
agonal /ˈag.əʊ.nəl/
alert /əˈlɜːt/
amount /əˈmaʊnt/
application /ˌæp.lɪˈkeɪ.ʃən/
artery /ˈɑːtəri/
beneficial /ˌben.ɪˈfɪʃ.əl/
benefit /ˈben.ɪ.fɪt/
blade /bleɪd/
blood /blʌd/ **pressure** /ˈpreʃ.ər/
bundle /ˈbʌn.dl̩/
C-spine, cervical /səˈvaɪ.kəl/ **spine** /spaɪn/
capable /ˈkeɪ.pə.bl̩/
cardiac /ˈkɑː.di.æk/
caring /ˈkeə.rɪŋ/
cartilage /ˈkɑː.təl.ɪdʒ/

catheter /ˈkæθɪtə/
cause /kɔːz/
clear /klɪər/
compliance /kəmˈplaɪ.ənt s/
compress /kəmˈpres/
considered /kənˈsɪd.əd/
contain /kənˈteɪn/
copious /ˈkəʊ.pi.əs/
course /kɔːs/
create /kriːˈeɪt/
cricoid /ˈkraɪ.kɔɪd/
cartilage /ˈkɑː.təl.ɪdʒ/
current /ˈkʌr.ənt/
damaged /ˈdæm.ɪdʒd/
deal with /dɪəl/
decompress /ˌdiː.kəmˈpres/
decompression /ˌdiː.kəmˈpreʃ.ən/
diffused /dɪˈfjuːst/
diffusion /dɪˈfjuː.ʒən/
digital /ˈdɪdʒ.ɪ.təl/
directly /daɪˈrekt .li/
director /daɪˈrek.tər/
drop /drɒp/
dyspnoea /dɪs.pniː.ə/
efficient /ɪˈfɪʃ.ənt/
eject /ɪˈdʒekt/
elasticity /ˌɪl.æsˈtɪs.ɪ.ti/
elderly /ˈel.dəl.i/
enroute /ˌɒnˈruːt/
epigastrium /ˌepɪˈgæs.tri.əm/
equal /ˈiːkwəl/
escape /ɪˈskeɪp/
exceed /ɪkˈsiːd/
excellent /ˈek.səl.ənt/
excretion /ɪkˈskriː.ʃən/
exert /ɪgˈzɜːt/
expiration /ˌek.spəˈreɪ.ʃən/
extraction /ɪkˈstræk.ʃən/
extubate /eks.tjʊ.beɪt/
facilitate /fəˈsɪl.ɪ.teɪt/
failure /ˈfeɪ.ljə/
faint /feɪnt/
finding /ˈfaɪndɪŋ/
found /faʊnd/
full /fʊl/

geriatric /ˌdʒer.iˈæt.rɪk/
glottic /ˈglɒt.ɪk/
gradually /ˈgræd.jʊ.li/
grunt /grʌnt/
hyperresonance /ˌhaɪ.pə.ˈrez.ən.əns/
hypertrophy /haɪˈpɜː.trə.fi/
impact /ˈɪm.pækt/
impending /ɪmˈpen.dɪŋ/
imperative /ɪmˈper.ə.tɪv/
improper /ɪmˈprɒp.ər/
improvement /ɪmˈpruː.v.mənt/
inadequate /ɪˈnæd.ɪ.kwət/
increasingly /ɪnˈkriː.sɪŋ.li/
indicate /ˈɪn.dɪ.keɪt/
infant /ˈɪnfənt/
injury /ˈɪndʒəri/
inspiration /ˌɪn.spɪˈreɪ.ʃən/
intercostal /ˌɪn.təˈkɒs.təl/
intermittent /ˌɪn.təˈmɪt.ənt/
intrathoracic /ˌɪn.trə.θɔːˈræs.ɪk/
jugular /ˈdʒʌg.jə.lər/ vein / veɪn/
lie /laɪ/
limited /ˈlɪm.ɪ.tɪd/
low-pitched /ˌləʊˈpɪtʃt/
lower /ˈləʊ.ə/ airways /ˈeə.weɪz/
midaxillary /mɪd.ækˈsɪl.ər.i/
mistaken /mɪˈsteɪ.kən/
needle /ˈniː.dḷ/
negative /ˈneg.ə.tɪv/
neutral /ˈnjuː.trəl/
nonrebreather /ˌnɒn.rəbrə.
ðər/ mask / mɑːsk/
notice /ˈnəʊtɪs/
observe /əbˈzɜːv/
occasional /əˈkeɪʒənəl/
opening /ˈəʊ.pən.ɪŋ/
oriented /ˈɔːrɪəntɪd/
orthostatic /ˌɔː.θəˈstætɪk/
partially /ˈpɑː.ʃəl.i/
past /pɑːst/
percussion /pəˈkʌʃ.ən/
pericardial /ˌper.ɪˈkɑː.di.əl/
pole /pəʊl/
posterior /pɒsˈtɪə.ri.ər/
precaution /prɪˈkɔː.ʃən/

produce /prə'djuːs/
prolonged /prə'lɒŋd/
pulsus /pʌls.əs/ **paradoxus/**
'pær.ə.dɒks.əs/
purpose /'pɜː.pəs/
pursed /pɜːsd/**-lip** /lɪp/
radial /'reɪ.di.əl/
receive /rɪ'siːv/
remain /rɪ'meɪn/
reposition /ˌriː.pə'zɪʃən/
respond /rɪ'spɒnd/
rib /rɪb/
scenario /sɪ'nɑː.ri.əʊ/
seal /siːl/
sentence /'sen.təns/
shift /ʃɪft/
short /ʃɔːt/ **of st**
sinus /'saɪ.nəs/
sniffing /snɪf.ɪŋ/
sodium bicarbonate /ˌsəʊ.
di.əm.baɪ'kɑː.bən.ət/
space /speɪs/
spinal /'spaɪ.nəl/ **cord** /kɔːd/
straight /streɪt/
strike /straɪk/ **(struck, struck)**
successfully /sək'ses.fə.li/
suffer /'sʌf.ər/
suspected /sə'spek.tɪd/
swiftly /'swɪft.li/
swollen /'swəʊ.lən/
syncope /'sɪŋ.kə.pɪ/
systolic /sɪs'tɑl.ɪk/
tamponade /tæm.pə'neɪd/
tension /'tent.ʃən/ **pneumothorax**
/ˌnjuː.mə'θɔː.ræks/
terminal /'tɜː.mɪ.nəl/
tidal /'taɪdəl/ **volume** /'vɒljuːm/
tolerate /'tɒl.ər.eɪt/
top /tɒp/
tracheobronchial /trə.kiː.ə'brɒŋ.ki.əl/
transport /'træn.spɔːt/
trap /træp/
under /'ʌn.dər/
underneath /ˌʌn.də'niːθ/
upon /ə'pɒn/

utilize /'juː.tɪ.laɪz/
vein /veɪn/
venous /'viː.nəs/ **return** /rɪ'tɜːn/
visualization /ˌvɪʒ.u.əl.aɪ'zeɪʃən/
vocal /'vəʊkəl/ **cords** /kɔːdz/
warning /'wɔː.nɪŋ/ **sign** /saɪn/
whimper /'wɪmpə/
withhold /wɪð'həʊld/
within /wɪ'ðɪn/

Hypocalcaemia results in decreased 2_____ and increased myocardial irritability.

Hypomagnesaemia results in increased myocardial 3_____.

a. contractility; b. irritability; c. MOST likely

Case study 3

The protective sac surrounding the heart is the:

- myocardium
- septum
- endocardium
- pericardium ◄

The pericardium is the fibroserous sac enclosing the heart that is composed of two layers, the 1_____ and the parietal 2_____. The 3_____ is the middle layer of the walls of the heart. The 4_____ is the inner walls of the heart that separate the right and left 5_____ of the heart from the ventricles. The endocardium is the 6_____ layer of the heart.

a. epicardium; b. myocardium; c. innermost; d. pericardium; e. septum; f. atria

Case study 4

In a patient experiencing chest pain, the presence of jugular venous distention while sitting at a 45° angle: indicates right heart compromise. ◄

The 1_____ _____ reflect the pressure within 2_____ circulation. Normally, the jugular veins are not 3_____ in a patient sitting or standing. JVD

Part 2
Cardiology

Unit 1
Case study 1

What is the correct 1_____ at which you should 2_____ chest compressions on an 3_____ victim of cardiac arrest? - 100 times per minute ◄

a. speed; b. adult; c. perform

Case study 2

Hypocalcaemia and hypomagnesaemia would 1____ _____ result in:

- decreased cardiac conduction
- increased myocardial irritability ◄
- decreased cardiac contractility
- decreased myocardial automacity

present at a 45° angle indicates that pressure in the right side of the heart is elevated and indicates right heart 4_____.

a. distended; b. systemic; c. compromise; d. jugular veins

Case study 5

Signs and symptoms asociated with 1_____ _____ include distant heart tones, JVD, and:

- pulse 2_____
- hypotension ◄
- wheezing
- delayed 3_____

_____

Beck's triad includes 4_____, distant heart tones, and JVD. This triad of symptoms can aid in the diagnosis of cardiac tamponade.

a. pericardial tamponade; b. hypotension; c. paradoxus; d. capillary refill

Case study 6

Which term best describes the following definition? Disease of arterial vessels marked by 1_____, 2_____, and loss of elasticity in the arterial walls

- atherosclerosis
- arterionecrosis
- arteriosclerosis ◄
- angina

3_____ is the most common form of arteriosclerosis, usually involving medium-sized and large arteries.

Arterionecrosis is destruction (4_____) of the arteriole.

Angina is chest 5_____ associated with a deficiency of oxygen supply to the heart muscle.

a. thickening; b. hardening; c. necrosis; d. discomfort; e. Atherosclerosis

Case study 7

The volume of blood 1_____ from the left 2_____ into the 3_____ system each minute is:

- preload
- cardiac output ◄
- afterload
- stroke volume

a. ventricle; b. arterial; c. ejected

Case study 8

The 1_____ against which the heart must pump is:

- afterload ◄
- blood pressure
- preload
- cardiac output

2_____ is defined as the pressure within the ventricles at the end of diastole.

Blood pressure is defined as pressure that 3__ _____ on the walls of arteries.

a. resistance; b. is exerted; c. Preload

Case study 9

The 1_____ of blood ejected from the heart in one cardiac 2_____ is:

- cardiac output
- stroke volume ◄
- preload
- 3_____

a. contraction; b. afterload; c. amount

Case study 10

Nitroglycerin has all of the following properties:

- prevents vasospasm ◄
- is a 1_____ ◄
- decreased preload ◄

2_____ is a vasodilator, it works against 3_____ and decreased preload.

a. Nitroglycerin; b. vasodilator; c. vasospasm

Case study 11

Your patient in ventricular tachycardia is lethargic, diaphoretic, and 1_____ and has vomited once. His vital signs are: BP 54/P, pulse 184, respirations 14. Describe your management of this patient: ABCs, high-flow oxygen, cardioversion. ◄

ABCs and high-flow oxygen are indicated for this patient and 2_____ needs to be performed because the patient is in 3_____ _____with a pulse.

a. cardioversion; b. ventricular tachycardia; c. pale

Case study 12

You respond to a 76-year-old man with syncope. He is sitting upright in the bathroom when you arrive. He stated that he was having a bowel movement when he 1_____ ___. Based on the information provided, you suspect the cause of the patient's syncope is:

- digitalis toxicity
- an atrial dysrhythmia
- vasovagal episode ◄
- underlying myocardial ischemia

Your patient's history should lead you to the 2_____ __ a vasovagal episode. Having a 3_____ _____ or bearing down to have a bowel movement can 4_____ the vagus nerve and slow down the heart rate enough to cause dizziness/syncope.

a. bowel movement; b. conclusion of; c. stimulate; d. blacked out

Case study 13

All of the following are considered anginal equivalents:

- diaphoresis, syncope, 1_____ ◄
- dyspnoea, palpitations, 2_____ ◄
- fatigue, dizziness, 3_____ ◄

a. dizziness; b. palpitations; c. syncope

Case study 14

You respond to a possible 1_____ ____. On arrival, you find bystander CPR in progress on a male patient in his thirties. Your first action should be: to stop bystander CPR to assess ABCs. ◄

Bystander CPR is a courageous effort to 2_ _____ and is important in the chain of survival but there are times when bystander perform CPR 3_____. As an EMS provider, you must 4____ _____ CPR and verify a patent airway, the absence of breathing, and pulselessness when you arrive on scene.

a. save a life; b. stop bystander; c. drowning call; d. inappropriately

Case study 15

All of the following are treatable causes of 1_____ _____ _____:

- hypothermia, hypovolemia, cardiac 2_____, acidosis ◄
- acidosis, 3_____ thrombosis, pulmonary 4_____ ◄
- 5_____ pneumothorax, hyperkalemia, coronary thrombosis ◄

Other 6_____ _____ of PEA: hypoxia, hypokalemia, drug overdose.

a. treatable causes; b. tension; c. coronary; d. pulseless electrical activity; e. tamponade; f. embolism

Case study 16

How often should you 1_____ rescue breaths for a child who is 2_____? – 12 to 20 breaths 3___ _____. ◄

a. per minute; b. provide; c. apnoeic

Case study 17

What is the 1_____ _____ of chest compressions to ventilations while 2_____ two-person CPR on an adult with an advanced airway in place? – 30 3_____ to 2 ventilations. ◄

a. compressions; b. performing; c. proper rate

Case study 18

You respond to a shopping mall for a possible cardiac arrest. When you arrive, you find a male patient in his seventies in 1_____ _____. The mall security officers have an 2___ _____. The AED is in the process of 3_____ _ _____. Your first response should be to: allow the AED to deliver the initial shock. ◄

The best treatment for a shockable rhythm is defibrillation. If an AED is in the process of delivering a shock, 4_____ it to do so.

a. delivering a shock; b. cardiac arrest; c. AED attached; d. allow

Case study 19

Which signs/symptoms are considered atypical presentation of myocardial ischemia?

- Lower extremity pain, 1_____ pain, abdominal pain ◄
- 2_____ pain, 3_____ pain, sharp or knifelike pain ◄
- nausea, dizziness, palpitations ◄

a. Shoulder; b. reproducible; c. epigastric

Case study 20

A dissecting aortic aneurysm may produce which of the following signs/symptoms?

- a ripping or tearing pain sensation ◄
- 1_____ in the abdomen
- the same 2_____
  _____ in each arm
- respiratory distress

A classic description of pain associated with a 3_____ _____ _____ is a ripping or tearing sensation.

a. dissecting aortic aneurysm; b. blood pressure; c. pain

Case study 21

You are evaluating a male patient with 1_____ __ a "tearing sensation" epigastric pain. He tells you that the pain began two hours ago after eating lunch. He says he has never 2_____ any pain like this. He rates the pain as a 10, and states that it is 3_____ into his back and shoulder. Based on the information provided, you suspect the pain may be the 4_____ __:

- a myocardial infarction
- a hiatal hernia
- an aortic aneurysm.◄
- gastric oesophageal reflux disease

a. result of; b. complaints of; c. radiating; d. experienced

Vocabulary 1

ABCs /ˌeɪ.biːˈsiː/
advanced /ədˈvɑːnt st/
AED, Automated /ˈɔː. tə.meɪ.tɪd/ **External** /ɪkˈstɜː.nəl/ **Defibrillator** /ˌdiːˈfɪb.rɪ.leɪ.tər/
afterload /ˈɑːf.tər.ˈləʊd/
allow /əˈlaʊ/
angina /ænˌdʒaɪ.nə/
anginal /ænˌdʒaɪ.nəl/
aortic /eɪˈɔː.tɪk/ **aneurism** /ˌæn.jʊə.rɪ.zəm/
arterial /ɑːˈtɪərɪəl/
arterionecrosis /ɑːˌtɪə.rɪə.neˈkrəʊ.sɪs/
arteriosclerosis /ɑːˌtɪə. ri.əʊ.skləˈrəʊ.sɪs/
atherosclerosis /ˌæθ.ə.rəʊ.skləˈrəʊ.sɪs/
atrium pl atria /ˈeɪ.tri.əm/
attach /əˈtætʃ/
atypical /ˌeɪˈtɪp.ɪ.kəl/
automacity /ɔːˈtɒm.ə.sɪt.i/
back /bæk/
bear /beər/ **down** /daʊn/
black out /ˈblæk.aʊt/
bowel /ˈbaʊ.əl/ **movement** /ˈmuː.v.mənt/
capillary /kəˈpɪl.ər.i/ **refill** /ˈriː. fɪl/ zpětné plnění kapilár
cardiac /ˈkɑː.dɪˌæk/ **output** /ˈaʊtˌpʊt/
cardioversion /ˌkɑː.di.əˈvɜː.ʃən/
chain /tʃeɪn/
composed /kəmˈpəʊzd/ **of**
compromise /ˈkɒmprəˌmaɪz/
conclusion /kənˈkluː.ʒən/
conduction /kənˈdʌk.ʃən/
contractility /ˌkən.trækˈtɪ.lə.ti/
coronary /ˈkɒr.ən.ər.i/
courageous /kəˈreɪ.dʒəs/
defibrillation /diːˌfɪb.rɪˈleɪ.ʃən/
deficiency /dɪˈfɪʃ.ənt .si/
diaphoresis /ˌdaɪ.ə.fəˈriː.sɪs/
diastole /daɪˈæs.tə.li/
digitalis /ˌdɪdʒ.ɪˈteɪ.lɪs/

discomfort /dɪˈskʌmp.fət/
dissecting /daɪˈsekt.ɪŋ/ aortic /eɪˈɔː.tɪk/ aneurysm /ˈæn.jʊə.rɪ.zəm/
distant /ˈdɪs.tənt/
drowning /ˈdraʊn.ɪŋ/
dysrhythmia /dɪsˈrɪθ.mɪə/
effort /ˈef.ət/
eject /ɪˈdʒekt/
elasticity /ˌɪl.æsˈtɪs.ɪ.ti/
elevated /ˈel.ɪ.veɪ.tɪd/
embolism /ˈem.bə.lɪzəm/
embolus pl emboli /ˈem.bə.ləs/
enclose /ɪnˈkləʊz/
endocardium /ˌen.dəˈkɑː.di.əm/
epigastric /ˌepɪˈgæs.trɪk/
episode /ˈep.ɪ.səʊd/
equivalent /ɪˈkwɪv.əl.ənt/
exert /ɪgˈzɜːt/
experience /ɪkˈspɪə.ri.ənt s/
fatigue /fəˈtiːg/
fibroserous /ˌfaɪ.brəˈsɪə.rəs/
harden /ˈhɑː.dən/
hiatal /haɪˈeɪ.təl/ hernia /ˈhɜː.ni.ə/
hiatus /haɪˈeɪ.təs/
hypocalcaemia /ˌhaɪ.pəʊ.kælˈsiː.mi.ə/
hypomagnesaemia /ˌhaɪ.pəʊ.ˌmæg.nəˈsiː.mi.ə/
hypotension /ˌhaɪ.pəʊˈten.t ʃən/
hypothermia /ˌhaɪ.pəʊ ˈθɜː.mi.ə/
inappropriately /ˌɪn.əˈprəʊ.pri.ət.li/
initial /ɪˈnɪʃəl/
inner /ˈɪn.ər/
irritability /ˌɪr.ɪ.təˈbɪl.ɪ.ti/
ischaemia /ɪsˈkiː.mɪ.ə/
jugular /ˈdʒʌg.jə.lər/
knife /naɪf/
layer /ˈleɪ.ə/
like /laɪk/
marked /mɑːkt/
medium /ˈmiː.di.əm/ -sized /saɪzd/
middle /ˈmɪd.l/
muscle /ˈmʌsəl/
myocardial /maɪ.əˌkɑː.di.əl/
myocardium /ˌmaɪ.əˈkɑː.di.əm/
necrosis /neˈkrəʊsɪs/

officer /ˈɒf.ɪ.sər/
OPA, Oropharyngeal /ˈɔː.rə.fəˈrɪn.dʒi.əl/ Airway /ˈeə.weɪ/
output /ˈaʊt.pʊt/
overdose /ˈəʊ.və.dəʊs/
parietal /pəˈraɪə.təl/
patent /ˈpeɪ.tənt/
pericardial /ˌper.ɪˈkɑː.di.əl/
pericardium /ˌper.ɪˈkɑː.di.əm/
pneumothorax /ˌnjuːməʊˈθɔː.ræks/
preload /ˌpriːˈləʊd/
presence /ˈprez.ənt s/
proper /ˈprɒpə/
protective /prəˈtek.tɪv/
pulseless /ˈpʌls.ləs/
pulselessness /ˈpʌls.ləs.nəs/
radiate /ˈreɪ.di.eɪt/
rate /reɪt/
reflect /rɪˈflekt/
reflux /ˈriː.flʌks/
reproducible /ˌriː.prə.djuːsɪ.bl/
rip /rɪp/
sac /sæk/
security /sɪˈkjʊə.rɪ.ti/
sensation /senˈseɪ.ʃən/
separate /ˈsep.ər.ət/
septum /ˈsep.təm/
sharp /ʃɑːp/
shockable /ˈʃɒk.ə.bl/
shopping /ˈʃɒp.ɪŋ/ mall /mɔːl/
shoulder /ˈʃəʊl.dər/
state /steɪt/
stroke /strəʊk/ volume /ˈvɒl.juːm/
supply /səˈplaɪ/
surround /səˈraʊnd/
survival /səˈvaɪ.vəl/
systemic /sɪˈstem.ɪk/
tearing /ˈteər.ɪŋ/
tension /ˈtent ʃən/
thicken /ˈθɪk.ən/
thrombosis /θrɒmˈbəʊ.sɪs/
toxicity /tɒkˈsɪs.ɪ.ti/
treatable /ˈtriːt.ə.bl/
underlying /ˌʌndəˈlaɪ.ɪŋ/
upright /ˈʌp.raɪt/

vagus /ˈvəɪ.gəs/ pl **gi**
vasodilator /ˌveɪ.zə.daɪˈleɪ.tər/
vasospasm /ˌveɪ.zəʊˈspæzm/
vasovagal /ˌveɪ.zəʊˈvæg.əl/
ventricle /ˈven.trɪ.kl̩/
vomit /ˈvɒm.ɪt/

Unit 2

Case study 1

Before providing rescue breathing to an 1_____ victim, you must check for breathing. You do this by: looking, listening, and feeling the 2_____ through the victim's nose or mouth ◄

When performing CPR an an adult in 3_____ _____ it is important to: allow the chest to fully recoil between 4_____. ◄

a. airflow; b. compressions; c. unresponsive;
d. cardiac arrest

Case study 2

You are performing 1___ on an elderly woman in cardiac arrest. After the patient has been 2_____ and proper ET tube placement has been confirmed, you should: 3_____ asynchronous CPR while ventilating the patient at a rate of 8 to 10 breaths/minute. ◄

After an advanced airway is placed, "cycles" of CPR are no longer delivered. Give 4_____ chest compressions without pauses for breaths. Give 8 to 10 breaths per minute.

a. intubated; b. perform; c. continuous;
d. CPR

Case study 3

Stimulation of the vagus nerve may result in:

- vasodilatation
- an inrease in heart rate
- a decrease in heart rate ◄
- an increase in cardiac output

Stimulation of the 1_____ nerve can occur in many ways. When 2_____, a decrease in 3_____ _____ may be observed.

a. vagus; b. stimulated; c. heart rate

Case study 4

A rapid heart rate or 1_____ heart beat may cause the patient to experience a sensation 2_____ _____ as:

- palpitations ◄
- dysrhythmia
- fainting
- anxiety

Another common term to describe this 3_____ is "fluttering".

a. commonly known; b. irregular; c. sensation

Case study 5

Your patient is complaining of back and flank pain described as a tearing sensation. Inspection of the abdomen reveals a pulsatile mass. Treatment includes: gentle handling and rapid transport. ◄

1____ ___ _____ pain described as a tearing sensation and a 2_____ abdominal mass are classic signs of an abdominal 3_____ _____. Gentle handling and rapid transport to the hospital is essential once the diagnosis is made.

> a. Back and flank; b. pulsating; c. aortic aneurysm

Case study 6

The presence of pulmonary congestion indicated by abnormal lung sounds such as crackles (rales) in a patient complaining of chest pain may indicate:

- hypotension
- increased vagal tone
- increased stroke volume
- left ventricular failure ◄

Left ventricular failure occurs when the heart fails as an effective forward pump, which causes 1____ _____ of blood into pulmonary 2_____. When the backpressure becomes high enough, it forces the blood into the capillaries of the alveoli resulting in 3_____ _____. Adventitious lung sounds such as crackles are commonly present in 4_____ ventricular failure.

> a. back pressure; b. pulmonary congestion; c. left; d. circulation

Case study 7

An unwanted 1____ _____ of dopamine administration includes:

- increased myocardial oxygen demand◄
- 2_____ depression

- ventricular 3_____
- dilation of renal 4_____ at high doses

> a. respiratory; b. dysrhythmias; c. vessels; d. side effect

Case study 8

A 70-year-old woman remains in 1_____ following 10 minutes of well-coordinated 2____, intubation, IV and several rounds of 3_____. There are no obvious causes that would explain her cardiac arrest. At this point, it would be MOST appropriate to: consider ceasing resuscitative efforts ◄

> a. CPR; b. medications; c. asystole

Case study 9

You arrive on the scene of a 56-year-old male patient who developed chest pain while mowing the lawn on a hot August day. He states the pain has subsided after a few minutes of 1____. Your assessment shows that he is alert, and 2_____, BP 148/92, pulse 48, respiration of 20. His skin is warm and moist. He has no past medical history and takes no medications. Treatment should include: transport for evaluation. ◄

Transport for evaluation must be considered for this patient. A 3_____ ____ of 48 while mowing the lawn on a hot August day should be a concern. With the presence of chest pain, you should suspect an 4_____ cardiac origin and transport.

a. rest; b. oriented; c. underlying;
d. bradycardic rate

Case study 10

Your patient is a 47-year-old male who is experiencing paroxysmal junctional tachycardia. He called EMS because of a sensation of 1_____ ____ _____. There is no previous history of heart disease. The ventricular rate is approximately 130 per minute, BP is 100/70 and falling, and respirations are 32 and shallow. What should you do? – Attempt vagal manoeuvres to slow the heart rate down. ◄

Because the patient does not seem to be tolerating the rapid heart rate well, vagal 2_____ should be attempted first, followed by 3_____ _____ if necessary. If the heart rate increases or the patient becomes 4_____, synchronized 5_____ may be indicated.

a. cardioversion; b. manoeuvres; c. unstable;
d. palpitations and lightheadedness;
e. pharmacological therapy

Case study 11

What is the effect of parasympathetic stimulation on the heart?

- A decreased rate and increased stroke volume. ◄

Parasympathetic stimulation through the 1_____ _____ acts to decrease the heart rate; this paradoxically 2_____ stroke volume because the longer time interval between contractions allows the 3_____ to fill more efficiently.

a. increases; b. ventricles; c. vagus nerve

Case study 12

What does pulse pressure refer to? – 1_____ between the systolic and diastolic readings.◄

Pulse pressure 2_____ ___ the difference between the 3_____ ____ _____ blood pressure readings. A 4_____ pulse pressure indicates increasing diastolic pressure and decreasing systolic pressure. 5_____will stop once blood pressures come together.

a. Perfusion; b. narrowing; c. diastolic and systolic; d. Difference; e. refers to

Case study 13

The presence of pulmonary congestion indicated by abnormal lung sounds such as crackles (rales) in a patient complaining of chest pain may indicate: left ventricular failure. ◄

Left ventricular failure occurs when the heart fails as an effective forward pump, which causes 1____ _____ of blood into pulmonary 2_____. When the backpressure becomes high enough, it forces the blood into the capillaries of the alveoli resulting in 3_____ _____. Adventitious lung sounds such as crackles are commonly present in 4_____ ventricular failure.

a. back pressure; b. pulmonary congestion;
c. left; d. circulation

a. CHF patients; b. permanent damage;
c. acute episode; d. congestive heart failure

Case study 14

Cardiogenic shock can result in all of the following: 1_____, respiratory failure, an elevated heart rate. ◄

2_____ _____ is the most severe form of pump 3_____ that often results in dysrhrythmias, hypotension, respiratory failure, and possibly organ failure. The heart rate is initially elevated as the body attempts to 4_____ for the shock.

a. compensate; b. Cardiogenic shock;
c. failure; d. dysrhrythmias

Case study 15

This patient is exhibiting the signs and symptoms of which of the following diseases?

- chronic bronchitis
- emphysema
- congestive heart failure ◄
- status asthmaticus

This patient is exhibiting the classic signs and symptoms of 1_____ _____ _____. His history of AMI indicates that he may have 2_____ _____ to the heart and raises the possibility that he is now having an 3_____ _____ of failure.

What medication should be used for this patient? – Morphine sulphate. ◄

Oxygen, morphine, nitroglycerin, and furosemide are all used in the treatment of 4___ _____.

Case study 16

What does a prolonged sinus tachycardia accompanying an acute 1_____ _____ suggest?

- Cardiogenic shock may develop. ◄
- Damage of the heart is minimal.
- Hypervolaemia is the 2_____ _____.
- The diagnosis of MI is incorrect.

In a patient with acute MI, sinus tachycardia 3_____ that cardiogenic shock may develop.

a. suggests; b. underlying cause;
c. myocardial infarction

Case study 17

How should you 1_____ the patient to check for jugular vein distention?

- 2_____ flat on his or her back
- 3_____ upright near 90°
- 4_____ up in anatomical position
- seated at a 45° angle ◄

Check for jugular vein distention with the patient 5_____ at a 45° angle. Most patients will have observable jugular veins when supine.

a. elevated; b. position; c. sitting; d. lying;
e. standing

Case study 18

What does a prolonged sinus tachycardia accompanying an acute 1_____

_____ suggest?

- Cardiogenic shock may develop. ◀
- Damage of the heart is minimal.
- Hypervolaemia is the 2_____ _____.
- The diagnosis of MI is incorrect.

In a patient with acute MI, sinus tachycardia 3_____ that cardiogenic shock may develop.

> a. suggests; b. underlying cause;
> c. myocardial infarction

Case study 19

What does a carotid artery bruit indicate?

- good peripheral 1_____
- obstruction of blood flow ◀
- jugular vein 2_____
- congestive heart failure

3_ _____, noisy blood flow in a vessel, indicates partial obstruction due to 4_____ buildup or the presence of an 5_____

> a. embolus; b. plaque; c. A bruit; d. perfusion;
> e. distention

Case study 20

1____ _____ are used to treat: paroxysmal supraventricular tachycardia. ◀

Paroxysmal supraventricular 2_____ (PSVTs) may be 3_____ by vagal manoeuvres, such as the Valsalva manoeuvre or ice-water 4_____.

> a. managed; b. Vagal manoeuvres;
> c. immersion; d. tachycardia

Case study 21

In which situation would you 1_____ having the patient perform a Valsalva manoeuvre to slow the heart rate?

- male, age 34, paroxysmal junctional tachycardia ◀
- male, age 68, idioventricular escape rhythm
- female, age 74, 2_____ ventricular contrations
- female, age 39, ventricular tachycardia

When PJT is caused by stress or excessive 3_____ _____ in a patient with no history of heart disease, the Valsalva manoeuvre can be successful at 4_____ the heart rate.

> a. caffeine intake; b. slowing; c. premature;
> d. consider

Vocabulary 2

adventitious /ˌæd.vənˈtɪʃ.əs/
airflow /ˈeə.fləʊ/
alveolus pl **alveoli** /ˌæl.viˈəʊ.ləs/
anxiety /æŋˈzaɪ.ə.ti/
asynchronous /eɪˈsɪŋ.krə.nəs/
asystole /ə.sɪs.tə.lɪ/
backpressure /ˌbækˈpreʃ.ər/
beat /biːt/
bruit /bruːt/

buildup /ˈbɪld.ʌp/
caffeine /ˈkæf.iːn/
capillary /kəˈpɪl.ər.i/
cardioversion /ˌkɑː.di.əˈvɜː.ʃən/
carotid artery /kəˌrɒt.ɪdˈɑː.tər.i/
cease /siːs/
commonly /ˈkɒm.ən.lɪ/
compensate /ˈkɒm.pən.seɪt/
confirmed /kənˈfɜːmd/
congestion /kənˈdʒes.tʃən/
congestive /kənˈdʒes.tɪv/
continuous /kənˈtɪn.ju.əs/
CPR, Cardiopulmonary /
ˌkɑː.di.əʊˈpʊl.mə.nə.ri/
Resuscitation /rɪˌsʌs.ɪˈteɪ.ʃən/
demand /dɪˈmaːnd/
diastolic /daɪˈæs.tə.lɪk/
dopamine /ˈdəʊ.pə.mɪːn/
effective /ɪˈfek.tɪv/
effort /ˈef.ət/
embolus pl emboli /ˈem.bə.ləs/
emphysema /ˌemp.fəˈsiː.mə/
escape /ɪˈskeɪp/
essential /ɪˈsen.tʃəl/
evaluation /ɪˌvæl.juˈeɪ.ʃən/
fail /feɪl/
failure /ˈfeɪ.ljə/
faint /feɪnt/
fall /fɔːl/ (fell, fallen)
flank /flæŋk/
flat /flæt/
flutter /ˈflʌt.ər/
force /fɔːs/
forward /ˈfɔː.wəd/
gentle /ˈdʒen.tl/
handling /ˈhænd.lɪŋ/
heart /hɑːt/ rate /reɪt/
hypervolaemia /ˌhaɪ.pəˌvoˈliː.mi.ə/
idioventricular /ˌɪd.i.əʊ.venˈtrɪk.jə.lər/
immersion /ɪˈmɜː.ʃən/
intake /ˈɪn.teɪk/
junction /ˈdʒʌŋk.ʃən/
junctional /ˈdʒʌŋk.ʃən.əl/
tachycardia /ˌtæk.ɪˈkɑː.di.ə/
lightheadedness /ˌlaɪtˈhed.ɪd.nəs/

manoeuvre /məˈnuː.vər/
moist /mɔɪst/
observable /əbˈzɜː.vəbəl/
obvious /ˈɒb.vi.əs/
paradoxically /ˌpær.əˈdɒk.sɪ.kəl.i/
parasympathetic /ˈpær.ə.sɪm.pəˈθet.ɪk/
paroxysmal /ˌpær.ɒk.ˈsɪz.məl/
past /pɑːst/
perform /pəˈfɔːm/
perfusion /pəˈfjuː.ʒən/
plaque /plɑːk/, /plæk/
premature /ˈprem.ə.tʃər/
pulmonary /ˈpʊl.mə.nə.ri/
congestion /kənˈdʒes.tʃən/
pulsatile /ˈpʌlsə.taɪl/ mass /mæs/
reading /ˈriː.dɪŋ/
recoil /rɪˈkɔɪl/
refer /rɪˈfɜːr/
renal /ˈriː.nəl/
round /raʊnd/
sensation /senˈseɪ.ʃən/
shallow /ˈʃæl.əʊ/
side /saɪd/ effect /ɪˈfekt/
status /ˈsteɪ.təs/ asthmaticus /æsθˈmæt.ɪk.əs/
stroke /strəʊk/ volume /ˈvɒl.juːm/
subside /səbˈsaɪd/
supine /ˈsuː.paɪn/
supraventricular /ˈsuːprə.venˈtrɪk.jə.lər/
systolic /sɪsˈtɑl.ɪk/
treatment /ˈtriːt.mənt/
unstable /ʌnˈsteɪ.bl/
unwanted /ʌnˈwɒn.tɪd/
vagal /ˈveɪ.gəl/
Valsalva /vælˈsæl.və/
manoeuvre /məˈnuː.vər/
vasodilatation /ˌveɪ.zə.daɪ.ləˈteɪ.ʃən/
ventricular /venˈtrɪk.jə.lər/
vessel /ˈves.əl/

Part 3
Medical
emergencies

Respiratory; neurology;
endocrinology; allergies/
anaphylaxis; gastroenterology;
urology; environmental;
behavioural; toxicology

Unit 1
Case study 1

A sharp type of pain
that travels along a definitive
neural route is termed:

- peritonitis
- somatic pain ◄
- referred pain
- visceral pain

Dull, 1_____ _____
pain that originates in the walls
of the 2_____ _____ is
termed: visceral pain. ◄

Pain that originates in a
3_____ other than where it is
felt is known as: referred pain ◄

a. poorly localized; b. region; c. hollow organs

Case study 2

In a patient with 1_____
_____, assessment of the
abdomen should be performed
in the following order: inspect,
auscultate, palpate, percuss ◄
2_____ is the obvious
first step since you are going
to look before you do anything.
3_____ may not provide
much useful information but if
you are going to auscultate, it must
be performed before palpation.
4_____ is the third step.
You can gain a lot of information
through palpation. 5_____ (if
performed) is the last assessment step.

a. Auscultation; b. Percussion; c. Palpation; d. Inspection; e. abdominal pain

Case study 3

When ventilating a patient
via an 1_____ _____, the
amount of air flowing into the
lungs will be reduced if: there is
increased airway resistance. ◄
Airway resistance resulting
from 2_____, bronchoconstriction,
or increased 3_____ production
can cause increased 4_____
_____, resulting in a
decrease in the amount of air
flowing into the 5_____.

a. mucus; b. oedema; c. airway resistance;
d. endotracheal tube; e. lungs

Case study 4

One 1_____ of Glasgow
Coma Scale 2_____ is:

- pupillary response and size
- respiratory rate
- heart rate
- motor response ◄

The Glasgow Coma Scale
measures eye opening, and verbal
response, and 3_____ _____.

a. motor response; b. measures; c. area

Case study 5

1_____ injuries are tissue
2_____ that occur directly
at the point of 3_____:

- concussion
- contrecoup
- coup ◄
- epidural

a. disruptions; b. impact; c. Coup

Case study 6

Why is important to limit
the time 1____ _____
a patient's airway?

- The 2_____ _____
  level will decrease. ◄
- Bradycardia can develop. ◄

Suctioning removes oxygen
from the airway and can cause
vagal stimulation resulting in
3_____. Adults should
not be suctioned for longer than
10-15 seconds. 4_____
patients should not be suctioned
for longer that 5 seconds.

a. for suctioning; b. Paediatric; c. bradycardia;
d. blood oxygen

Case study 7

A syndrome that develops as a
complication of an illness such as
multisystem 1_____, severe sepsis,
or 2_____ _____ is termed:

- adult respiratory
  syndrome (3_____) ◄
- pneumonia syndrome (PS)
- chronic obstructive
  pulmonary disease (COPD)
- congestive heart
  failure (CHF)

ARDS is a form of 4_____
_____ that occurs as a response to
a wide variety of lung injury insults.

a. toxic inhalation; b. ARDS; c. pulmonary
oedema; d. trauma

Case study 8

An expression of
1_____ _____ of
abnormal lung cells is best termed:

- pulmonary disease
- chronic bronchitis
- lung cancer ◄
- viral pneumonia

2____ _____ is an
excessive and uncontrolled growth
of 3_____ _____.

a. Lung cancer; b. cancerous cells;
c. uncontrolled growth

Case study 9

A 49-year-old male with COPD is tired, confused, and in severe respiratory distress. His 1_____ _____ _____ is most likely caused by:

- carbon dioxide excretion
- hypoxia ◄
- tachypnoea

2_____ can affect the 3_____ at the cellular level resulting in a decreased mental status.

a. brain; b. altered mental status; c. Hypoxia

Case study 10

A diagnostic device for measuring forced 1_____ is a:

- pulse oximeter
- capnometer
- peak flow meter ◄
- end-tidal CO_2 detector

The peak 2_____ _____ _____ measures the amount of air a patient can forcefully exhale with 3____ _____.

a. respiratory flow meter; b. one breath; c. exhalation

Case study 11

Which device would be most effective in determining if an endotracheal tube is placed in the stomach? – End-tidal CO_2 detector ◄

This instrument measures the 1_____ __ _____ of carbon dioxide in the sampled gas at the tip of the 2_____ _____.

It can be used as an assessment tool to help determine proper endotracheal tube 3_____.

a. endotracheal tube; b. placement; c. presence or absence

Case study 12

The process of 1___ _____ between that alveoli and the pulmonary capillary bed is termed:

- ventilation
- diffusion ◄
- perfusion
- osmosis

2_____ is the process of gas molecules moving across a 3____ _____ from a 4_____ _____ of molecules to a lower concentration.

a. higher concentration; b. Diffusion; c. gas exchange; d. cell membrane

Case study 13

1____ _____ of albuterol administration include:

- hypotension and bradycardia
- pallor and sedation
- tachycardia and tremor ◄
- respiratory depression

Administration of albuterol can stimulate the 2_____ nervous system resulting in an increased 3____ _____ and 4_____.

a. tremor; b. Side effects; c. sympathetic; d. heart rate

Case study 14

Upper respiratory infections
(1____) are more severe in:

- patients with asthma
  or COPD ◄
- patients with HIV
  infection ◄

Patients with 2____-_____
respiratory disease or who
are 3_____
are more prone to URI.

> a. immunocompromised; b. pre-existing;
> c. URI

Case study 15

Predisposing factors
1_____ to the
development of pneumonia are:

- alcoholism ◄
- cigarette smoking ◄
- extremes of age ◄

Chest pain may be a
symptom of a problem but is not
a 2_____ _____ in
itself. The very young and old,
cigarette smokers, and alcoholism
are all predisposing factors to the
3_____ __ pneumonia.

> a. predisposing factor; b. development of;
> c. contributing

Case study 16

A patient is anxious and has been
breathing rapidly and deeply for the
past 45 minutes. You can expect his
blood 1_____ _____ level to be:

- elevated

- decreased ◄
- normal
- acidotic

Rapid, deep breathing can
result in 2_____ _____
of carbon dioxide leading to
3_____ _____.

> a. respiratory alkalosis; b. excess elimination;
> c. carbon dioxide

Case study 17

When the entire lobe of a
lung is filled with infection and
cellular debris, it is termed:

- pleuric disease
- mild aspiration
- consolidation ◄
- haemoptysis

The 1_____, 2_____,
and 3_____ can fill up the
lung creating consolidation.

> a. infection; b. debris; c. fluid

Case study 18

You find a morbidly obese
42-year-old patient lying 1_____ in
his bed. He is in marked respiratory
distress and is able to speak only
in two-word sentences. What
should you do FIRST? – Sit him
up or place him on his side. ◄

Morbidly obese patients in
respiratory distress should be sat
up or placed 2__ _____ ____.
When a morbidly obese patient is
supine, his/her own 3_____ _____
can often impair the mechanics of

4_____. This is known as Pickwickian syndrome.

a. respiration; b. body weight; c. on their side; d. supine

Case study 19

You are called to attend to an 18-year-old male who is having a severe asthma attack. He is awake and alert but appears very tired. His vital signs are blood pressure 158/90, pulse 132, respiratory rate 32 and extremely laboured. Upon auscultation of his chest you note breath sounds heard only in the 1_____ _____ with very little wheezing 2_____.

- This is significant because it shows: bronchoconstriction with air trapping. ◄

This 3_____ _____ results in decreased 4____ _____ in the lungs and can lead to profound hypoxia.

- His fatigue is significant in that it tells you: he is in danger of respiratory failure. ◄

5_____ in this situation indicates that the patient is becoming tired. This is an ominous sign of 6_____ respiratory failure and the development of 7_____ _____. He is tachycardic at a rate of 132 beats per minute and has pale and diaphoretic skin.

- What is causing these signs? – Hypoxia, and release of epinephrine and norepinephrine. ◄

Both hypoxia and anxiety cause activation of the 8_____ nervous system and the 9_____ of epinephrine and norepinephrine, which causes diaphoresis, elevation of the heart rate (tachycardia), and peripheral vasoconstriction (pale skin).

- Why is he able to talk only in 10_____, _____ _____? – His tidal volume is inadequate for him to speak in full sentences. ◄

Because of the air trapping, he does not have enough air (tidal volume) available to speak.

- Which 11_____ will assist 12 __ _____ his airways? – Administration of a nebulized beta-2 agonist. ◄

A nebulized beta-2 agonist (such as albuterol) delivered by mask or hand-held device using 5-10 LPM of oxygen can assist in bronchodilation.

- What medication can be administered into the subcutaneous tissues to help 13_____ his respiratory distress? – Epinephrine 1:1,000, 0.3 mg. ◄

14_____ epinephrine is an option to treat cases of severe asthma because of its beta-2 agonist properties.

a. air exchange; b. alleviate; c. release;
d. Subcutaneous; e. serious condition; f. upper
lobes; g. respiratory arrest; h. bilaterally;
i. pending; j. intervention; k. short; broken
phrases; l. in dilating; m. sympathetic;
n. Fatigue

Case study 20

A disease that results from
the 1_____ of the walls
of the 2_____ and lessens
the amount of surface area for
3___ _____ is termed:

- emphysema ◄
- chronic bronchitis
- asthma
- pneumonia

a. gas exchange; b. alveoli; c. destruction

Vocabulary 1

acidotic /əˈsɪd.ə.tɪk/
activation /ˌæk.tɪˈveɪ.ʃən/
alcoholism /ˈæl.kə.hɒl.ɪ.zəm/
alkalosis /ˌælkəˈləʊ.sɪs/
alleviate /əˈliː.vi.eɪt/
altered /ˈɔːltəd/
appear /əˈpɪər/
aspiration /ˌæspɪˈreɪʃən/
assist /əˈsɪst/
attend /əˈtend/
auscultate /ˈɔː.skəl.teɪt/
auscultation /ˌɔː.skəlˈteɪ.ʃən/
bed /bed/
beta-2 agonist /ˈbiː.tə.tuː/
agonists /ˈæg.ə.nɪsts/
bilaterally /ˌbaɪˈlæt.ər.ə.li/
blood /blʌd/
bradycardia /ˌbræd.ɪˈkaːdi.ə/
break /breɪk/ **(broke broken)**
bronchoconstriction /ˌbrɒŋ.kəʊ.kənˈstrɪk.ʃən/
cancer /ˈkænt.sər/

cancerous /ˈkæn.sər.əs/
capillary /kəˈpɪl.ər.i/ **bed** /bed/
capnometer /kæpˈɒm.ɪ.tər/
capnometry /kæpˈnɒm.ə.tri/
cell /sel/
cellular /ˈsel.jʊ.lər/
concussion /kənˈkʌʃ.ən/
confused /kənˈfjuːzd/
consolidation /kənˌsɒl.ɪˈdeɪ.ʃən/
contrecoup /ˈkɒn.trə.kuːp/
contribute /kənˈtrɪb.juːt/
COPD, Chronic /ˈkrɒnɪk/ **Obstructive** /əbˈstrʌk.tɪv/ **Pulmonary** /ˈpʊl.mə.nə.ri/ **Disease** /dɪˈziːz/
coup /kap/
debris /ˈdeb.riː/, /ˈdeɪ.briː/
deeply /ˈdiːp.li/
definitive /dɪˈfɪn.ɪ.tɪv/
destruction /dɪˈstrʌk.ʃən/
development /dɪˈvel.əp.mənt/
device /dɪˈvaɪs/
diaphoretic /ˌdaɪ.ə.fəˈret.ɪk/
diffusion /dɪˈfjuː.ʒən/
disruption /dɪsˈrʌp.ʃən/
distress /dɪˈstres/
dull /dʌl/
elevate /ˈel.ɪ.veɪt/
end /end/ **-tidal** /ˈtaɪ.d əl/
entire /ɪnˈtaɪə/
epidural /ˌepɪˈdjʊərəl/
epinephrine /ˌepɪˈnef.riːn/
exchange /ɪksˈtʃeɪndʒ/
excretion /ɪkˈskriː.ʃən/
exhale /eksˈheɪl/
expression /ɪkˈspreʃ.ən/
extreme /ɪkˈstriːm/
fatigue /fəˈtiːg/
fill /fɪl/
forced /fɔːst/
forcefully /ˈfɔːs.fəl.i/
gain /geɪn/
gas /gæs/
Glasgow /ˌglɑːz.gəʊ/ **Coma** /ˈkəʊ.mə/ **Scale** /skeɪl/
growth /grəʊθ/

haemoptysis / hiː'mɒ.ptɪ.sɪs/
hand-held /'hændheld/
hollow /'hɒl.əʊ/
hypoxia /haɪ'pɒk.siə/
immunocompromised /ˌim.
jə.nəʊ'kɒm.prə.maɪzd/
impact /'ɪm.pækt/
impair /ɪm'peər/
inhalation /ˌɪn.hə'leɪ.ʃən/
inspect /ɪn'spekt/
inspection /ɪn'spek.ʃən/
insult /'ɪn.sʌlt/
intact /ɪn'tækt/
laboured /'leɪ.bəd/
lessen /'les.ən/
lobe /ləʊb/
localized /'ləʊ.kəl.aɪzd/
look /lʊk/
measure /'meʒ.ər/
mechanic /mɪ'kænɪk/
mechanics /mə'kæn.ɪks/
membrane /'mem.breɪn/
mental /'men.təl/ status /'steɪtəs/
mild /maɪld/
molecule /'mɒl.ɪ.kjuːl/
morbidly /ˌmɔː'bɪd.ɪ.ti/
motor /'məʊ.tər/
moving /'muː.vɪŋ/
multisystem /'mʌl.tɪ'sɪs.təm/
nebulized /'neb.jə.laɪzd/
neural /'njʊə.rəl/
norepinephrine /nɔrˌep.ə'nef.rɪn/
occur /ə'kɜːr/
oedema /ɪ'diː.mə/
ominous /'ɒmɪnəs/
option /'ɒpʃən/
order /'ɔː.dər/
originate /ə'rɪdʒ.ɪ.neɪt/
osmosis /ɒz'məʊ.sɪs/
oxygen /'ɒk.sɪ.dʒən/
pallor /'pæl.ər/
palpate /'pæl.peɪt/
palpation /pæl'peɪ.ʃən/
peak /piːk/ flow /fləʊ/ meter /m.ɪ.tər/
pending /'pen.dɪŋ/

percuss /pə'kʌs/
percussion /pə'kʌʃ.ən/
perfusion /pə'fjuː.ʒən/
Pickwickian /pɪk'wɪk.i.ən/
syndrome /'sɪndrəʊm/ Pickwikův
placement /'pleɪs.mənt/
pleuric /'plʊə.rɪk/ disease /dɪˌziːz/
point /pɔɪnt/ to /tə/
poorly /'pɔː.li/
pre-existing /ˌpriː.ɪg'zɪs.tɪŋ/
predispose /ˌpriː.dɪ'spəʊz/
proper /'prɒpə/
property /'prɒp.ə.ti/
pulse /pʌls/ oximeter /'ɒk.sɪ.m.ɪ.tər/
pupillary /pjuː.pɪl.ər.i/
referred /rɪ'fɜːd/ pain /peɪn/
region /'riː.dʒən/
release /rɪ'liːs/
remove /rɪ'muːv/
resistance /rɪ'zɪs.tənt s/
response /rɪ'spɒns/
route /ruːt/
sample /sɑːmpl/
sedation /sɪ'deɪˌʃən/
sepsis /'sep.sɪs/
size /saɪz/
somatic /sə'mæt.ɪk/
subcutaneous /ˌsʌb.kjʊ'teɪ.ni.əs/
surface /'sɜː.fɪs/
sympathetic /ˌsɪm.pə'θet.ɪk/
syndrome /'sɪn.drəʊm/
tachypnoea /ˌtæk.ɪp.'niː.ə/
tired /'taɪəd/
tissue /'tɪʃ.uː/, /'tɪs.juː/
tool /tuːl/
trap /træp/
tremor /'trem.ər/
uncontrolled /ˌʌn.kən'trəʊld/
variety /və'raɪə.ti/
ventilation /ˌven.tɪ'leɪ.ʃən/
via /'vaɪə/
visceral /'vɪs.ər.əl/ v
weight /weɪt/

Unit 2
Case study 1

Patients with chronic obstructive pulmonary disease (1_____) often breathe through pursed lips to increase pressure in the lungs. This method of breathing helps in: preventing alveolar collapse. ◄

2_____-___ breathing technique helps 3_____ _____ within the airways (even during exhalation) to support 4_____ _____ that have been damaged as a result of disease. In COPD, changes in the bronchioles that can result in significant air trapping include:

- inflammation ◄
- bronchospasm ◄
- increased mucus production ◄

All of these pathologies impair the flow of air through the 5_____ _____.

a. bronchial tree; b. maintain pressure;
c. Purse-lip; d. bronchial walls; e. COPD

Case study 2

A 64-year-old male presents with increased dyspnoea. He has a barrel chest, is thin, and is pink in colour. Clubbing of the fingers is present. Wheezes and rhonchi are present bilaterally in 1___ _____, and pursed lip breathing is noted. Vital signs are: blood pressure 162/92, pulse 118 beats per minute, respiratory rate 22.

- This patient's 2_____ suggests that he is most likely suffering from: COPD ◄
- The wheezes auscultated bilaterally indicate: narrowing of the airways ◄

Oedema and bronchoconstriction are examples of problems that can 3_____ ___ _____.

- The rhonchi 4_____ bilaterally indicate: excessive mucus in the larger airways. ◄

5_____ are rattling sounds with a low pitch and "snoring quality" that is usually associated with 6_____ mucus or other material in the larger airways.

- The clubbing of the fingers is associated with: respiratory disease ◄

7_____ is a deformity produced by the growth of soft tissue about the 8_____ __ _____. It is associated with 9_____ cardiac or respiratory disease.

- The 10____ _____ of this patient's skin is a result of: an excess of circulating red blood cells. ◄

As a part of the body's own 11_____ _____, a chronic state of low blood oxygen levels will cause an increased production of 12____ _____ _____ (polycythemia) that give the patient's skin a pink colour.

a. fingers or toes; b. Rhonchi; c. red blood cells; d. "pink" colour; e. all lobes; f. compensatory mechanism; g. appearance; h. Clubbing; i. chronic; j. excessive; k. auscultated; l. narrow the airway

Case study 3

A 19-year-old male is found breathing very rapidly. His roommate tells you he has been having a stressful time lately and recently lost his job. The patient is 1_____, alert, and very anxious. You note that he has spasms of his 2_____ ___ _____. Vital signs are blood pressure 130/78, pulse rate 116, respiratory rate 44 and regular. He takes no medications and has no past medical problems.

Hyperventilation resulting from pure anxiety leads to:

- respiratory acidosis
- respiratory alkalosis ◄
- a decreasing blood pH
- hepatic failure

Hyperventilation can result in an excess elimination of 3_____ _____ leading to respiratory alkalosis.

- Spasms of the hands and feet is termed: carpopedal spasms ◄

4_____ decreases blood calcium levels, which leads to hypocalcaemia. This results in 5_____ ___ _____ of the feet and hands.

- In this situation, it is important to: consider that he has a serious medical problem ◄

Since hyperventilation 6___ _____ a true medical emergency such as a 7_____ _____, it is important to consider that this patient has a serious medical problem.

a. fingers and feet; b. can mask; c. pulmonary embolism; d. cramping and spasms; e. Alkalosis; f. carbon dioxide; g. awake

Case study 4

Your EMS team is dispatched to care for a 39-year-old female with difficulty breathing. She is awake and appears 1_____ and _____. She tells you she had sudden onset of shortness of breath, and a "sense of doom" while typing on her computer keyboard. Her vital signs are: blood pressure 148/92, radial pulse is strong at 124 beats per minute, respiratory rate 36 per minute and shallow. Her skin is pale, cool, and dry. She denies having chest pain or any health problems.

- Your patient's 2_____ _____ reading is 89% on room air. This indicates: that she has hypoxemia. ◄

3_ _____ _____ is used as an assessment tool. A patient with a pulse oximetry value of less than 90% with no apparent cause or past medical history is considered to be moderately hypoxic and needs 4_____-____ _____ administration.

- What is significant about her apprehension and sense of doom? – It may indicate a threat to life. ◄

A patient who alerts you to his or her "sense of doom" should be taken 5_____ _____. There are numerous reports of patients who have "sensed" a problem and later suffered a catastrophic event including a 6_____ __ ____.

During your interview, you find that the patient takes 7_____ _____ pills and has had left calf 8_____ for two days with no history of trauma to the area.

- This information leads you to suspect: a pulmonary embolus ◄

A history of taking birth control pills combined with signs and symptoms that include a 9_____ ___ _____ lower extremity suggest deep vein thrombosis. This predisposes the patient to developing 10_____ _____.

- You interpret her cardiac rhythm as atrial 11_____ with a rapid ventricular response. ◄

Management of her condition would include all of the following:

- being on alert for 12_____ arrest ◄
- monitoring the cardiac rhythm ◄

- 13_____ intravenous access ◄

a. very seriously; b. threat to life; c. tenderness; d. fibrillation; e. establishing; f. pulse oximetry; g. high-flow oxygen; h. pulmonary embolus; i. A pulse oximeter; j. birth control; k. painful, and inflamed; l. cardiac; m. restless and apprehensive

Case study 5

A 23 year-old healthy male who has been 1_____ by another person has a pulse rate of 146 and a respiratory rate of 32.

- These vital signs 2_____ that his: sympathetic nervous system is activated.◄

Sympathetic nervous system 3_____ causes pupillary dilation and will 4_____ the pulse and respiratory rate.

a. stimulation; b. increase; c. threatened; d. indicate

Case study 6

Stroke, or 1_____ _____, can be compared to a heart attack in that:

- In both cases, 2_____ _____ causes tissue damage. ◄
- 3_____can be beneficial in treating certain heart and brain attacks. ◄

Both heart attack and brain attack cause organ tissue damage due to the interruption of blood flow. Studies show that thrombolytic agents used to treat heart attack patients can be effective in treating occlusive strokes.

> a. brain attack; b. Thrombolytics; c. oxygen deprivation

Case study 7

A 30-year-old suddenly developed a two- to three-minute grand mal seizure. On scene you find an 1_____ ____ _____ patient. After the insertion of an oropharyngeal airway, applying high-flow oxygen, and assisting ventilations with a bag-valve mask, the patient's pulse oximetry reading is 90%. His skin is pale and moist. It is important to consider:

- a paralyzed diaphragm
- transport to a hospital
- endotracheal intubation ◄
- placement of a nasopharyngeal airway

A 2_____ _____ reading of 90% in a person who is on high-flow oxygen indicates 3_____ _____. Intubation should be considered.

> a. moderate hypoxia; b. pulse oximetry; c. unconscious and unresponsive

Case study 8

A 30-year-old suddenly developed a two- to three-minute grand mal seizure. On scene you find an unconscious and unresponsive patient with the following vital signs: BP 178/100, pulse 50 and regular, respiratory rate 32 and irregular. He has no history of

substance abuse but has complained of headaches for the past two weeks. His blood glucose registers 110.

You suspect that his problem is most likely the result of:

- hypoglycaemia
- a structural lesion ◄
- hyperglycaemia
- atrial fibrillation

1_____ _____, such as brain tumours and intracerebral bleeds, can press on and 2_____ brain tissue. This can cause seizures and a number of other illnesses.

Two minutes after the insertion of an 3_____ _____, applying high-flow oxygen, and assisting his ventilations with a 4___-_____ _____, the patient's pulse oximetry reading is 90%. His skin is pale and moist.

- It is important to consider: immediate endotracheal intubation ◄

A pulse oximetry 5_____ __ 90% in a person who is on high-flow oxygen indicates moderate hypoxia. Intubation should 6__ _____.

- It is important to avoid excessive hyperventilation because it can: decrease the blood PaO2 to dangerously low levels. ◄

Excessive 7_____ of a patient with increasing

intracranial pressure can decrease the blood arterial carbon dioxide to dangerous levels.

The patient is now exhibiting decorticate posturing to 8_____ _____.

- These signs indicate: a lesion at or above the upper brainstem. ◄

Decorticate posturing (9_____) indicates a lesion at or above the 10_____. Decerebrate posturing (11_____), however, results from a lesion within the brainstem.

a. Structural lesions; b. brainstem; c. painful stimuli; d. oropharyngeal airway; e. flexion; f. extension; g. hyperventilation; h. reading of; i. be considered; j. bag-valve mask; k. destroy

Case study 9

A 27-year-old patient is complaining of persistent headache, fatigue and pain upon flexion of his neck. He has had a chronic fever of 100°F (37,8°C) for the past two days.

- His complaints lead you to suspect: meningitis. ◄

Headache with fever, fatigue, and pain 1____ _____ of the neck are all 2_____ signs and symptoms of meningitis.

- In treating this patient you would: wear gloves and place a mask on yourself and the patient. ◄

Universal 3_____ include use of 4_____ ___ _ _____ by the care provider as well as putting a mask on the patient, which significantly reduces the chance of exposure to the pathogen.

a. precautions; b. gloves and a mask; c. upon flexion; d. suspicious

Case study 10

You have a patient with metastatic brain cancer. He opens his eyes 1__ _____, and answers questions with 2_____ _____. When you start an IV in his left arm, he withdraws from the IV needle piercing the skin.

- You would 3_____ his Glasgow Coma Scale: 9 ◄

You should always have a Glasgow Coma Scale chart available 4__ _____ in your 5___ _____. This patient has a GCS score of 9 – eye opening = 2, verbal response = 3, motor response = 4.

a. calculate; b. incomprehensible sounds; c. EMS practice; d. to reference; e. to pain

Case study 11

Which of the following are signs/symptoms of an acute cerebral vascular accident:

- 1_____ of the speech ◄
- facial 2_____ ◄
- drooling ◄
- weak 3_____ _____ on the affected side ◄

a. slurring; b. motor response; c. droop

Case study 12

You are called to a local restaurant for a patient exhibiting bizarre behaviours and shouting obscenities. He is pale, diaphoretic, and 1_____ any past 2_____ _____.

- Which intervention should be most appropriate?
  – Fingerstick to check blood glucose. ◀

A 3_____ _____ is a quick 4____ to rule out hypoglycaemia, which could be the cause of this patient's 5_____. Any patient with an 6_____ _____ of consciousness should be tested for hypoglycaemia.

a. altered level; b. glucose fingerstick;
c. denies; d. behaviour; e. medical problems;
f. tool

Case study 13

You are called to assist a 25-year-old known Type I diabetic patient who is complaining of abdominal pain, 1_____, and 2_____. His glucometer reading is 510.

- The highest 3_____ _____ for this patient is to: correct fluid volume deficit. ◀

This patient has diabetic 4_____ and is likely to be profoundly 5_____ because excess glucose acts as an osmotic diuretic. Fluid replacement with normal saline should be started 6_____.

a. dehydrated; b. ketoacidosis;
c. immediately; d. vomiting; e. lethargy;
f. treatment priority

Case study 14

A patient's 1_____ reads 66. You may encounter all of the following symptoms of hypoglycaemia:

- 2_____ mental status ◀
- bizarre behaviour ◀
- hunger ◀

The signs and symptoms of hypoglycaemia are many and varied. Altered mental state including 3_____, bizarre behaviour, or 4_____ is often the most important and early 5_____ of a problem. Other signs/symptoms may include diaphoresis, tachycardia, 6_____ and headache. 7____ may be present in severe cases.

a. glucometer; b. agitation; c. Coma;
d. irritability; e. altered; f. indicator;
g. weakness

Case study 15

You receive a call to the home of a 66-year-old male with a 1_____ ___ weakness. The patient is cooperative but continues to ask you the same questions over and over again. You are concerned because he has developed 2_____ _____ over the past five minutes and is now diaphoretic.

- Your next action is to: establish IV and obtain a 3_____ _____ for a blood glucose test. ◄

With a presentation of confusion and diaphoresis you should be thinking of 4_____.

> a. Blood sample; b. hypoglycaemia;
> c. increased confusion; d. complaint of

Case study 16

When the body is not able to use glucose as a 1_____ _____ __ _____: adipose cells begin 2_____ _____ resulting in ketoacidosis. ◄

This 3___-_____ metabolism results in a rise of blood ketones, which can lead to 4_____.

> a. ketoacidosis; b. breaking down; c. primary source of energy; d. fat-based

Case study 17

Signs and symptoms of Graves' disease include agitation, emotional changes, insomnia, 1___ _____, weight loss, and 2_____. ◄

You must be familiar with signs and symptoms of the most common 3_____ _____. Graves' disease is the result of thyrotoxicosis (excessive thyroid hormones).

> a. endocrine disorders; b. heat intolerance;
> c. exophthalmos

Case study 18

A male patient has ingested 30 levothyroxine that belonged to his mother. You recognize this medication as a thyroid replacement hormone. You attach the ECG monitor and observe a sinus tachycardia of 140 with a corresponding pulse rate.

- Treatment would include: expedited transport for definitive care. ◄

1_____ _____ is a true medical emergency that requires 2_____ _____ to definitive care. Drug therapy that will block the effects of the 3_____ _____ of thyroid hormone is required.

> a. expedited transport; b. toxic level;
> c. Thyroid storm

Case study 19

A patient with Cushing's 1_____ would MOST likely present with:

- ketoacidosis
- hypoglycaemia ◄
- decreased urination
- acute hyperactivity

2_____ is associated with Cushing's syndrome due to 3_____ cortisol levels.

> a. excessive; b. Hypoglycaemia; c. syndrome

Case study 20

You are caring for a 78-year-old female patient who has a long history of 1_____ (Cushing's syndrome). She is complaining of left side weakness. You are assigned to establish an

IV line and obtain a blood sample
for 2_____ _____ testing.

- You should: take great
  care with venipuncture
  in this patient because
  hyperadrenalism leads
  to easy bruising and a
  delay in healing. ◄

Long term effects of
hyperadrenalism lead to paper
thin (almost transparent) skin
that can be easily 3_____ __
____. The disease process also
results in 4_____ _____.

a. hyperadrenalism; b. delayed healing;
c. bruised or torn; d. blood glucose

Vocabulary 2

abuse /əˈbjuːz/
access /ˈæk.ses/
accident /ˈæksɪdənt/
act /ækt/
adipose /ˈæd.ɪ.pəʊs/, /-pəʊz/
affect /əˈfekt/
agitation /ˌædʒ.ɪˈteɪ.ʃən/
alveolar /ˌæl.viˈəʊ.lər/
apparent /əˈpær.ənt/
appearance /əˈpɪə.rənt s/
apprehension /ˌæp.rɪˈhen.ʃən/
atrial /ˈeɪ.tri.əl/ fibrillation /ˌfaɪ.brɪˈleɪ.ʃən/
attach /əˈtætʃ/
barrel /ˈbær.əl/
behaviour /bɪˈheɪ.vjə/
beneficial /ˌben.ɪˈfɪʃ.əl/
birth /ˈbɜːθ/ control /kənˈtrəʊl/ pill /pɪl/
bizarre /bɪˈzɑːr/
blade /bleɪd/
bleed /bliːd/

blood /blʌd/ sample /ˈsɑːm.pl /
brainstem /ˈbreɪn.stem/
break /breɪk/ down /daʊn/
bronchial /ˈbrɒŋ.ki.əl/ tree /triː/
bronchiole /ˈbrɒŋ.ki.əʊl/
bronchospasm /ˌbrɒŋ.kəʊ.ˈspæz.əm/
bruise /bruːz/
calcium /ˈkæl.si.əm/
calculate /ˈkælkjʊˌleɪt/
calf /kɑːf/
care /keə/
care /keə/ provider /prəˈvaɪ.dər/
carpopedal /ˌkɑː.pəˈpɪː.d.əl/
case /keɪs/
catastrophic /ˌkæt.əˈstrɒf.ɪk/
chart / tʃɑːt/
check /tʃek/
clubbing /ˈklʌb.ɪŋ/
collapse /kəˈlæps/
coma /ˈkəʊ.mə/
compare /kəmˈpeər/
compensatory /ˌkɒm.pənˈseɪt.ə ri/
concern /kənˈsɜːn/
confusion /kənˈfjuː.ʒən/
cool /kuːl/
cooperative /kəʊˈɒp.ər.ə.tɪv/
corresponding /ˌkɒr.ɪˈspɒn.dɪŋ/
cortisol /ˈkɔː.tɪ.sɒl/
cramp /kræmp/
decerebrate /diˌser.əˈbreɪt/
posturing /ˈpɒs.tʃər.ɪŋ/
decorticate /ˌdi.kɔːˈti ˈkeɪt/
posturing /ˈpɒs.tʃər.ɪŋ/
deep /diːp/
definitive /dɪˈfɪn.ɪ.tɪv/
dehydrated /ˌdiː.haɪˈdreɪ.tɪd/
delay /dɪˈleɪ/
deny /dɪˈnaɪ/
diabetic /ˌdaɪəˈbet.ɪk/ ketoacidosis /ˈkiːtəʊˌæs.ɪˈdəʊ.sɪs/
diaphoresis /ˌdaɪ.ə.fəˈriː.sɪs/
diaphragm /ˈdaɪ.ə.fræm/
dilation /daɪˈleɪˌʃən/
dispatch /dɪˈspætʃ/
diuretic /ˌdaɪ.jʊəˈret.ɪk/

doom /duːm/
drool /druːl/
droop /druːp/
emergency /ɪˈmɜː.dʒənt .si/
emotional /ɪˈməʊ.ʃən.əl/
encounter /ɪnˈkaʊntə/
endocrine /ˈen.də.krɪn/
establish /ɪˈstæb.lɪʃ/
event /ɪˈvent/
exhibit /ɪɡˈzɪb.ɪt/
exophthalmos /ˌeks.ɒfˈθæl.məs/
expedite /ˈek.spə.daɪt/
extension / ɪkˈsten.t ʃən/
facial /ˈfeɪ.ʃəl/
familiar /fəˈmɪl.i.ər/ **with** /wɪð/
fat-based /fæt.beɪst/
fibrillation /ˌfaɪ.brɪˈleɪ.ʃən/, /ˌfɪb.rɪˈleɪ.ʃən/
fingerstick /ˈfɪŋ.gə.stɪk/
flexion /flek.ʃən/
glucometer /ˌgluː.kəˈm.ɪ.tər/
grand mal /ˌgrɑːndˈmæl/
Graves' /greɪvz/ **disease** /dɪˈziːz/
heal /hiːl/
hepatic /hepˈæt.ɪk/
hyperactivity /ˌhaɪ.pərˈæk.tɪv.ɪ.ti/
hyperadrenalism /ˌhaɪ.pər.ædˈriː.nəl.ɪzm/
hypocalcaemia /ˌhaɪ.pəʊ.kælˈsiː.mi.ə/
hypoxaemia /ˌhai.pɒkˈsiː.mi.ə/
immediate /ɪˈmiː.di.ət/
incomprehensible /ɪnˌkɒm.prɪˈhen.sɪ.bl̩/
inflamed /ɪnˈfleɪmd/
inflammation /ˌɪn.fləˈmeɪ.ʃən/
insertion /ɪnˈsɜː.ʃən/
insomnia /ɪnˈsɒm.ni.ə/
interruption /ˌɪn.təˈrʌp.ʃən/
intolerance /ɪnˈtɒl.ər.ənt s/
intracerebral /ˌɪn.trəˈser.ə.brəl/
intravenous /ˌɪn.trəˈviː.nəs/
irritability /ˌɪr.ɪ.təˈbɪl.ɪ.ti/
IV, intravenous /ˌɪn.trəˈviː.nəs/
ketoacidosis /ˈkiː.təʊ.æ.ɪˈdəʊ.sɪs/
ketone /ˈkiː.təʊn/

lesion /ˈliː.ʒən/
levothyroxine /lev.ɒ.θaɪˈrɒk.sɪn/
management /ˈmænɪdʒmənt/
mask /mɑːsk/ maska, maskovat
meningitis /ˌmen.ɪnˈdʒaɪ.tɪs/
mental /ˈmen.təl/ **status** /ˈsteɪtəs/
metastatic /ˌmet.əˈstæt.ɪk/
moderately /ˈmɒd.ər.ət.li/
moist /mɔɪst/
narrow /ˈnær.əʊ/
nasopharyngeal /ˌneɪ.zə.fəˈrɪn.dʒi.əl/
note /nəʊt/
obscenity /əbˈsen.ɪ.ti/
obtain /əbˈteɪn/
occlusive /ɒˈkluː.sɪv/
oedema /ɪˈdiː.mə/
onset /ˈɒn.set/
osmotic /ɒzˈmɒt.ɪk/ **pressure** /ˈpreʃ.ər/
painful /ˈpeɪn.fəl/
paralyze /ˈpær.əl.aɪz/
part /pɑːt/
pathogen /ˈpæθ.ə.dʒən/
pathology /pəˈθɒl.ə.dʒi/
persistent /pəˈsɪs.tənt/
pH /ˌpiːˈeɪtʃ/
pierce /pɪəs/
pill /pɪl/
polycythaemia /ˌpɒl.ɪ.saɪˈθiːm.ɪ.ə/
postural /ˈpɒst.ʃər.əl/
posture /ˈpɒs.tʃər/
practice /ˈpræk.tɪs/
predispose /ˌpriː.dɪˈspəʊz/
profoundly /prəˈfaʊnd.li/
pupillary /pjuː.pɪl.ər.i/
pure /pjʊər/
pursed /pɜːsd/**-lip** /lɪp/
radial /ˈreɪ.di.əl/
rattle /ˈræt.l̩/
recognize /ˈrekəg.naɪz/
red /red/ **blood** /blʌd/ **cell** /sel/
reference /ˈref.ər.ənt s/
replacement /rɪˈpleɪs.mənt/
restless /ˈrest.ləs/
rhonchus /rong'kəs/ pl. **-chi**
rise /raɪz/

48

roommate /ˈrʊm.meɪt/
rule /ruːl/ out /aʊt/
saline /ˈseɪ.laɪn/
seizure /ˈsiː.ʒə/
sense /sens/
shouting /ˈʃaʊ.tɪŋ/
show /ˈʃəʊ/
slur /slɜːr/
snore /snɔːr/
soft /sɒft/
source /sɔːrs/
speech /spiːtʃ/
state /steɪt/
structural /ˈstrʌktʃərəl/
substance /ˈsʌb.stənt s/
sudden /ˈsʌd.ən/
suspicious /səˈspɪʃ.əs/
sustain /səˈsteɪn/
tenderness /ˈten.də.nəs/
thin /θɪn/
threat /θret/
thrombolytic /θrɒm.bəˈlɪt.ɪk/
thyroid /ˈθaɪə.rɔɪd/ storm /stɔːm/
thyroid gland /ˈθaɪə.rɔɪd ˌglænd/
thyrotoxicosis /ˌθaɪˈrəˌtɒksiˈkəʊ.sɪs/
toe /təʊ/
torn /tɔːn/
transparent /trænˈspær.ənt/
tumour /ˈtjuː.mər/
unconscious /ʌnˈkɒnʃəs/
unresponsive /ˌʌn.rɪˈspɒnt .sɪv/
urination /ˌjʊə.rɪˈneɪ.ʃən/
value /ˈvæl.juː/
varied /ˈveə.rɪd/
vascular /ˈvæs.kjʊ.lər/
vein /veɪn/
venipuncture /ˌve.niˈpʌŋk.tʃər/
weakness /ˈwiːk.nəs/
weight /weɪt/ loss /lɒs/
wheeze /wiːz/
withdraw /wɪðˈdrɔː/
within /wɪˈðɪn/

Unit 3

Case study 1

Hyperadrenalism is: associated with a high incidence of atherosclerosis including hypertension and stroke. ◀

1_____ is associated with high incidence of atherosclerosis hypertension and 2_____, which are all risk factors for 3_____.

---

a. stroke; b. Hyperadrenalism; c. diabetes

Case study 2

A patient experiencing Addisonian crisis may display these signs/symptoms: cardiovascular collapse, hypotension, hypoglycaemia. ◀

Presentation of 1_____ _____ (Addisonian crisis) may include cardiovascular 2_____, hypotension, and 3_____. These serious signs/symptoms are attributed to 4_____ _____ in the water and electrolyte 5_____ within the body.

---

a. Major disturbances; b. collapse; c. adrenal insufficiency; d. hypoglycaemia; e. balance

---

Case study 3

You have a patient who presents with a whole body rash. There is no complaint of shortness of breath.

- What history findings lead you to conclude that 1___ _____ is the result of a delayed hypersensitivity

reaction? – History of
taking a new medication
for the past seven days. ◄

A 2_____ hypersensitivity
reaction may occur several hours
or even days 3_____ _____.
Common causes are 4_____
__ _____. A patient may
very well present with the signs/
symptoms of allergic reaction several
day after starting a new medication.

a. after exposure; b. medications and
chemicals; c. the rash; d. delayed

Case study 4
Urticaria, is defined as:
raised areas or wheals on the skin
due to histamine release ◄
Raised areas or wheals on the
skin associated with 1_____
reaction and 2_____ _____
are known as urticaria (3_____).

a. hives; b. histamine release; c. allergic

Case study 5
You are called to an elementary
school. On arrival, you are directed
to a teacher. The class is holding a
birthday party for Austin, who turned
10 today. His mom baked brownies
for the party that contained nuts.
The teacher is 1_____ __
nuts. She ate brownies five minutes
ago. She complaints of 2_____
in her chest that is 3_____
_____ to breathe. She is not
able to talk in 4_____ _____.

• Given this information,
you suspect the patient

is experiencing: a severe
allergic reaction. ◄

Her respiratory distress is
5_____ _____. Her blood
pressure is 74/48, pulse 140,
respirations 40. You decide to
administer epinephrine.

• The correct 6____ ___
_____ are: 3-5ml of
1:10,000 solution IV ◄

Because this patient is
demonstrating pending cardiovascular
and respiratory 7_____, the
administration of 8_____
epinephrine is indicated.

a. dose and route; b. collapse; c. making
difficult; d. intravenous; e. full sentences;
f. allergic to; g. becoming worse; h. tightness

Case study 6
A patient with severe vomiting
presents with the 1_____ of
his eyes dramatically blood red.
This is most likely the result of:

• hyphema
• subconjunctival
haemorrhage ◄
• conjunctivitis
• blunt trauma

A 2_____
_____ involves rupture
of small blood vessels in the
subconjunctival space resulting in
the "white" of the eye becoming
3_____ ___. This may occur after a
4_____ _____ or 5_____
_____. While it looks dramatic,

this type of haemorrhage usually clears without 6_____ and rarely causes any residual problems.

a. strong sneeze; b. intervention; c. scleras; d. excessive vomiting; e. subconjunctival haemorrhage; f. blood red

Case study 7

You arrive on scene of a 30-year-old male lying on the ground. According to a bystander, the patient was on top of a ladder changing a light bulb. After he stuck his hand in the light fixture, he was attacked by yellow jackets that had a nest in the fixture. The patient then jumped from the top of the ladder to escape the bees. You estimate his fall to the ground to be 8 feet. He has numerous yellow jacket 1_____ on his left arm and neck.

The patient is unconscious and 2_____. As you assess his airway and breathing, you observe a respiratory rate of 8 per minute with deep 3_____ respirations, 4_____ muscle use, and obvious inspiratory stridor with each breath.

- Management of this patient's airway would include: c-spine immobilization, assist ventilations, immediate endotracheal intubation. ◀

With the possibility of spine injury proper precautions must be taken.

Assessment of the chest reveals no obvious trauma. You note

equal but distant lung sounds with 5_____ on auscultation.

- You suspect the respiratory distress to be from: bronchial constriction 6_____ __ anaphylactic reaction. ◀

Based on the presence of bee stings, and the absence of obvious 7_____ _____ causing the respiratory distress, you should suspect severe 8_____ _____ secondary to anaphylactic shock.

a. accessory; b. stings; c. gasping; d. wheezing; e. bronchial constriction; f. unresponsive; g. secondary to; h. chest trauma

Case study 8

You are assessing a patient with acute right lower quadrant pain. You suspect acute appendicitis.

- A 1_____ _____ of pain from 2_____ located one or two inches above the anterior iliac crest in a direct line with the umbilicus is known as: McBurney's point. ◀
- The presence of 3_____ _____ in this patient represents: peritoneal irritation. ◀

Rebound tenderness is pain on release of the examiner's hand, allowing the patient's abdominal wall to return to its normal position and is usually associated with 4_____ _____. This assessment finding can be present in other abdominal conditions and is not 5_____ ___ appendicitis.

> a. specific to; b. rebound tenderness; c. common site; d. appendicitis; e. peritoneal irritation

Case study 9

Your patient states that he has experienced right upper quadrant pain and right shoulder pain for the last seven days.

The patient is 1_____, 2_____, and in obvious discomfort. He has a bounding pulse rate of 132. He states that this episode of pain began after eating fried onion rings with hot mustard sauce.

- You suspect his 3_____ ____ ____ is caused by: stress response to the body and sympathetic nervous system activation. ◄

You notice that he has pain with 4_____ under the right costal margin.

- This is known as: Murphy's sign. ◄

Murphy's sign is pain caused when an 5_____ _____ is palpated by pressing under the right costal margin.

With the information gathered you suspect:

- pancreatitis
- appendicitis

- cholecystitis (inflammation of the gallbladder). ◄
- diverticulitis

> a. elevated heart rate; b. inflamed gallbladder; c. palpation; d. pale; e. diaphoretic

Case study 10

A 39-year-old male patient is lying on a couch, covered with several blankets. He has a garbage can next to him that has a small amount of vomitus in it. He has a past 1_____ _____ of alcoholism.

The patient 2_____ __ severe epigastric pain that 3_____ into his back and shoulders. His 4_____ is softly distended and he will not allow you to palpate it due to the pain. He states that he took his temperature 30 minutes ago and it was 104.2° F (40.1°C) BP is 86/42, pulse 138, respirations 20.

- You suspect the patient is 5_____ _____: pancreatitis. ◄

His history of alcoholism and presentation should lead you to suspect severe 6_____. Eighty percent of all cases of pancreatitis are associated with alcoholism.

- You suspect his vital signs are a result of: septic shock from the disease process. ◄

His BP of 86/42 and pulse of 138 lead you to believe a 7_____ _____ is present. His temperature of 104.2°

F (40.1°C) may indicate 8_____.
Severe pancreatitis is associated with septic shock, and when present it has a high 9_____ _____.

> a. suffering from; b. abdomen; c. mortality rate; d. medical history; e. sepsis; f. pancreatitis; g. complains of; h. radiates; i. shock state

Case study 11

You respond to a 21-year-old male with a complaint of vomiting after he drank an excessive amount of alcohol. He is 1_____, 2_____ and experiencing excessive dry heaves at this time. You note the presence of specks of blood on the toilet. He has no history of GI problems and takes no medications.

- You suspect the 3_____ is: the result of a Mallory-Weis tear ◄

An 4_____ ____ or laceration that 5_____ _____ excessive vomiting is known as a Mallory-Weis tear. While you may suspect this type of injury, it is difficult to be 100% certain. Do not 6____ ___ more serious causes of upper GI bleeding.

> a. bleeding; b. alert; c. results from; d. oriented; e. rule out; f. oesophageal tear

Case study 12

Maroon or tarry-coloured 1_____ indicates:

- peritonitis

- bowel obstruction
- the presence of partially digested blood ◄
- alcoholism

2_____ is dark, tarry, 3____-_____ stool that indicates the presence of 4_____ _____ blood.

> a. partially digested; b. stool; c. Melena; d. foul-smelling

Case study 13

1_____ and 2_____ following an overaggressive dialysis treatment are MOST indicative of:

- hypovolemia
- hypokalemia ◄
- hyperkalemia
- air embolism

3_____ _____ treatment can lead to a reduction of 4_____ (hypokalemia). This is likely to be seen immediately after dialysis treatment.

> a. potassium; b. overaggressive dialysis; c. Bradycardia; d. hypotension

Case study 14

What treatment for the care of a patient who is suffering from complications of dialysis is correct?
– To prevent 1_____ of the problem, start an IV only if ordered by medical control. ◄
Fluid administration in dialysis patients should be under the 2_____ _____ of medical control.

Dysrhythmias are 3_____ and if present, are generally caused by electrolyte 4_____. To prevent accidental damage to the shunt, a BP should never be assessed on the arm with the 5_____.

a. imbalances; b. direct authority; c. common; d. shunt; e. exacerbation

Case study 15

You arrive on scene of a 54-year-old female patient who is unable to urinate. She states that she had outpatient surgery in which she received anaesthesia. She presents in severe discomfort and has a 1_____ _____ bladder that is noticeable on inspection of the abdomen.

- This patient's situation is: a true medical emergency. ◄

The 2_____ __ _____ is a true medical emergency because a full, distended bladder is 3_____ _____ for the patient. Definitive care usually requires insertion of a 4_____ _____, which is not common in the prehospital setting. EMS treatment is primarily supportive.

a. inability to urinate; b. urethral catheter; c. firmly distended; d. extremely painful

Case study 16

A 42-year-old male presents with severe pain in the left flank area with no history or signs of trauma. The patient has excruciating 1_____ pain with intermittent vomiting.

What problem would you suspect as the cause of the patient's discomfort?

- abdominal aortic aneurysm
- appendicitis
- gallbladder attack
- renal calculi ◄

Renal calculi 2_____ _____ of flank pain, excruciating colicky pain, and 3_____ are considered classic signs and symptoms of 4_____ _____ (kidney stones)

- Treatment for this patient would be: IV fluids and morphine. ◄

5_____ ____ should be focused on comfort and support. Give nothing by mouth and establish IV line for medication administration. An antiemetic may be indicated, and 6____ _____ is important.

Note: While there may be concern about the use of pain medication in "undiagnosed" abdominal pain or that administration of pain medication may 7____ _____ and make in-hospital assessment more difficult, the use of morphine is not 8_____ in renal calculi.

a. vomiting; b. Sudden onset; c. mask symptoms; d. contraindicated; e. pain management; f. renal calculi; g. colicky; h. Prehospital care

Case study 17

You are transporting a patient who is 1_____ ____ _____

of methamphetamine. The patient, who is clearly anxious, has a BP 176/92, a pulse of 146, and respiration of 24. The patient suddenly becomes 2_____ and begins thrashing around, trying to 3___ ___ the stretcher.

- You should: administer intramuscular haloperidol. ◀

A benzodiazepine such as a haloperidol should be used to control anxiety caused by 4_____ _____. Chemical restraints are a widely accepted prehospital treatment.

a. stimulant abuse; b. get off; c. violent; d. under the influence

Case study 18

A skin rash, a metallic taste in the mouth and explosive diarrhoea are MOST indicative of:

- lead poisoning
- cyanide poisoning
- arsenic poisoning ◀
- mercury poisoning

1_____ is the second leading cause of acute 2_____ _____. Symptoms are a metallic taste in the mouth, explosive 3_____, and severe 4_____ pain.

a. abdominal; b. diarrhoea; c. Arsenic; d. metal poisoning

Case study 19

You are called to attend to a 61-year-old female complaining of headache, vomiting, abdominal pain, and 1___ __ _____.

She has recently been using a gas home-heating device to warm up her bedroom. Her sister lives next door and they always eat every meal together. The patient cannot get out of bed saying she is 2___ _____. She appears to be sleeping now.

Upon assessing the patient you note that she can speak clearly, slowly moves all extremities, and has a blood pressure of 164/86, pulse regular at 104, respiratory rate at 18 with normal effort. She has not eaten since last evening when she ate dinner with her sister. Her sister, however, feels fine.

- The patient's condition suggests: carbon monoxide poisoning ◀

The 3____-_____ _____ in the bedroom, the patient's signs and symptoms, and the fact that her sister is not sick should lead you to suspect carbon monoxide poisoning. Her pulse oximetry is 99%.

- This can be misleading because: pulse oximetry is inaccurate in certain cases of 4_____. ◀

Because carbon monoxide binds readily with the 5_____ molecule, the 6_____ _____ reading can read normal even though the patient may be hypoxic.

- What treatment is most important? – provide high flow oxygen ◀

7_____ high flow oxygen is essential in patients with 8_____ _____ poisoning.

> a. loss of coordination; b. carbon monoxide; c. Providing; d. poisoning; e. haemoglobin; f. home-heating device; g. too tired; h. pulse oximetry

Case study 20

Physical assessment findings, signs, or symptoms that support your suspicion that a patient is 1_____ ___ _____ of alcohol or drugs include: chest pain and dysrhythmias, confusion and polyuria, dilated pupils and anxiety, constricted pupils and respiratory depression.◄

Chest 2_____ and dysrhythmias are a typical sign/symptom of cocaine abuse.

3_____ and polyuria represent alcohol use.

Dilated 4_____ and anxiety represent evidence of hallucinogens.

5_____ pupils and respiratory depression are the result of opiates.

> a. Confusion; b. Constricted; c. under the influence; d. pain; e. pupils

Vocabulary 3

abrupt /əˈbrʌpt/
accessory /əkˈses.ər.i/
accumulate /əˈkjuː.mjʊ.leɪt/
Addison's disease /ˈæd.ɪ.sənz.dɪˌziːz/
allow /əˈlaʊ/
anaphylactic /ˌæn.ə.frˈlæk.tɪk/
aneurysm /ˌæn.jʊə.rɪ.zəm/
anterior /ænˈtɪə.ri.ər/
anti-emetic /ˌæn.tɪ.ɪˈmet.ɪk/
appendicitis /əˌpen.dɪˈsaɪ.tɪs/

arsenic /ˈɑː.sən.ɪk/
asymmetrical /ˌeɪ.sɪˈmet.rɪk.əl/
attack /əˈtæk/
attribute /ˈæt.rɪ.bjuːt/
awareness /əˈweə.nəs/
balance /ˈbæl.əns/
bee /biː/
bind /baɪnd/ **(bound, bound)**
bladder /ˈblæd.ər/
blood /blʌd/ **vessel** /ˈves.əl/
blunt /blʌnt/
bound /baʊnd/
brownie /ˈbraʊ.ni/
bulb /bʌlb/
C-spine, cervical /səˈvaɪ.kəl/ **spine** /spaɪn/
campus /ˈkæm.pəs/
carbon monoxide /ˌkɑː.bən.məˈnɒk.saɪd/
cessation /sesˈeɪ.ʃən/
chemical /ˈkem.ɪ.kəl/
cholecystitis /ˌkəʊ.lɪ.sɪˈstaɪ.tɪs/
colicky /ˈkɒl.ɪ.ki/
comfort /ˈkʌm.fət/
complaint /kəmˈpleɪnt/
conclude /kənˈkluːd/
conditioning /kənˈdɪʃ.ən.ɪŋ/
conjunction /kənˈdʒʌŋk.ʃən/
conjunctivitis /kənˌdʒʌŋk.tɪˈvaɪ.tɪs/
constricted /kənˈstrɪkt.ɪd/
copperhead /ˈkɒp.ər.hed/
costal /ˈkɒs.təl/
cottonmouth /ˈkɒt.ən.maʊθ/
Crohn's disease /ˈkrəʊnz.dɪˌziːz/
cyanide /ˈsaɪə.naɪd/
daydream /ˈdeɪ.driːm/
delayed /dɪˈleɪd/
demonstrate /ˈdem.ən.streɪt/
direct /daɪˈrekt/
disc /dɪsk/
discomfort /dɪˈskʌmp.fət/
discontinuation /ˌdɪs.kənˌtɪn.juˈeɪ.ʃən/
distant /ˈdɪs.tənt/
distend /dɪˈstend/
disturbance /dɪˈstɜː.bənts/

diverticulitis /ˌdaɪ.vəˌtɪk.jʊˈlaɪ.tɪs/
dose /dəʊs/
drizzle /ˈdrɪz.əl/
drowsy /ˈdraʊ.zi/
dysphasia /disˈfeɪ.zɪə/
electrolyte /ɪˈlek.trə.laɪt/
equal /ˈiːkwəl/
escape /ɪˈskeɪp/
essential /ɪˈsen.tʃəl/
estimate /ˈes.tɪ.meɪt/
exacerbation /ɪgˌzæsəˈbeɪʃən/
examiner /ɪgˈzæm.ɪ.nər/
excruciating /ɪkˈskruː.ʃi.eɪ.tɪŋ/
expectorate /ɪkˈspek.tər.eɪt/
experience /ɪkˈspɪə.ri.ənt s/
eyebrow /ˈaɪ.braʊ/
fibrillate /ˈfaɪ.brɪ.leɪt/
finding /ˈfaɪndɪŋ/
fire fighter /ˈfaɪəˌfaɪ.tər/
fixture /ˈfɪks.tʃər/
focused /ˈfəʊkəst/
foul /faʊl/
frown /fraʊn/
gallbladder /ˈgɔːlˈblæd.ər/
garbage /ˈgɑː.bɪdʒ/ can /kæn/
gasp /gɑːsp/
gather /ˈgæð.ər/
goblet /ˈgɒb.lət/
goof /guːf/ around /əˈraʊnd/
ground /graʊnd/
haemorrhage /ˈhem.ər.ɪdʒ/
hallucinogen /həˈluː.sɪ.nə.dʒen/
heave /hiːv/
histamine /ˈhɪs.tə.miːn/
hives /haɪvz/
humidity /hjuːˈmɪd.ɪ.ti/
hyperkalaemia /ˌhaɪ.pə.kæˈliː.mi.ə/
hypersensitivity /ˌhaɪ.pə.ˌsen.sɪˈtɪv.ɪ.ti/
hyphaema /haɪ.θe.mə/
hypokalaemia /ˌhaɪ.pəʊ.kæˈliː.mi.ə/
hypovolaemia /ˌhaɪpəʊ.vəˈlːːmi.ə/
iliac /ˈɪl.i.æk/ crest /krest/
imbalance /ˌɪmˈbæl.ənt s/
immobilization /ɪˌməʊ.bəl.aɪˈzeɪ.ʃən/

inaccurate /ɪˈnæk.jʊ.rət/
inattentiveness /ˌɪn.əˈten.tɪv.nəs/
incidence /ˈɪnt.sɪ.dənt s/
influence /ˈɪnfluəns/
inguinal /ˈɪŋ.gwɪ.nəl/
insertion /ɪnˈsɜː.ʃən/
inspiratory /ɪnˈspaɪə.rə.tər.i/
insufficiency /ˌɪn.səˈfɪʃ.ən.si/
intermittent /ˌɪn.təˈmɪt.ənt/
intervention /ˌɪn.təˈven.ʃən/
intramuscular /ˌɪn.trəˈmʌs.kjʊ.lər/
irritation /ˌɪr.ɪˈteɪ.ʃən/
ladder /ˈlæd.ər/
lead /led/
light-headed /ˌlaɪtˈhed.ɪd/
major /ˈmeɪ.dʒə/
Mallory-Weis /ˈmæl.ər.i-vaɪs/
syndrome /ˈsɪn.drəʊm/
margin /ˈmɑː.dʒɪn/
maroon /məˈruːn/
medication /ˌmed.ɪˈkeɪ.ʃən/
melaena /məˈliːn.ə/
mercury /ˈmɜː.kjʊ.ri/
metallic /məˈtæl.ɪk/
methamphetamine /ˌmeθ.æmˈfet.ə.miːn/
mimic /ˈmɪm.ɪk/
misleading /ˌmɪsˈliː.dɪŋ/
mortality /mɔːˈtæl.ə.ti/
Murphy's /ˈmɜː.fiz/ sign /saɪn/
mustard /ˈmʌs.təd/
nerve /nɜːv/
nest /nest/
nondiscernible /ˌnɒn.dɪˈsɜː.nɪ.bl̩/
note /nəʊt/
noticeable /ˈnəʊ.tɪ.sə.bl̩/
numerous /ˈnjuː.mə.rəs/
obvious /ˈɒb.vi.əs/
onion /ˈʌn.jən/
onset /ˈɒnˌset/
outermost /ˈaʊ.tə.məʊst/
outpatient /ˈaʊt.peɪ.ʃənt/
outpouching /ˈaʊt.paʊtʃ.ɪŋ/
palsy /ˈpɔːl.zi/
pancreatitis /ˌpæŋ.kri.əˈtaɪ.tɪs/

partially /'pɑː.ʃəl.i/
pending /'pen.dɪŋ/
peritoneal /ˌper.ɪ.tə'ni.əl/
peritonitis /ˌper.ɪ.tə'naɪ.tɪs/
periumbilical /ˌper.ɪ.ʌm'bɪl.ɪ.kəl/
petit mal /ˌpə'ti'mæl/
phlegm /flem/
pill-rolling /'pɪlˌrəʊ.lɪŋ/ tremor /'trem.ər/
pit viper /'vaɪpə/
polyuria /ˌpɒl.ɪ'jʊə.ri.ə/
potassium /pə'tæs.i.əm/
precaution /prɪ'kɔː.ʃən/
presume /prɪ'zjuːm/
pupil /'pjuː.pəl/
radiate /'reɪ.di.eɪt/
raise /reɪz/
rash /ræʃ/
rebound /ˌriː'baʊnd/
tenderness /'ten.dər.nəs/
release /rɪ'liːs/
renal /'riː.nəl/ calculi /'kæl.kjʊ.laɪ/
residual /rɪ'zɪd.ju.əl/
restraint /rɪ'streɪnt/
reveal /rɪ'viːl/
ring /rɪŋ/
rough /rʌf/
route /ruːt/
rule /ruːl/ out /aʊt/
rupture /'rʌp.tʃər/
sclera /'sklɪə.rə/
search /sɜːtʃ/ for /fɔː/
secondary /'sek.ən.dri/
sheet /ʃiːt/
shunt /ʃʌnt/
side /saɪd/
site /saɪt/
slipper /'slɪp.ər/
snake /sneɪk/
sneeze /sniːz/
soaked /səʊkt/
soccer /'sɒk.ər/
specific /spə'sɪf.ɪk/
speck /spek/
spell /spel/

stagnate /stæg'neɪt/
state /steɪt/
stick /stɪk/ (stuck, stuck)
sting /stɪŋ/
stonelike /'stəʊn.laɪk/
stool /stuːl/
strenuous /'stren.ju.əs/
stretcher /'stretʃə/
stridor /straɪd.ər/
subconjunctival /ˌsʌbˌkɒn.dʒaŋk.'tɪ.vəl/
succession /sək'seʃ.ən/
suffer /'sʌf.ər/
supportive /sə'pɔː.tɪv/
surgery /'sɜː.dʒər.i/
suspect /sə'spekt/
suspicion /sə'spɪʃən/
tarry /'tær.i/
tear /teər/
telephone /'tel.ɪ.fəʊn/
temporal /'tem.pər.əl/
tepid /'tep.ɪd/
thrash /θræʃ/
tightness /'taɪt.nəs/
umbilicus /ʌm'bɪl.ɪ.kəs/
unaware /ˌʌn.ə'weər/
urethra /jʊə'riː.θrə/
urinate /'jʊə.rɪ.neɪt/
urticaria /ˌɔː.tɪ'keə.ri.ə/
valuable /'væl.jʊ.bl̩/
varix /veə.rɪks/ pl varices /'vær.ɪ.siːz/
vertebral /'vɜː.tɪ.brəl/
violent /'vaɪələnt/
voluntary /'vɒləntərɪ/
wheal /wiːl/
white /waɪt/
yellow jacket /'jel.oʊˌdʒæk.ɪt/

Unit 4

Case study 1

These statements about delirium tremens are true:

- DTs can occur from either an 1_____ discontinuation or 2_____ of alcohol after prolonged use.◄
- DTs are characterized by a decreased level of consciousness and 3_____. ◄
- There is 4_____ _____ associated with Dts. ◄

a. significant mortality; b. abrupt; c. ingestion; d. hallucinations

Case study 2

All of the following are signs and symptoms of 1_____ _____:

- salivation ◄
- lacrimation ◄
- urination ◄

SLUDGE is a helpful mnemonic to remember signs of poisoning – S = salivation, L = lacrimation, U = urination, D =2_____, G = GI (3_____) upset, E =4_____. Other symptoms of organophosphate poisoning include 5_____, bradyardia, anxiety, and 6_____ _____.

a. Bronchoconstriction; b. defecation; c. visual disturbances; d. organophosphate poisoning; e. emesis; f. gastrointestinal

Case study 3

The patient is conscious but slow to respond and appears highly intoxicated. He asks for help and falls to the floor. His appearance is pale and diaphoretic with a blood pressure of 90/64, pulse 144, respiration of 36. You note that the porch is covered in coffee-ground emesis.

- This patient is most likely suffering from: ruptured oesophageal varices ◄

The patient's past 1_____ _____ and 2_____ should lead you to the conclusion of ruptured 3_____ _____.

- His appearance and vital signs indicate: shock ◄

This patient 4__ _____ shock as evidences by his 5_____ pulse rate (144), evidence of 6_____ (pale and moist skin), and his ability to maintain his 7_____ _____.

- Treatment of this patient should include: close monitoring of airway 8_____, administration of 9_____ oxygen, establishing intravenous access, and treatment for shock. ◄

As always, the airway is your priority. You must protect the airway and prevent 10_____ of emesis. Supplemental oxygen, 11_____ intravenous access, and treatment for shock are required.

During transport to the hospital, your patient has several additional episodes of vomiting. It starts as coffee-ground 12_____ that quickly changes to bright red blood. He is less responsive with intermediate periods of 13_____. Blood pressure is 82/64, pulse 148, respirations 40.

You know that: his vital signs and change in mental status indicate decompensated shock.

- His condition is 14_____ and rapid transport is necessary. ◀

a. is experiencing; b. blood pressure;
c. medical history; d. supplemental; e. emesis;
f. aspiration; g. patency; h. establishing;
i. serious; j. syncope; k. elevated;
l. vasoconstriction; m. presentation;
n. oesophageal varices

Case study 4

The MOST common and 1_____ ____ of pit viper 2_____ is: rapidly developing oedema around the bite area.◀

Pit vipers include rattlesnakes, copperheads, and cottonmouths. Rapidly developing oedema around the 3____ ____ can occur in as little as 15 minutes.

a. envenomation; b. bite area; c. reliable sign

Case study 5

Minute respiratory 1_____ is best described as: the 2_____ __ ____ moved in and out of the 3_____ during one minute ◀

a. lungs; b. volume; c. amount of air

Case study 6

You respond to the local college campus soccer field for a 20-year-old female patient with a complaint of severe muscle cramps. The temperature is 88°F (31.1°C) with high humidity. The patient had just finished a strenuous workout when the cramps began. Her skin is hot to touch and she is sweating profusely.

You suspect this patient is suffering:

- heatstroke
- heat exhaustion
- heat cramps ◀
- exercise-induced fatigue

1___ _____ are acute painful spasms of the voluntary muscles following 2_____ activities in a 3___ _____.

- Treatment should include: oral hydration if the patient is able to take fluids. ◀

Treatment for heat cramps include 4_____ the patient from the hot environment and administration of oral 5_____ _____ or sport drinks for hydration. If oral fluids cannot be administered because of nausea, 6__ __ ____ of normal saline may be needed.

a. removing; b. Heat cramps; c. an IV line; d. strenuous; e. saline solution; f. hot environment

Case study 7

Your ambulance is assigned to stand by at a building fire. The outside temperature is 103°F (39.4°C) and the 1_____are wearing full protective clothing. Approximately 30 minutes into the incident, a firefighter has collapsed and you are 2_____ to care for him.

The patient is a 36-year-old male in good physical condition. He appears anxious and complains of nausea and a headache. He is 3_____ profusely with cool clammy skin. BP is 116/48, radial pulse is 150 and weak, respirations are 36 and shallow, temperature is 101.2° F (38.3° C).

This patient's signs/symptoms indicate:

- heatstroke
- heat exhaustion ◄
- heat stress
- heat fatigue

Profuse sweating with cool and clammy skin, tachycardia, rapid, shallow respiration, and a body temperature over 99.8° F (37.7° C) indicates 4_____ _____.

- Treatment for this patient should include: removing clothing, establishing IV of normal saline, placing in air conditioning. ◄

The patient is now apprehensive. 5_____ reveals a BP of 78/30, pulse 154, respirations 36

and shallow. You are unable to take another temperature because he is not cooperating. His skin is extremely hot to touch and has stopped sweating. Online medical control has requested that you start rapid active cooling.

- This can be achieved by: covering the patient in a sheet that has been soaked in tepid water. ◄

This patient has progressed from 6___ _____ to 7_____ as indicated by severe apprehension, hypotension, hot skin, and the cessation of sweating.

- Overcooling of a heatstroke patient: may cause a reflex hypothermia, shivering may result which can lead to a rise in core temperature, 102° F should be used as a target temperature to prevent overcooling. ◄

a. heat exhaustion; b. Reassessment; c. sweating; d. heat exhaustion; e. firefighters; f. assigned; g. heatstroke

Case study 8

You are called for a 62-year-old male with a 1_____ __ severe abdominal pain. He is lying as still as possible in his bed.

- Upon inspection of the abdomen you find 2_____ in the periumbilical area. This is known as: Cullen's sign. ◄

- This 3_____ finding may indicate: intraabdominal haemorrhage ◄

a. assessment; b. ecchymosis; c. complaint of

Case study 9

You are called by the local police department to help search for an elderly man with Alzheimer's s disease who wandered away from his home. It is 11.30 p.m. and he has been missing for three hours. It is 3°C outside with a light drizzle. The man is wearing pyjamas and slippers. At 4.30 a.m. the patient is located lying behind a pile of wood, five blocks from his home. He is unconscious, unresponsive, apnoeic, and pulseless. His skin is cold to the touch and his muscles are 1_____. His core body temperature is 32°C

- Initial treatment should include: CPR ◄

CPR is indicated even if 2_____ __ _____ are present. Hypothermic patients cannot be presumed dead until a core body temperature of 34°C has been achieved and 3_____ _____ are still unsuccessful.

- You are considering the administration of cardiac medication for this patient: IV medication may be administered, but space at longer than standard intervals. ◄

4___ _____ is reduced so administered medication such as epinephrine or lidocaine 5___ _____ to toxic levels. In addition, administered drugs may retain in the 6_____ _____. When the patient is rewarmed and peripheral circulation resumes, a large toxic bolus of medication may be delivered to the central circulation.

- Care during transportation for this patient should include all of the following: avoiding rough handling due to cardiac irritability, protection against further 7____ _____, transporting in a horizontal position. ◄

a. heat loss; b. resuscitation efforts; c. Drug metabolism; d. may accumulate; e. peripheral circulation; f. signs of death; g. rigid

Case study 10

You are called to attend to a patient who fell 7 feet (2.13 m) from a porch and landed on his head. He is 1_____, has erratic respirations, and is bleeding from a 2___ _____. Your first action to manage the airway would be:

- nasotracheal intubation
- head-tilt, chin-lift
- jaw thrust ◄
- to initiate in-line traction with intubation

The modified 3___ _____ is the easiest and safest method to manage the airway immediately.

a. jaw thrust; b. head wound; c. unresponsive

Case study 11

You are having lunch with your nephew J. and his friend S. You notice that S. appears to have periods of inattentiveness and daydreaming. During these spells, his eyelids 1_____ and he appears to be 2_____ __ his surroundings. You ask J. if he has ever noticed this before. J. says he has been "goofing around" like this for a week now.

- These signs indicate S. may have: petit mal seizure disorder. ◄

3_____ ____, or absence, seizure is characterized by a brief loss of awareness for 10-30 seconds. This type of seizure occurs in 4_____ and usually disappears after 20 years of age.

a. childhood; b. unaware of; c. flutter; d. Petit mal

Case study 12

A 58-year-old female has a history of smoking two packs of cigarettes per day. She suffers from frequent upper respiratory infections with a 1_____ _____ and expectorates white, thick 2_____. She most likely is suffering from:

- asthma
- congestive heart failure
- chronic bronchitis ◄
- bronchiolitis

Years of exposure to 3_____ _____ (e.g. cigarettes) can result in an increase in the number of goblet cells in the bronchial system with an increased 4_____ __ _____.

a. production of mucus; b. toxic irritation; c. productive cough; d. phlegm

Case study 13

A 66-year-old female, is unable to get out of bed. She responds to verbal stimuli with clear speech, her smile is asymmetrical, she cannot move her left leg, and weakly moves her left harm. Her skin is warm but pale. Vital signs are: BP 162/88, pulse 110 beats per minute and irregular, respiratory rate 22 per minute with lung sounds clear bilaterally. A blood glucose reading is 130 mg/dl. The cardiac monitor shows a very irregular, narrow complex tachycardia with no identifiable P waves.

Damage of what body system 1__ _____ movement of the left side of her body?

- cardiovascular system
- central nervous system ◄
- pulmonary system
- endocrine system

An asymmetrical smile in conjunction with the inability to move her left leg and weakness of her left arm indicate injury to the patient's 2_____ _____ _____ (CNS)

- The patient's 3_____ smile is

63

most likely a direct result of: damage to cranial nerve VII.

- A patient's ability to smile, 4_____, lift eyebrows, and 5_____ ____ _____ is controlled by cranial nerve VII. ◄
- Why was it important to obtain a blood glucose reading on this patient? – Hypoglycaemia can mimic stroke. ◄

Patients who are hypoglycaemic can exhibit signs and symptoms similar to a stroke.

- Her cardiac rhythm is: atrial fibrillation ◄

6_____ _____ is an irregular, narrow complex rhythm with nondiscernible P waves.

This cardiac rhythm makes her more prone to the development of:

- diabetes
- emboli ◄
- brain tumours
- cardiogenic shock

As the atria fibrillate, they also dilate. This allows for blood to 7_____ in the atria and can lead to 8____ _____.

A family member states that she was fine one hour ago when he talked to her on the telephone.

- This is important information because: it establishes a reference point for the onset of symptoms. ◄

Studies suggest that there is a three-hour window between the time of onset of symptoms and time of thrombolytic intervention for treatment to be 9_____. Establishing a 10_____ _____ for the onset of symptoms is critical.

a. is affecting; b. Atrial fibrillation; c. reference point; d. asymmetrical; e. effective; f. central nervous system; g. stagnate; h. clot formation; i. frown; j. wrinkle the forehead

Case study 14

You are called to attend to a 51-year-old male who fell in his living room. His wife states that he has been very depressed and has not eaten or drunk anything for the past 24 hours. You notice the patient has a stonelike face, 1_____ _____, and is exhibiting "pill-rolling" 2_____.

These are all signs of:

- multiple sclerosis
- Bell's palsy
- Parkinson's disease ◄
- vertebral disc disease
- In managing this patient, it is important to: start an intravenous line, determine a blood glucose level, and apply a cardiac monitor. ◄

Starting an intravenous line will allow access for medications if necessary, 3_____ the blood glucose level will show if the altered mental status is due to hypoglycaemia, and applying a

4_____ _____ will determine if there is a rhythm disturbance.

> a. cardiac monitor; b. determining; c. muscular rigidity; c. movements

Case study 15

Your EMS Unit is called to attend to a 79-year-old female who experienced an abrupt onset of facial drooping, dysphasia, and marked 1_____. Upon examination, she is now alert and oriented, 2_____ clear, and moves all extremities well. Vital signs are normal.

- Your assessment findings 3____ ____ to suspect: transient ischemic attack. ◀

Since her signs and symptoms 4_____ _____, and she has no neurological deficit, she most likely suffered a 5_____ ischemic attack. TIA is considered a significant 6_____ ____ for the development of a 7_____.

> a. stroke; b. hemiparesis; c. warning sign; d. disappeared rapidly; e. lead you; f. speech; g. transient

Case study 16

Ecchymosis in the 1_____ ____ associated with intraabdominal 2_____ is known as:

- peritonitis
- Cullen's sign
- Mallory-Weiss 3____
- Grey-Turner's sign ◀

> a. sign; b. flank area; c. haemorrhage

Case study 17

Small outpouchings of mucosal and submucosal tissue that push through the outermost layer of the 1_____ is known as:

- Crohn's 2_____
- inguinal hernia
- 3_____ colitis
- diverticulitis ◀

> a. disease; b. ulcerative; c. intestine

Case study 18

A peak flow value of 100 (litres/min) shows:

- normal 1_____
- mild severity
- moderate 2_____
- severe respiratory compromise ◀

A 3____ ____ of 100 (litres/min) is very low; 400-650 litres/min is the normal range.

> a. peak flow; b. value; c. severity

Case study 19

In differentiating between syncope and a grand mal seizure, you know that syncope:

- often begins in a standing position ◀
- presents with jerking motions during 1_____
- causes the patient to remain drowsy following the event
- is often 2_____ by aura

3_____ usually occurs when the person is in the 4_____ _____. It can begin with dizziness or feeling light-headed, or can occur without warning.

> a. standing position; b. Syncope;
> c. unconsciousness; d. preceded

Case study 20

A seizure characterized by a rapid 1____ _____ or auras that include unusual smells, tastes, or sounds is termed:

- a simple partial seizure disorder
- 2____ ___ seizure disorder
- pseudoseizure 3_____
- complex partial seizure disorder ◄

A complex partial seizure disorder can present in many ways since they usually 4_____ in the temporal lobe of the brain. They are usually of 5____ _____ and while patients experience a loss of contat with their surroundings, they do not lose motor tone.

> a. short duration; b. originate; c. disorder;
> d. mood change; e. petit mal

Case study 21

Your EMS team is called to a patient in her mid-thirties who is having a generalized motor seizure. Bystanders inform you that she hase been seizing continually for the past 10 minutes. You note that the patient 1__ _____ violently, is diaphoretic, and slightly cyanotic.

This prolonged seizure is specifically termed:

- petit mal seizure disorder
- grand mal seizure disorder
- complex seizure disorder
- status epilepticus ◄

2_____ _____ is two or more generalized motor seizures occuring in succession and is a life threatening emergency situation.

- The most valuable early intervention is to: use bag-valve mask assistance with 100% oxygen. ◄

Air exchange is poor during a generalized motor seizure. It is extremely important to protect the airway from obstruction and deliver 100% oxygen using a bag-valve mask for 3_____ _____.

Administration if the medication terminated her seizure activity. Now you should be alert for which of the following side effects?

- respiratory depression ◄
- hyperglycaemia
- hypertension
- fever

Valium (4_____) is a sedative and anticonvulsant that depresses seizure activity in the brain. A side effect of Valium is respiratory depression.

> a. Status epilepticus; b. respiratory assistance;
> c. diazepam; d. is shaking

Vocabulary 4

abrupt /əˈbrʌpt/
accumulate /əˈkjuː.mjʊ.leɪt/
asymmetrical /ˌeɪ.sɪˈmet.rɪk.əl/
awareness /əˈweə.nəs/
campus /ˈkæm.pəs/
cessation /sesˈeɪ.ʃən/
colitis /kə.lɪ.tɪs/
conclude /kənˈkluːd/
conditioning /kənˈdɪʃ.ən.ɪŋ/
conjunction /kənˈdʒʌŋk.ʃən/
copperhead /ˈkɒp.ər.hed/
daydream /ˈdeɪ.driːm/
discontinuation /ˌdɪs.kənˌtɪn.juˈeɪ.ʃən/
disturbance /dɪˈstɜː.bənt s/
diverticulitis /ˌdaɪ.vəˌtɪk.jʊˈlaɪ.tɪs/
drizzle /ˈdrɪz.əl/
drowsy /ˈdraʊ.zi/
dysphasia /disˈfeɪ.zɪə/
expectorate /ɪkˈspek.tər.eɪt/
experience /ɪkˈspɪə.ri.ənt s/
eyebrow /ˈaɪ.braʊ/
fibrillate /ˈfaɪ.brɪ.leɪt/
fire fighter /ˈfaɪəˌfaɪ.tər/
frown /fraʊn/
goblet /ˈɡɒb.lət/
goof /ɡuːf/ around /əˈraʊnd/
humidity /hjuːˈmɪd.ɪ.ti/
inattentiveness /ˌɪn.əˈten.tɪv.nəs/
inguinal /ˈɪŋ.ɡwɪ.nəl/
intervention /ˌɪn.təˈven.ʃən/
irritation /ˌɪr.ɪˈteɪ.ʃən/
jerk /dʒɜːk/
light-headed /ˌlaɪtˈhed.ɪd/
mimic /ˈmɪm.ɪk/
nondiscernible /ˌnɒn.dɪˈsɜː.nɪ.bl̩/
onset /ˈɒnˌset/
outermost /ˈaʊ.tə.məʊst/
outpouching /ˈaʊt.paʊtʃ.ɪŋ/
palsy /ˈpɔːl.zi/
partially /ˈpɑː.ʃəl.i/
petit mal /ˌpəˈtiˈmæl/
phlegm /flem/

pill-rolling /ˈpɪlˌrəʊ.lɪŋ/ tremor /ˈtrem.ər/
pit viper /ˈvaɪpə/
polyuria /ˌpɒl.ɪˈjʊə.ri.ə/
presume /prɪˈzjuːm/
rough /rʌf/
search /sɜːtʃ/ for /fɔː/
sheet /ʃiːt/
slipper /ˈslɪp.ər/
soaked /səʊkt/
soccer /ˈsɒk.ər/
spell /spel/
stagnate /stæɡˈneɪt/
state /steɪt/
stonelike /ˈstəʊn.laɪk/
strenuous /ˈstren.ju.əs/
succession /səkˈseʃ.ən/
temporal /ˈtem.pər.əl/
tepid /ˈtep.ɪd/
unaware /ˌʌn.əˈweər/
urinate /ˈjʊə.rɪ.neɪt/
valuable /ˈvæl.jʊ.bl̩/
varix /ˈveə.rɪks/ pl varices /ˈvær.ɪ.siːz/
vertebral /ˈvɜː.tɪ.brəl/
voluntary /ˈvɒləntərɪ/
workout /ˈwɜːkˌaʊt/
wrinkle /ˈrɪŋkəl/

Part 4
Trauma

Assessment; recognition; and treatment of various traumatic injuries

Unit 1
Case study 1

You arrive on the scene of a patient who has been stabbed with a knife in the right side of the back. The patient presents with left-sided hemiparalysis and sensory loss. Despite another stab wound to the the right abdomen, the patient denies pain. What type of 1_____ _____ injuries do you suspect?

- compression
- transection
- neurogenic shock
- Brown-Sequard's syndrome ◄

2_____-_____ syndrome is caused by a 3_____ injury that affects one side of the spinal cord. The damage to the one side results in 4_____ ___ _____

loss to that side of the body because of the switching of the associated nerves as they enter the spinal cord.

a. sensory and motor; b. spinal cord; c. penetrating; d. Brown-Sequard's

Case study 2

Describe the effects of pericardial tamponade. – Cardiac output is reduced, and central venous pressure rises. ◄

In pericardial 1_____, the pericardial sack fills with fluid and compresses 2____ _____. This impairs 3_____ _____. The result is a decrease in 4_____ _____ (the left ventricle cannot effectively fill and pump) and an increase in central venous pressure (venous blood returning to the heart is impaired and the 5_____ _____ cannot fill or pump effectively).

a. right ventricle; b. cardiac output; c. ventricular filling; d. tamponade; e. the heart

Case study 3

Your patient rolled a farm tractor over a hill. He has a large puncture wound to his right neck, above the clavicle. It appears that the wound is from a tree branch. Moderate bleeding is present.

Care for the puncture wound would include:

- application of direct pressure with a bulky trauma dressing
- application of an occlusive dressing ◄

- application if a
  sterile dressing
- needle decompression

a. air embolism; b. decreased blood flow;
c. entering; d. highly vascular; e. airway
structures; f. haematoma; g. aspiration;
h. occlusive dressing

Application of an 1_____
_____ is necessary because this
is a highly vascular area. An occlusive
dressing will prevent air from
2_____ an injured vessel and the
development of an 3___ _____.

Which transport position would
be appropriate for this patient?

- Trendelenburg position ◄
- left lateral recumbent
- right lateral recumbent
- prone

The Trendelenburg position
would be appropriate to decrease
the potential for air 4_____
into an injured vessel.

A major concern with
this type of injury is:

- rib fracture
- clavicle fracture
- flail chest
- oedema ◄

Oedema is a serious concern
because injury to this 5_____
_____ area of the neck can lead
to a rapidly expanding 6_____.
This haematoma can put pressure
on other blood vessels resulting in
7_____ _____ ____ to the
brain or put pressure on nearby
8_____ _____ resulting in
an airway management nightmare!

Case study 4

You perform a rapid trauma
survey on an MBC (motorbike
collision) victim and find him
1_____ and very pale,
with 2____ and 3_____ skin.
He has contusions, 4_____,
and diminished breath sounds
on the right side of the chest. BP
74/50, pulse of 140 centrally, no
peripheral pulse found at this time,
and respirations 32 and shallow.

- What is the most likely
  cause of these findings? –
  Haemopneumothorax ◄

With the information
given, 5_____, absent
peripheral pulses, diminished
breath sounds on the right with
chest trauma on the right, a
6_____ is likely.

- An 7_____ _____
  and rapid trauma survey
  should be completed in
  what length of time? – Less
  than three minutes. ◄

This patient received an initial
assessment and rapid trauma survey
to identify all 8____ _____.
It is recommended that these
assessment steps be 9_____
in two or three minutes or less.

a. initial assessment; b. performed; c. life threats; d. haemopneumothorax; e. cool; f. clammy; g. crepitus; h. lethargic; i. hypotension

Case study 5

Which of the following would you expect to cause the greatest 1_____?

- A hunting knife
- A bullet from a handgun
- A bullet from a rifle ◄
- An arrow

Ballistics is the study of projectiles in motion. Studies suggest that wounds from 2_____ _____ are two to four times 3____ _____ than handgun bullets due to mass energy and 4_____.

a. velocity; b. more lethal; c. rifle bullets; d. cavitation

Case study 6

The next three questions are based on the following scenario:

You have arrived on scene where you find a 50-year-old male who has a large jagged laceration from a chain saw on his medial left upper thigh. Bright red blood is spurting from the wound. Your patient is alert, 1_____, and anxious, with pale, 2_____ skin.

- What is the priority of care for this patient? – Apply a pressure dressing while elevating the left leg. ◄

This patient is alert and oriented, so he has an 3_____ airway and is breathing.

Your priority for this patient is "circulation", which includes 4_____ major haemorrhage. Applying a 5_____ _____ and elevation are necessary.

Your rapid 6_____ _____ reveals an isolated upper leg laceration that is seven inches (17.8 cm) in length and 7_____ bright red blood freely. His BP is 110/60, peripheral pulse 128, respiratory rate 24, and his GCS is 15. Several components of the circulatory system are essential for adequate 8_____. These are components of the 9_____ _____:

- stroke volume and the Frank-Starlings mechanism ◄
- preload and afterload ◄
- the pump, the fluid, and the container ◄

Bleeding has been controlled and your patient is enroute to the trauma centre. You instruct your partner to 10_____ __ _____ and deliver fluid resuscitation.

- The most appropriate treatment is: a bolus of normal saline or Ringer's lactate solution. ◄

a. pressure dressing; b. oriented; c. diaphoretic; d. intact; e. stopping; f. circulatory system; g. profusion; h. trauma assessment; i. pumping; j. establish IV access

Case study 7

The next four questions are based on the following scenario:

You are on duty at your EMS service when you are called to respond to a car that struck a light pole. As you arrive on scene, you notice that power lines are down on top of the car. The driver is hanging halfway out of the driver's side window, unconscious, with slow, snoring-type respirations.

- What is your first priority? – Calling the power company for assistance prior to starting patient care. ◄

Your safety is the 1_____ _____. Do not approach the car until you are notified by the proper officials that the power has been 2_____ ___.

After the patient is removed from the car, a rapid trauma 3_____ shows a GCS of 9, BP 178/100, pulse 56, and respirations 34 and irregular.

What is your differential diagnosis from this assessment?

- hypoglycaemia
- hyperglycaemia
- Cushing's syndrome ◄
- CVA

Cushing's or herniation syndrome __ 4_____ __ hypertension, bradycardia, and erratic respirations.

- To manage the airway of this patient appropriately you would: intubate and hyperoxygenate with BVM at a rate of 24 breaths per minute. ◄

Intubation and 5_____ _____ are essential. You would hyperventilate this patient because he exhibits signs/symptoms of 6_____ _____ _____ (Cushing's syndrome).

You have established two large-bore IVs of normal saline.

- The appropriate rate is: enough fluid to maintain stable vital signs. ◄

The objective of prehospital fluid resuscitation is 7__ _____ vital signs until the patient arrives at the hospital.

a. is manifested by; b. turned off; c. to stabilize; d. supplemental oxygen; e. first priority; f. survey; g. increased intracranial pressure

Case study 8

Please state the best clue 1___ _____ possible injuries that may be sustained in a motor vehicle collision (2___):

- length of skid marks
- debris at the scene
- 3_____ symptoms
- mechanism of injury ◄

a. for determining; b. patient; c. MVC

Case study 9

A 42-year-old male is the victim of a house fire. He has reddened and blistered areas over most of the anterior chest, abdomen, and anterior surfaces of both arms.

- Using the rule of nines, estimate what percent of BSA he has burned: 27% (Chest = 9%, abdomen = 9%, anterior surfaces of both arms = 9%.) ◄
- Initial treatment for this burn patient would include: covering the burn area with dry bulky 1_____ and keeping the patient warm. ◄

Manage the burns by 2_____ them with a dry bulky dressing. A dressing reduces air movement past sensitive partial thickness burns, thus reducing pain. Damaged skin loses temperature 3_____ _____ so it is important to keep the patient covered, even if the environment is not cold.

- Medical control has asked that you initiate 4_____ _____ enroute to the hospital: two large-bore catheters are introduced and a bolus of 0.5 ml of normal saline (NS) for every kilogram of the patient's weight multiplied by the percentage of BSA is initiated. ◄

Current fluid resuscitation recommends that two large-bore catheters 5__ _____. When EMS transport time is less than 1 hour a bolus of 0.5 ml of 6_____

_____ (NS) for every kilogram of the patient's weight multiplied by the percentage of BSA should be initiated.

While transporting your burn patient to the 7____ _____, you notice that his voice now sounds 8_____ and he is making "crowing" sound on inspiration.

- What is the most likely cause? – 9_____ for help while standing inside the burning house. ◄

Risk factors for inhalation injuries associated with burns include standing in the burn environment (10___ _____ rise), screaming or yelling in the hot 11_____ (the 12____ _____ allows toxic gases to enter the lower airway), and being trapped in a closed burn environment.

a. normal saline; b. environment; c. hot gases; d. regulation capacity; e. dressings; f. fluid therapy; g. covering; h. Risk factors; i. open glottis; j. hoarse; k. be introduced; l. Screaming; m. burn centre

Case study 10

A burn victim with suspected thermal or chemical airway burns needs close monitoring for signs of 1_____ _____.

- Appropriate management would include: 2_____ high-flow oxygen by 3_____ mask at 15 litres per minute once the airway has been secured. ◄

a. nonrebreather; b. respiratory compromise; c. Providing

Case study 11

These statements regarding electrical injuries are true:

- Until the power is off, nobody should 1 __ _____ to approach the electrical burn patient. ◄
- Patients in cardiac arrest because of 2_____ have a high 3_____ _____ if prehospital intervention is prompt. ◄
- When treating a victim of a recent lightning strike the rescuer: need not be grounded to prevent electrical shock. ◄

By the time the victim of a 4_____ _____ is reached, the electricity will have dissipated. While you may be concerned as long as the storm remains nearby, there is 5__ _____ of electrical shock from 6_____ the victim of a lightning strike.

a. survival rate; b. electrocution; c. be allowed; d. no danger; e. lightning strike; f. touching

Case study 12

The next two questions are based on the following scenario:

You are called to the scene of a 22-year old man who was playing in a softball tournament. He was hit in the eye with a hard-hit line-drive softball.

According to his teammates he was knocked to the ground and had a brief 1_____ __ _____ that lasted approximately seven seconds.

While assessing the injured eye you notice a collection of blood in front of the patient's pupil and iris. What is your differential diagnosis?

- Raccoon's eye
- retinal detachment
- hyphema ◄
- corneal laceration

2_____ is a collection of blood in the 3_____ _____ of the eye due to trauma. This type of injury is a potential threat to the patient's 4_____ and requires 5_____ by an ophthalmologist.

- How would you transport this patient to the hospital? – Immobilized on a 6_____ with the head of backboard elevated. ◄

A c- spine injury should be suspected with any injury to the head. Treatment of this patient would include 7___ _____ _____. The preferred position of transport of a hyphema is with the head elevated, therefore, you should 8_____ the head of the backboard.

a. Backboard; b. anterior chamber; c. full body immobilization; d. elevate; e. Hyphema; f. evaluation; g. vision; h. loss of consciousness

Case study 13

You arrive on scene to find a pickup truck that struck a utility pole head on. The patient is ambulatory on-scene. He is alert and oriented to person and place but slow to respond. You note the smell of alcohol on the patient as you speak with him.

You are sent to evaluate the damage to the truck. Which finding would lead you to believe the patient may have a life-threatening injury?

- a deformed dashboard
- a deformed steering wheel. ◀
- the airbag did not deploy
- significant front end damage

The amount of energy required to deform a steering wheel is significant. Possible 1_____-_____ injuries from the body striking a steering wheel include: flail chest, 2_____ contusion, 3_____ _____, tracheal or vascular injuries, 4_____ contusion, pneumothorax, solid and hollow organ injury. Bilateral femur fractures may result in an "up-and-over" path occurred.

- It is important to remember that when dealing with an 5_____ _____ your assessment must be thorough because: alcohol can mask signs and symptoms of injury. ◀

Alcohol is a central nervous system 6_____. Because of this, alcohol can 7_____ signs and symptoms of injury. It is important to assess all trauma patients 8_____, but be especially meticulous when you suspect drug/alcohol use.

a. aortic tear; b. pulmonary; c. depressant; d. intoxicated patient; e. thoroughly; f. mask; g. life-threatening; h. myocardial

Case study 14

You are called to the scene of a patient who was involved in an altercation at the local pool hall. You find one victim in the back alley anxious and screaming for your assistance. You notice immediately that he has clammy skin and a dusky appearance. He has a respiratory rate of 40 and his breathing is shallow. He tells you that he has been hit multiple times in the 1_____, 2_____, and 3____ with a pool stick by "two big guys."

While assessing his chest you notice multiple contusions to the right side with diminished respirations on the right.

What would you suspect?

- cardiac tamponade
- haemothorax
- ruptured diaphragm
- pneumothorax ◀

With a history of chest trauma, diminished breath sounds, agitation, increased respiratory rate, along with 4_____ colour, you should suspect 5_____.

While enroute to the local trauma centre with this patient, you notice that his level of consciousness has decreased and his colour has not improved despite 100% 0_2 by nonrebreather mask. He is becoming 6_____ and his pulse rate is 140. Respiratory rate remains at 40 and his breathing is still shallow. Ongoing assessment reveals 7_____ neck veins and hyperresonant percussion on the right chest.

- Your next course of action would be: needle decompression between the second and the third intercostal space anterior chest. ◄

The above symptoms are classic for tension pneumothorax, which is a serious and immediate 8_____ _____ that requires immediate 9_____ _____.

---

a. life threat; b. chest; c. abdomen; d. back;
e. hypotensive; f. dusky; g. pneumothorax;
h. chest decompression; i. distended

Case study 15

A 22-year-old male is found in an alley with multiple stab wounds to the extremities, abdomen, and chest. BP is 82/40, pulse 142 weak, respirations 10.

- Your exam reveals distended neck veins, equal breath sounds, and a radial pulse that disappears during

inspiration. You suspect: cardiac tamponade. ◄

The diagnosis of cardiac tamponade often relies upon symptoms. Hypotension, distended neck veins, and 1_____ heart sounds are classic symptoms of cardiac tamponade and are known as Beck's triad. If the patient loses his or her 2_____ _____ during inspiration, it is suggestive of 3_____ _____ and the presence of cardiac tamponade.

As you log-roll the patient to place him on the long spine board, you inspect his back and discover another stab wound just below the right scapula. You observe blood bubbling out of the wound with each breath.

- You suspect: an open pneumothorax. ◄

An open pneumothorax (sucking chest wound) includes a 4_____ or bubbling sound as air moves in and out of the chest wall. 5_____ is usually present and frothing of the blood may occur as the 6___ ___ _____ combine.

- Priority care for this patient would include: closure of the chest wall with an occlusive dressing taped on three sides. ◄

Treatment of an open pneumothorax includes 7_____ the chest wall 8___ _____ of an occlusive dressing that is 9_____ on three sides.

a. by application; b. muffled; c. taped; d. Bleeding; e. closing; f. air and blood; g. pulsus paradoxus; h. peripheral pulse; i. sucking

Case study 16

You arrive on scene of a 34-year-old male who was struck by a car. Bystanders tell you the patient was standing on the sidewalk when his neighbour, who was backing out on the driveway, struck him. Your patient is sitting in the yard with an obvious open tibia/fibula fracture on the right leg.

As you 1_____ his right upper chest, you notice the patient guarding his shoulder. Closer exam reveals a fractured 2_____. Complications associated with a fractured clavicle include injury to the:

- carotid artery
- subclavian vein. ◄
- descending aorta
- inferior vena cava

Physical exam concludes that the right clavicle fracture and open right tibia/fibula fracture are his only obvious injuries but you are concerned because his level of consciousness 3___ _____ and his heart rate has increased 30 beats per minute. Although his abdomen was unremarkable upon examination, you know that an

4_____ of severe abdominal trauma is the presence of:

- absent bowel sounds
- back pain
- referred pain to the clavicle
- unexplained shock.◄

When assessment of a trauma patient does not reveal significant injury, the presence of 5_____ _____ should lead you to suspect serious 6_____/_____ trauma.

a. clavicle; b. indicator; c. unexplained shock; d. abdominal/thorax; e. auscultate; f. is deteriorating

Case study 17

A high velocity bullet passes through the body. Besides the direct damage caused by the 1_____what other related condition could cause harm to the patient?

- the type of 2_____ used to make the bullet
- the internal opening created by cavitation ◄
- the 3_____ residue
- the length of the bullet

Cavitation caused by the pressure wave of the bullet s forces creates both 4_____ and 5_____ openings within the tissues. Tremendous forces are transferred from the 6_____ of the bullet to the tissues, causing damage.

a. permanent; b. metal; c. bullet; d. gunpowder; e. temporary; f. velocity

Vocabulary 1

agitation /ˌædʒ.ɪˈteɪˌʃən/
air bag, airbag /ˈeə.bæg/
alley /ˈæl.i/
altercation /ˌɔːltəˈkeɪʃən/
ambulatory /ˌæm.bjəˈleɪ.tər.i/
approach /əˈprəʊtʃ/
arrow /ˈær.əʊ/
backboard /ˈbæk.bɔːd/
ballistics /bəˈlɪs.tɪks/
be /biː/ trapped /træpd/
bilateral /baɪˈlæt.ər.əl/
blister /ˈblɪs.tər/
bowel /ˈbaʊ.əl/
Brown-Sequard's /braʊn-sei.
kahr/ syndrome /ˈsɪn.drəʊm/
bubble /ˈbʌb.l/
bulky /ˈbʌl.ki/
bullet /ˈbʊl.ɪt/
cardiac /ˈkɑːdɪˌæk/ output /ˈaʊtˌpʊt/
cavitation /ˌkæv.ɪˈteɪ.ʃən/
chain /tʃeɪn/
chamber /ˈtʃeɪm.bə/
chest /tʃest/
clammy /ˈklæm.i/
clavicle /ˈklævɪkəl/
closure /ˈkləʊ.ʒə/
collection /kəˈlekʃən/
collision /kəˈlɪʒ.ən/
component /kəmˈpəʊnənt/
conclude /kənˈkluːd/
container /kənˈteɪ.nər/
contusion /kənˈtjuːˌʒən/
corneal /kɔːˈniː.əl/
crepitus /ˈkrep.ɪ.təs/
crow /krəʊ/
current /ˈkʌr.ənt/
dashboard /ˈdæʃˌbɔːd/
deal with /dɪəl/
debris /ˈdeb.riː/, /ˈdeɪ.briː/
decompression /ˌdiːˌkəmˈpreʃ.ən/
deny /dɪˈnaɪ/
deploy /dɪˈplɔɪ/
depressant /dɪˈpres.ənt/

descend /dɪˈsend/
detachment /dɪˈtætʃmənt/
deteriorate /dɪˈtɪə.ri.ə.reɪt/
diagnosis /ˌdaɪ.əgˈnəʊ.sɪs/
diaphragm /ˈdaɪ.ə.fræm/
differential /ˌdɪf.əˈren.t ʃəl/
disappear /ˌdɪs.əˈpɪər/
dissipate /ˈdɪs.ɪ.peɪt/
down /daʊn/
dress /dres/
driveway /ˈdraɪvˌweɪ/
dusky /ˈdʌs.ki/
duty /ˈdjuːtɪ/
electrocution /ɪˌlek.trəˈkjuːˌʃən/
elevation /ˌel.ɪˈveɪʃən/
enroute /ɒnˈruːt/
erratic /ɪˈræt.ɪk/
expand /ɪkˈspænd/
femur pl femora /ˈfiːˌmər/
fibula pl -ae /ˈfɪb.jʊ.lə/
fibula, kost lýtková
finding /ˈfaɪndɪŋ/
flail /fleɪl/ chest /tʃest/
flail /fleɪl/
force /fɔːs/
Frank-Starlings mechanism
/ˈmekəˌnɪzəm/
froth /frɒθ/
glottis /ˈglɒt.ɪs/ pl glotides
grounded /graʊnd.ɪd/
guard /gɑːd/
gunpowder /ˈgʌnˌpaʊ.dər/
haematoma pl haematomata /
ˌhiː.məˈtəʊ.mə/
haemopneumothorax /ˈhiː.
məˌnjuːˌməˈθɔːˌræks/
handgun /ˈhændˌgʌn/
hang /hæŋ/
hanging /ˈhæŋɪŋ/
harm /hɑːm/
head on /ˌhedˈɒn/
hemiparalysis /ˌhem.ɪ.pəˈræl.ə.sɪs/
hemiparesis /ˌhem.ɪ.pəˈriːˌsɪs/
herniation /ˌhɜːˌniːˈeɪˌʃən/
hit /hɪt/ (hit, hit)

hoarse /hɔːs/
hollow /'hɒl.əʊ/
hunting /'hʌn.tɪŋ/ knife /naɪf/
hyperglycaemia /ˌhaɪ.pə.glaɪ'siː.mi.ə/
hyperresonant /ˌhaɪ.pə.'rez.ən.ənt/
hyperventilate /haɪ.pə'ven.tɪ.leɪt/
hyphaema /haɪ.θe.mə/
indicator /'ɪn.dɪ.keɪ.tər/
inferior /ɪn'fɪə.ri.ər/ vena
cava /ˌviː.nə'keɪ.və/
initial /ɪ'nɪʃ.əl/
intact /ɪn'tækt/
intercostal /ˌɪn.tə'kɒs.təl/
iris /'aɪrɪs/
jagged /'dʒæg.ɪd/
knock /nɒk/
laceration /ˌlæsə'reɪʃən/
large /lɑːdʒ/ bore /bɔː/
lateral /'læt.rəl/
lethal /'liː.θəl/
lightning /'laɪt.nɪŋ/
line /laɪn/ -drive /draɪv/
log /lɒg/ -roll /rəʊl/, logroll
maintain /meɪn'teɪn/
mark /mɑːk/
meticulous /mə'tɪk.jʊ.ləs/
motion /'məʊʃən/
motor /'məʊ.tər/
muffle /'mʌf.l̩/
multiple /'mʌl.tɪ.pl̩/
multiply /'mʌltɪplaɪ/
nightmare /'naɪt.meər/
nonrebreather /ˌnɒn.rəbrə.
ðər/ mask /mɑːsk/
notify /'nəʊtɪˌfaɪ/
occlusive /ɒ'kluː.sɪv/
dressing /'dres.ɪŋ/
oedema /ɪ'diː.mə/
official /ə'fɪʃəl/
partial /'pɑː.ʃəl/
path /pɑːθ/
pericardial /ˌper.ɪ'kɑːdi.əl/
physical /'fɪz.ɪ.kəl/
pickup /pɪkʌp/
pole /pəʊl/

pool /puːl/ hall /hɔːl/
pool /puːl/ stick /stɪk/
potential /pə'ten.ʃəl/
power /'paʊə/ line /laɪn/
power /'paʊə/
power /paʊər/ company /'kʌm.pə.ni/
pressure /'preʃ.ə/ dressing /'dres.ɪŋ/
profusion /prə'fjuː.ʒən/
projectile /prə'dʒek.taɪl/
prompt /prɒmp t/
prone /prəʊn/
puncture /ˈpʌŋk.tʃə/
raccoon /rə'kuːn/ eyes /aɪz/
recognition /ˌrek.əg'nɪʃ.ən/
recumbent /rɪ'kʌm.bənt/
redden /'red.ən/
rescuer/'res.kjuː.ər/
residue /'rez.ɪ.djuː/
retinal /'ret.ɪ.nəl/
rib /rɪb/
rifle /'raɪ.fl̩/
roll /rəʊl/ over /'əʊ.vər/
saline /'seɪ.laɪn/
saw /sɔː/
scapula /'skæp.jʊ.lə/ pl -ae
scream /skriːm/
sensory /'sent.sər.i/
skid /skɪd/
snore /snɔːr/
solid /'sɒl.ɪd/
spine /spaɪn/ board /bɔːd/
spurt /spɜːt/
stab /stæb/
stable /'steɪ.bl̩/
steering /'stɪər.ɪŋ/ wheel /wiːl/
stick /stɪk/
storm /stɔːm/
strike /straɪk/ (struck, struck)
strike /straɪk/
subclavian /sʌb'kleɪv.i.ən/
suck /sʌk/
supplemental /ˌsʌp.lɪ'men.təl/
surface /'sɜː.fɪs/
survey /'sɜː.veɪ/
survival /sə'vaɪ.vəl/

sustain /səˈsteɪn/
switch /swɪtʃ/
tamponade /tæm.pəˈneɪd/
tape /teɪp/
teammate /ˈtiːm.meɪt/
tear /teər/
temporary /ˈtempərərɪ/
tension /ˈtentʃən/ **pneumothorax**
/ˌnjuːməˈθɔː.ræks/
thickness /ˈθɪknɪs/
thigh /θaɪ/
thorax /ˈθɔː.ræks/
tibia /ˈtɪb.i.ə/ pl. -ae
touching /ˈtʌtʃ.ɪŋ/
transection /ˌtrænˈsek.ʃən/
transfer /trænsˈfɜːr/
tremendous /trɪˈmen.dəs/
Trendelenburg /tren.del.ˈen.
berg/ **position** /pəˈzɪʃ.ən/
truck /trʌk/
turn /tɜːn/ **off** /ɒf/
unremarkable /ˌʌn.rɪˈmɑː.kə.bl̩/
utility /juːˈtɪl.ɪ.ti/
vascular /ˈvæs.kjʊ.lər/
velocity /vɪˈlɒsɪtɪ/
voice /vɔɪs/
wave /weɪv/
yell /jel/

Unit 2

Case study 1

You respond to a 25-year-old male involved in an industrial accident. Upon arrival, you see that your patient is trapped in a machine. He has suffered a partial amputation of the right leg just above the knee that is bleeding profusely.

- Your first action is to: stabilize the machinery. ◄

Stabilizing the machinery serves two purposes. First, it assures your 1_____, and second it will prevent 2_____ _____ to the patient.

The patient remains 3_____ in the machine. He is awake, alert, and anxious. His blood pressure is 96/44, pulse 142, respiration 26. His skin is pale and moist.

- He is in what state of shock: Compensated. ◄

This patient is in 4_____ _____. His elevated pulse rate (142) and evidence of vasoconstriction (5____, _____ ____) is able to maintain his blood pressure despite continued blood loss.

The patient has been freed from the machinery. Direct pressure and elevation do not stop the haemorrhage.

- The next step would be to apply: pressure at an arterial point proximal to the injury. ◄

If bleeding still persists after direct pressure and elevation, the next step is to find an 6_____ _____ _____ proximal to the wound and apply firm pressure.

Despite all efforts to control the bleeding, you are not successful. His pulse is now 52 and very weak. His respirations are 6 and laboured. Blood pressure is 78/30.

- This shock state indicates: decompensated shock ◄

7_____ _____ is when the body can 8__ _____ respond to the 9_____ blood loss. This is evident in the scenario by a decreased pulse rate, respirations, and blood pressure.

a. Decompensated shock; b. continued; c. compensated shock; d. arterial pulse point; e. safety; f. additional injury; g. pale; moist skin; h. trapped; i. no longer

Case study 2

You are caring for a 24-year-old male who wrecked his all-terrain vehicle. He states that his handlebar struck him in the stomach. He has 1_____ ____ _____ in the abdomen and you suspect bowel rupture.

- This condition can lead to peritonitis and the development of serious complications.◄

Rupture of the 2_____ or small bowel that allows digestive enzymes to enter the peritoneal cavity can cause 3_____, which can lead to infection and 4_____ _____.

a. serious complications; b. peritonitis; c. bruising and tenderness; d. stomach

Case study 3

You are called to the scene of a stabbing. You find one victim lying supine on the ground in a large pool of blood with multiple

lacerations to the abdomen. The scene is secure. Your initial assessment finds a patient responding only to pain with no peripheral pulse and respiratory rate of 8.

- Priority care of this patient would be: intubation and fluid resuscitation. ◄

Priority for this patient who presents with respiratory compromise and hypovolemia is 1_____ _____ and 2_____ _____.

While transporting this patient to the hospital, a large section of bowel protrudes through one of the lacerations.

- Your management would be: to gently cover the area with 3_____ _____ and nonadherent material as a dressing. ◄

Intestines should never be 4_____ ____ into the abdominal compartment. A moist nonadherent dressing should be gently placed over the bowel to prevent it from "drying out" because of the risk of 5_____ _____.

a. irreversible damage; b. moistened gauze; c. airway support; d. fluid resuscitation; e. pushed back

Case study 4

You respond to a "man down" call. When you arrive, you find a 52-year-old male lying on the ground next to a ladder. It is unclear if he was placing the ladder against the house when he came into contact with power lines or if he fell from the top of the ladder.

Examination shows the patient to be unresponsive. He has a rapid 1_____ _____ and snoring respirations of 8, BP is 88/42.

- Treatment should include: 2_____ the airway with a 3____ _____ manoeuvre and ventilation with a bag-valve device.◄

It is unclear if this patient fell, so you 4_____ _____ trauma and c-spine injury. A jaw thrust manoeuvre and bag-valve mask ventilation is the 5____ _____.

a. jaw thrust; b. best choice; c. must suspect; d. irregular pulse; e. opening

Case study 5

There are anatomic differences in 1_____ _____ compared to adults.

- When using the rule of nines for 2_____ _____, what is a correct 3_____ for a child? – The head of a child is 18% compared to 9% of an adult. ◄

a. calculating burns; b. modification; c. paediatric patient

Case study 6

Your patient is a 44-year-old female who was burned when a high temperature water pipe exploded. She has 1_____ to the chest, abdomen, 2_____ right arm, and 3_____ __ ___ right leg.

- According to the rule of nines, this patient 4____ _____: 36 percent burns. ◄

Chest = 9%, abdomen = 9%, entire arm = 9%, front of the leg = 9%.

a. blisters; b. entire; c. has sustained; d. front of the

Case study 7

The next three questions are based on the following scenario:

You are called to the scene of a 60-year-old woman who fell down a flight of stairs. The patient is found to be 1_____ and oriented, with warm, dry, and pink skin. She is 2_____ __ a headache and upper back pain. Her vital signs are BP 90/62, pulse 60, and respiration rate 20.

- Which would be your 3_____ _____? – Neurogenic or distributive shock.◄

4_____ or distributive shock is recognized by hypotension, bradycardia, and a normal initial appearance.

During your rapid trauma survey you find that the patient has no sensation below the border of the rib cage.

- This would suggest 5_____ _____: between T4 – T10. ◄

You would suspect injury at the thoracic level.

You have started a large-bore IV normal saline on this patient.

- Choose the appropriate solution and rate: normal saline at a rate to maintain a systolic BP of 90. ◄

The objective of prehospital fluid resuscitation is to stabilize vital signs until the patient arrives at the hospital. This patient requires close observation since neurogenic shock does not allow the body's normal 6_____ _____ to work.

```
a. Neurogenic; b. compensatory mechanisms;
c. initial impression; d. spinal pathology;
e. complaining of; f. alert
```

Case study 8

You are called to the scene of a mass casualty incident where you are responsible for the triage 1_____ _____.
Which of the following patients would be the first to be transported to the local trauma centre?

- A 50-year-old man complaining of knee and ankle pain
- An 18-year-old female with a five-minute lapse of consciousness after being struck in the head ◄
- A 25-year-old female, eight months pregnant with partial thickness burns on her arms and legs covering 5% of her BSA (body surface area)
- A 32 -year-old male with a large piece of metal impaled in his left foot

Of the choices listed, the patient with a possible 2_____ _____ should be transported first. Others are all 3_____ _____ that do not pose an immediate 4_____ _____ a head injury is capable of.

```
a. life threat; b. isolated injuries;
c. transportation decision; d. head injury
```

Case study 9

Your patient was struck in the head with a six-inch-diameter (15 cm) tree branch while trimming a tree. He complained of dizziness immediately after the incident but states he "feels fine" now. The next day, he complains of 1_____ ___ _____.

- You suspect a: subdural haematoma. ◄

A 2_____ _____ is usually due to rupture of 3_____ _____ _____. This type of bleeding is slow and the 4_____ of symptoms 5____ _____ several hours to develop after the injury.

a. onset; b. subdural haematoma; c. small venous vessels; d. may take; e. dizziness and vomiting

Case study 10

Which head injury will likely result in immediate neurological signs/symptoms with rapid deterioration?

- concussion
- contusion
- subdural haematoma
- epidural haematoma ◄

An 1_____ _____ involves 2_____ _____. Because the bleeding is arterial, 3_____ _____ builds rapidly, compressing the 4_____ and increasing pressure within the skull. As the pressure rapidly builds, the patient will immediately display 5_____ _____/_____.

a. neurological signs/symptoms; b. cerebrum; c. arterial vessels; d. epidural haematoma; e. intracranial pressure

Case study 11

Cushing's reflex includes a sudden 1_____ in systolic pressure, 2_____, and:

- erratic (3_____ _____) respirations. ◄
- irregular pulse
- increased respirations
- pupil dilation

a. bradycardia; b. increase; c. usually slow

Case study 12

You are called to the scene of a single-car MVC involving a 25-year-old female who is 30 weeks pregnant.

- What normal physiological alterations take place during pregnancy that may affect your assessment of this patient? – Decreased blood pressure and increased pulse. ◄

Normal physiological changes to vital signs during the 1_____ _____ of pregnancy include 2_ _____ in blood pressure 1m-15 mm Hg due to a reduction in peripheral vascular resistance. The 3_____ _____ will increase 10-20 beats per minute due to an increased maternal blood volume. Note: The blood pressure will rise back to baseline in the third trimester. Keep these 4_____ _____ in mind when assessing a pregnant trauma patient.

You ascertain that this patient needs to be transported to the local trauma centre for evaluation.

- What would be the best technique for the transport? – Properly secured to backboard and tilted to left side. *

The backboard must be tilted on its 5_____ _____ 10-15 degrees to prevent 6_____ _____ syndrome. Tilting the board will allow 7____ _____ to displace to the left and 8_____ compression of the inferior vena cava.

- During what month of gestation does the uterus rise out of the pelvic cavity and become more susceptible to blunt trauma? – Fifth month. ◄

After the third month of gestation the foetus and uterus grow rapidly. After the fifth month of pregnancy, the uterus rises out of the pelvis and is more 9_____ to injury.

> a. normal changes; b. heart rate; c. supine hypotension; d. second trimester; e. prone; f. a drop; g. left side; h. the uterus; i. prevent

Case study 13

A 5-year-old boy fell 10 feet (3 metres) from a jungle gym at school, hitting his head on the ground. Your initial evaluation reveals a child who is lethargic and does not respond appropriately 1__ _____. His respirations are shallow, at a rate of 40 with a 2_____ ___ ____ radial pulse.

- What is your first priority? – Rapid c-spine control and airway assistance with BVM and high-flow 0$_2$. ◄

Injured children can rapidly transition from a state of rapid and laboured breathing to a state of 3_____ _____ resulting in respiratory arrest. 4_____ _____ is essential.

- One of the most important prognostic indicators of potential CNS injury is: history of loss of consciousness. ◄

> a. Airway management; b. total exhaustion; c. rapid and weak; d. to commands

Case study 14

You are dispatched to a 77-year-old male patient who has fallen from a ladder while cleaning the gutters. He fell approximately 14 feet (4.3 metres) and struck the ground. He is awake and very anxious. He is having obvious trouble breathing. His pulse is 104, respirations 34, and blood pressure 122/76. His wife tells you that he struck his back on the riding lawn mower as he fell.

In your assessment, you find crepitus and instability to the left rib cage. 1____ _____ are present and equal. Closer assessment reveals paradoxical movement. You suspect:

- tension pneumothorax
- massive haemothorax
- flail chest ◄
- abdominal aneurysm

Flail chest is three or more 2_____ ____ that are fractured in two or more places. This segment of the chest is free to move with the pressure changes of respirations.

- Paradoxical movement is best described as chest wall movement that is: inward with inspiration and outward with expiration. ◄

Paradoxical chest wall movement associated with flail chest is defined as the motion of a flail segment 3_____ __ the normal motion of the chest wall.

Prehospital management for this patient includes:

- a needle decompression midclavicular line
- positive pressure ventilation ◄
- an occlusive dressing
- chest decompression midaxillary line

Positive pressure ventilation of the patient with a flail chest 4_____ the mechanism that causes the paradoxical chest wall movement, restores tidal volume, and reduces the pain of chest wall movement.

Your patient is in severe respiratory distress. Reassessment reveals absent lung sounds on the left, 5_____ _____ to the right, and SpO$_2$ reading of 82%.

- Immediate treatment must include: left side chest decompression. ◄

The signs and symptoms displayed by this patient are consistent with a left side 6_____ _____ and immediate chest decompression is required.

a. reverses; b. tracheal deviation; c. tension pneumothorax; d. Lung sounds; e. adjacent ribs; f. opposite to

Case study 15

One of the most common mechanisms of injury in the geriatric population is falls.

- This statement is true regarding the force required to 1_____ _ _____ in a geriatric patient: Less force is required than in other patients. ◄

2_____ is common in the geriatric population. This disease process makes bones much more 3_____ to hip and other fractures. In 4_____ _____, a simple action such as sneezing may 5_____ __ a fracture.

a. susceptible; b. severe cases; c. result in; d. break a bone; e. Osteoporosis

Case study 16

You are called to the scene of an assault on a 75-year-old woman. She is unresponsive, with blood coming from the back of her head and multiple contusions and skin tears to her knees and arms. She has snoring respirations, a strong radial pulse of 60 beats per minute, and a moderate amount of bright red blood from a large laceration and haematoma in her occipital region.

- What is your first priority? – Immediately 1_____ -_____ and open the airway. ◄

Airway and c-spine are always a priority before 2_____ _____.

Why would this patient be more
susceptible to severe 3____ _____?

- a history of Alzheimer's disease
- dehydration
- Pickwickian syndrome
- decreased size of the brain ◄

As part of the normal
physiologic changes 4____ _____,
a decrease occurs in brain weight
and size. By the age of 80, the
brain loses approximately 3.5
ounces (99 grams) in weight.

After completing your rapid
trauma assessment on your
patient, you find a blood pressure
of 99/54, heart rate of 50, and
respiratory rate of 14 and regular.

- What is your priority
  of care? – Careful fluid
  resuscitation. ◄

Fluid resuscitation needs to
be carefully administered due
to the decreased response of the
5_____ _____ with
age. Reduced circulation, loss of
circulatory defence responses,
coupled with increased presence
of ventricular dysfunction
produces a significant challenge in
6_____ _____ in the elderly.

a. managing shock; b. with aging; c. stabilize
the c-spine; d. other treatments; e. head
trauma; f. cardiovascular system

Vocabulary 2

additional /əˈdɪʃ.ən.əl/
adjacent /əˈdʒeɪ.sənt/

affect /əˈfekt/
age /eɪdʒ/
alert /əˈlɜːt/
all-terrain vehicle /ˌɔːl.tə.reɪnˈviː.ɪ.kl/
allow /əˈlaʊ/
alteration /ˌɒl.təˈreɪ.ʃən/
ankle /ˈæŋ.kl̩/
appropriately /əˈprəʊ.pri.ət.li/
arrest /əˈrest/
arterial /ɑːˈtɪə.ri.əl/
ascertain /ˌæs.əˈteɪn/
assault /əˈsɒlt/
assure /əˈʃɔːr/
baseline /ˈbeɪsˌlaɪn/
blunt /blʌnt/
border /ˈbɔː.dər/
bruising /ˈbruː.zɪŋ/
calculate /ˈkælkjʊˌleɪt/
capable /ˈkeɪ.pə.bl̩/
cerebrum /sɪˈriː.brəm/
challenge /ˈtʃæl.ɪndʒ/
clavicular /kləˈvɪkjʊlə/
command /kəˈmɑːnd/
compartment /kəmˈpɑːt.mənt/
compensatory /ˌkɒm.pənˈseɪt.ə ri/
complete /kəmˈpliːt/
compress /kəmˈpres/
concussion /kənˈkʌʃ.ən/
condition /kənˈdɪʃ.ən/
consistent /kənˈsɪs.tənt/ with /wɪð/
contusion /kənˈtjuː.ʒən/
couple /ˈkʌp.l̩/
decrease /dɪˈkriːs/
defence /dɪˈfent s/
despite /dɪˈspaɪt/
deterioration /dɪˌtɪə.ri.əˈreɪ.ʃən/
deviation /ˌdiː.vɪˈeɪʃən/
diameter /daɪˈæm.ɪ.tər/
digestive /daɪˈdʒes.tɪv/
dispatch /dɪˈspætʃ/
displace /dɪˈspleɪs/
distributive /dɪˈstrɪbjʊtɪv/
dizziness /ˈdɪz.ɪ.nəs/
epidural /ˌepɪˈdjʊərəl/
equal /ˈiː.kwəl/

evident /'ev.ɪ.dənt/
exhaustion /ɪgˈzɔːs.tʃən/
firm /fɜːm/
flight /flaɪt/ of stairs /steərz/
foetus /'fiː.təs/
free /friː/
gauze /gɔːz/
gently /'dʒent.li/
gestation /dʒesˈteɪ.ʃən/
gutter /'gʌt.ər/
handlebar /ˌhæn.dl̩.bɑː/
impale /ɪmˈpeɪl/
impression /ɪmˈpreʃ.ən/
indicator /'ɪn.dɪ.keɪ.tər/
initial /ɪˈnɪʃəl/
instability /ˌɪn.stəˈbɪl.ɪ.ti/
intestine /ɪnˈtes.tɪn/
inward /'ɪn.wəd/
irreversible /ˌɪr.ɪˈvɜː.sɪ.bl̩/
jungle /'dʒʌŋ.gl̩/ gym /dʒɪm/
laboured /'leɪ.bəd/
lapse /læps/
lawn mower /'lɔːnˌməʊ.ər/
maternal /məˈtɜː.nəl/
midaxillary /mɪd.ækˈsɪl.ər.i/
midclavicular /mɪd.kləˈvɪk.jʊ.lər/
mind /maɪnd/
moisten /'mɔɪsən/
motion /'məʊʃən/
nonadherent /ˌnɒn.ədˈhɪə.rənt/
occipital /ɒkˈsɪp.ɪ.təl/
osteoporosis /ˌɒs.ti.əʊ.pəˈrəʊ.sɪs/
outward /'aʊt.wəd/
paradoxical /ˌpær.əˈdɒk.sɪ.kəl/
persist /pəˈsɪst/
pipe /paɪp/
pregnancy /'preg.nən.si/
pregnant /'pregnənt/
profusely /prəˈfjuːs.li/
prognostic /prɒgˈnɒs.tɪk/
prone /prəʊn/ to /tə/
protrude /prəˈtruːd/
proximal /'prɒk.sɪ.məl/
push /pʊʃ/
reassessment /ˌriː.əˈses.mənt/

rib /rɪb/ cage /keɪdʒ/
section /'sek.ʃən/
secure /sɪˈkjʊə/
segment /'seg.mənt/
shock /ʃɒk/
skull /skʌl/
small /smɔːl/ bowel /'baʊ.əl/
subdural /sʌbˈdjʊ.ə.rəl/
supine /'suː.paɪn/
susceptible /səˈsep.tɪ.bl̩/
sustain /səˈsteɪn/
tenderness /'ten.də.nəs/
tilt /tɪlt/
transition /trænˈzɪʃ.ən/
triage /'traɪ.ɪdʒ/
trim /trɪm/
uterus /'juː.tər.əs/
vague /veɪg/
valve /vælv/
vasoconstriction /ˌveɪ.zə.kənˈstrɪk.ʃən/
wreck /rek/

Unit 3

Case study 1

You respond to an explosion at a local fireworks production factory. The explosion rocked the ground several blocks away. There are multiple patients.

The mechanism of injury from a blast or explosion can be from three factors, primary, secondary, and tertiary.

- The mechanism of injury of a patient who suffers injuries from being struck by material propelled by the blast force is considered: a secondary mechanism of injury. ◄

A 1_____ _____ of injury from a 2_____ __ _____ is defined as any injury sustained from being struck by material propelled by the blast force.

- The mechanism of injury of a patient being thrown and impacting the ground or other object is considered: a tertiary mechanism of injury. ◄

A tertiary mechanism of injury from a blast or explosion is defined as any injury sustained from 3_____ _____ and 4_____ ___ _____ or other objects.

Your first patient is a 43-year-old male with burns over the front of his right arm, upper chest, and the front of his right leg.

- Using the rule of nines, what percent of burns does this patient have? – 22.5% ◄
  Front of right arm = 4.5%, 5_____ _____ = 9%, front of right leg = 9%

This patient is hoarse, has singed nasal hair, is coughing up charcoal-coloured sputum, and has developed inspiratory stridor.

- Treatment should include: immediate endotracheal intubation. ◄

Your concern with this patient is complete 6_____ _____ secondary to 7_____ of the airway. Immediate endotracheal intubation is indicated.

a. impacting the ground; b. upper chest; c. swelling; d. secondary mechanism; e. blast or explosion; f. being thrown; g. airway obstruction

Case study 2
The following 1_____ regarding a Glasgow coma scale score 7 is true:

- a perfect GSC score is 15 and a score of 7 represents serious injuries ◄
- a score between 9 and 12 indicates 2_____ injury
- a score of 8 or below 3_____ severe head injury

a. moderate; b. represents; c. statement

Case study 3
You arrive at the scene of a trench collapse. There are three trapped victims who are buried to the midchest. The rescue will take several hours because they will need to be dug out by hand. Crushing syndrome is a significant concern because crush injuries release toxins into the central circulation that can cause:

- alkalosis
- increased renal function
- cardiac dysrhythmias ◄
- dyspnoea

1_____ _____ creates lactic acid due to 2_____ _____ that takes place within the crushed body part. One of the 3_____ _____ with releasing a body part that has been crushed for several hours is the release of the lactic acid and other 4_____ into the circulating 5_____ _____ that can lead to profound metabolic acidosis.

Sodium bicarbonate is indicated in the treatment of crushing syndrome.

a. Crush syndrome; b. major concerns; c. anaerobic metabolism; d. toxins; e. blood volume

Case study 4

You are called to a scene of a motor vehicle collision (MVC). During your initial assessment, you find an 1_____32-year-old male with multiple 2_____ to his face and head. He has 3_____ respirations and a weak, 4_____ peripheral pulse. Your first action would be:

- to control major bleeding
- rapid extrication
- to open the airway with a jaw thrust and immobilize the cervical spine ◄

Always remember ABCs.

a. contusions; b. snoring; c. unresponsive; d. thready

Case study 5

Which of the following statements is true regarding 1_____ _____?

- Always use 2_____ or neutralizing agents.
- Acid burns are typically more serious than 3_____ burns.
- Both acids and alkalis cause burns by disrupting cell membranes and damaging tissues on contact ◄
- Always 4_____ a chemical spill from downwind.
- Antidotes and neutralizing agents should 5_____ be used as they may cause a violent reaction with the contaminants.◄
- Alkali burns are typically more severe because of their liquefaction necrosis process.◄
- You should approach from up wind.◄

a. approach; b. chemical burns; c. antidotes; d. alkali; e. never

Case study 6

Beck's triad is often associated with pericardial tamponade. It includes distant heart tones, 1___ (jugular venous distention), and:

- 2_____ paradoxus
- hypotension ◄
- wheezing
- delayed capillary refill

Beck's triad includes 3_____, distant heart tones, and JVD. This triad of symptoms can aid in the diagnosis of 4_____ _____.

a. cardiac tamponade; b. pulse;
c. hypotension; d. JVD

a. motor response; b. opening; c. pinched;
d. sounds; e. speech

Case study 7

A stab wound to the stomach or small intestine would cause gastric contents to enter the peritoneal cavity. Presentation would include:

- a rapid onset of cramping pain
- referred pain to the left shoulder
- a gradual onset of pain throughout the 1_____
- a rapid onset of sharp pain, diffuse throughout the abdomen ◄

Injury to the stomach or small bowel that allows digestive enzymes to enter the 2_____ _____ can cause a rapid development of 3 _____ ____ throughout the abdomen. This is a serious concern because peritonitis can develop and lead to 4_____ complications.

a. serious; b. peritoneal cavity; c. sharp pain;
d. abdomen

Case study 8

Your trauma patient opens her eyes, pulls her hand away when 1_____, and speaks only in garbled 2_____.

- What is her Glasgow Coma Scale score? – 9.◄

The score is 9; 2 points for eye 3_____, 5 points for 4_____ _____, and 2 points for 5_____.

Case study 9

Your patient is a 34-year-old woman who has been in an automobile 1_____. Her respiratory rate is 34 with normal chest wall 2_____; systolic blood pressure is 78; capillary refill is 3_____; and her Glasgow Coma Scale score is 10.

- This patient Revised Trauma Score score is: 9. ◄

Using the 4_____ Trauma Score, 3 points for the GCS, 3 points for the 5_____ blood pressure, and 3 points for the respiratory rate.

a. Revised; b. delayed; c. systolic;
d. expansion; e. crash

Case study 10

You are caring for a female patient who 1____ _____ by an automobile. She opens her eyes to voice 2_____ only, localizes pain when you pinch her arm, and is 3_____ ____ _____.

- Her Glasgow coma scale is: 12 ◄

The GCS for this patient is 12: three points for opening her eyes to 4_____ _____, five points for 5_____ _____, and four points for speaking clearly although the 6_____ _____ is confused.

a. verbal stimuli; b. localizing pain; c. awake but confused; d. thought process; e. was struck; f. command

Case study 11

What is the Glasgow Coma Scale Score for a patient who opens her eyes 1__ _____ to pain, speaks 2_____, and 3_____ in response to pain? – 8. ◄

Eye opening = 2; verbal response = 2; motor response = 4.

a. withdraws; b. incomprehensibly; c. in response

Case study 12

Your patient, a middle-aged female, was a 1_____ struck by a car. She opens her eyes only in response to pain and makes 2__ _____ response, her best motor response is withdrawal in response to pain.

- The Glasgow Coma Scale score for this patient is: 7. ◄

Her score is 7 3__ _____ __ 2 points for pain, 1 point for verbal response, and 4 points for motor response.

a. is composed of; b. pedestrian; c. no verbal

Case study 13

With the START triage method, several 1_____ _____ are quickly assessed to determine the order to care for and transport patients. According to the START method, which of the following patients would receive 2_____ _____ to support haemodynamic status without further assessment?

- male, radial pulse present, skin warm and dry
- female, 3_____ _____ present, capillary refill time 1 sec
- male, radial pulse present, skin pale and cyanotic ◄
- female, radial pulse present, capillary refill time 0.5 sec

The START method quickly reviews 4_____ _____ to determine patient priority: respirations, pulse, and mental status. After respiratory status is assessed, the basis for judging a patient's haemodynamic status is presence or absence of a radial pulse or 5____ _____ and temperature.

a. vital signs; b. radial pulse; c. three categories; d. skin colour; e. immediate treatment

Case study 14

What does a red tag mean in the METTAG triage system:

- the 1_____ is dead
- the victim has critical injuries ◄
- the victim has2 _____ injuries
- the victim has 3_____ injuries

When using the 4_____ _____ a red tag indicates a patient with 5_____ injuries who needs rapid transport.

a. critical; b. serious; c. METTAG system; d. victim; e. minor

Case study 15

Patients who are found in a hazardous materials 1_____ should be initially treated in which containment zone? – Warm. ◄

Major decontamination and treatment for life-threatening 2_____ should be conducted by properly protected personnel in the 3____ ____.

---

a. incident; b. conditions; c. warm zone

Case study 16

You respond to a 41-year-old male who has been injured in an explosion at an illegal chemistry (drug) laboratory. During assessment, you notice a spinal deformity and a possible closed head injury. Your patient also has ruptured tympanic membranes and signs sinus injuries.

Which of the following is not a phase of blast injury?

- alpha ◄
- primary
- secondary
- tertiary impact

1_____ _____ _____ is divided into three phases: primary, secondary, and tertiary. The primary phase occurs during the initial air blast and 2_____ ____. The secondary phase occurs when the patient is 3____ __ _____ propelled by the overpressure of the blast wave. The tertiary phase occurs when the victim is 4_____ ____ from the blast into the ground or other hard objects.

This patient's sinus injuries most likely occurred during which blast phase?

- alpha
- primary ◄
- secondary
- tertiary impact

During the primary blast, forces from the pressure wave and initial air blast result in 5_____ of air-containing organs such as the sinuses, auditory canals, stomach, lungs, and intestines.

Your victim has first- and second-degree burns to his face. These are flash burns from the 6_____. Witnesses deny that the patient's clothes were 7__ _____. You should suspect what injury?

- extensive lung tissue burns
- extensive airway burns
- aspiration pneumonia
- limited airway burns ◄

Often, burns are 8_____ to the oro- and nasopharynx in the upper airway. 9_____ stridor or 10_____ indicates that oedema is developing, which may lead to 11_____ _____. Flash burns rarely result in 12_____ airway or lung tissue burns. Aspiration pneumonia is an infectious process that develops following the introduction of a foreign body into the lungs. It is unlikely in this scenario, and if it has occurred, there will be no signs of infection yet.

During your assessment, you notice a rigid, very tender abdomen. If this injury occurred in the secondary phase, it would be due to which of the following?

- thermal burns to the stomach
- flying debris and propelled objects ◄
- deceleration impact with a hard surface
- compression of air-containing organs

Compression of air-containing organs is common in the 13_____ _____ _____. Deceleration injuries 14_____ during the tertiary phase and 15_____ _____ can occur during any phase of the blast, depending upon whether the 16_____ _____ is superheated, if flaming objects are striking the patient, or if the patient is thrown into a burning area. A 17_____, _____ abdomen indicates there are 18_____ _____ under the skin, and not surface injuries to the dermis from 19_____. This injury was most likely caused by flying debris or propelled objects 20_____ the patient.

---

a. internal injuries; b. primary blast phase; c. striking; d. occur; e. thermal burns; f. pressure wave; g. rigid, tender; h. burns; i. Worsening; j. limited; k. extensive; l. airway compromise; m. hoarseness; n. on fire; o. explosion; p. Blast injury impact; r. thrown away; s. hit by debris; t. pressure wave; u. compression

---

Case study 17

This statement about the vital signs of a patient with an 1___ is correct. –Vital signs vary greatly since they are related to the area and extent of cardiac damage. ◄

Vital signs in MI patients depend on the 2_____ ___ _____ of underlying heart 3_____ and the patient's response to the insult.

---

a. damage; b. location and extent; c. AMI

Vocabulary 3

acid /ˈæs.ɪd/
airway /ˈeə.weɪ/
alkali /ˈæl.kəl.aɪ/
alkalosis /ˌælkəˈləʊ.sɪs/
antidote /æn.tɪ.dəʊt/
aspiration /ˌæspɪˈreɪʃən/
auditory /ˈɔːdɪtərɪ/
awake /əˈweɪk/
away /əˈweɪ/
Beck's triad /ˈtraɪ.æd/
blast /blɑːst/
burn /bɜːn/
bury /ˈber.i/
canal /kəˈnæl/
capillary /kəˈpɪl.ər.i/ **refill** /ˈriː.fɪl/
cell /sel/
charcoal /ˈtʃɑːr.koʊl/
chemistry /ˈkem.ɪ.stri/
clearly /ˈklɪə.li/
command /kəˈmɑːnd/
complete /kəmˈpliːt/
composed /kəmˈpəʊzd/
compression /kəmˈpreʃən/
concern /kənˈsɜːn/
conduct /kənˈdʌkt/
confused /kənˈfjuːzd/
containment /kənˈteɪn.mənt/
contaminant /kənˈtæm.ɪ.nənt/
content /kənˈtent/

contusion /kənˈtjuː.ʒən/
cramp /kræmp/
crash /kræʃ/
critical /ˈkrɪt.ɪ.kəl/
crush /krʌʃ/ syndrome /ˈsɪn.drəʊm/ ·
dead /ded/
debris /ˈdeb.riː/, /ˈdeɪ.briː/
deceleration /diːˌseləˈreɪʃən/
decontamination /ˌdiː.kən.tæm.ɪˈneɪ.ʃən/
deformity /dɪˈfɔː.mɪ.ti/
deny /dɪˈnaɪ/
dermis /ˈdɜː.mɪs/
determine /dɪˈtɜː.mɪn/
diffuse /dɪˈfjuːz/
disrupt /dɪsˈrʌpt/
distant /ˈdɪs.tənt/
distension /dɪˈsten.tʃən/
downwind /ˌdaʊnˈwɪnd/
due /djuː/ to /tʊ/
dig /dɪg/ out /aʊt/
dyspnoea /dɪs.pniː.ə/
expansion /ɪkˈspæn.tʃən/
explosion /ɪkˈspləʊ.ʒən/
extrication /ˌek.strɪˈkeɪ.ʃən/
fireworks /ˈfaɪəˌwɜːk/
flaming /ˈfleɪ.mɪŋ/
flash /flæʃ/
flying /ˈflaɪ.ɪŋ/
force /fɔːs/
foreign /ˈfɒr.ən/ body /ˈbɒd.i/
garbled /ˈgɑː.bļd/
gradual /ˈgræd.jʊ.əl/
ground /graʊnd/
haemodynamic /ˌhiːmə.daɪˈnæm.ɪk/
hoarseness /ˈhɔːsnɪs/
illegal /ɪˈliː.gəl/
impact /ˈɪm.pækt/
incomprehensibly /ɪnˌkɒm.prɪˈhen.sɪ.bļi/
initially /ɪˈnɪʃ.əl.i/
injury /ˈɪndʒərɪ/
intestine /ɪnˈtes.tɪn/
judge /dʒʌdʒ/
jugular /ˈdʒʌg.jə.lər/

lactic /ˈlæk.tɪk/ acid /ˈæs.ɪd/
limited /ˈlɪm.ɪ.tɪd/
liquefaction /ˌlɪkwɪˈfækʃən/
localize /ˈləʊ.kəl.aɪz/
lung /lʌŋ/
major /ˈmeɪ.dʒə/
mean /miːn/
membrane /ˈmem.breɪn/
METTAG, Medical /ˈmed.ɪ.kəl/
Emergency /ɪˈmɜː.dʒənt.si/
Triage /ˈtraɪ.ɪdʒ/ Tag /tæg/
mid /mɪd/
middle /ˈmɪd.l/ age /eɪdʒ/
minor /ˈmaɪ.nə/
motor /ˈməʊ.tər/
nasopharynx /ˌneɪ.zəˈfær.ɪŋks/
necrosis /neˈkrəʊsɪs/
object /ˈɒb.dʒɪkt/
obstruction /əbˈstrʌk.ʃən/
oedema /ɪˈdiː.mə/
oropharynx /ˈɔː.rə ˈfær.ɪŋks/
overpressure /ˌəʊ.vəˈpreʃ.ər/
paradoxus /ˈpær.ə.dɒk.səs/
pedestrian /pɪˈdestrɪən/
peers /pɪərz/
perfect /ˈpɜː.fekt/
phase /feɪz/
pinch /pɪntʃ/
pinna /pin.ə/
point /pɔɪnt/
presentation /ˌprez.ənˈteɪ.ʃən/
profound /prəˈfaʊnd/
propelled /prəˈpeld/
properly /ˈprɒp.əl.i/
pull /pʊl/
radial /ˈreɪ.di.əl/
rarely /ˈreə.li/
referred /rɪˈfɜːd/ pain /peɪn/
release /rɪˈliːs/
renal /ˈriː.nəl/
response /rɪˈspɒns/
revise /rɪˈvaɪz/
rigid /ˈrɪdʒ.ɪd/
rock /rɒk/
rupture /ˈrʌp.tʃər/

score /skɔː/
serious /ˈsɪə.ri.əs/
singe /sɪndʒ/
sinus /ˈsaɪ.nəs/
snore /snɔːr/
sodium bicarbonate /ˌsəʊ.di.əm.baɪˈkɑː.bən.ət/
sound /saʊnd/
speech /spiːtʃ/
spill /spɪl/
spinal /ˈspaɪ.nəl/
sputum /ˈspjuː.təm/
statement /ˈsteɪt.mənt/
stimulus /ˈstɪm.jʊ.ləs/ pl **stimuli**
stomach /ˈstʌm.ək/
stridor /straɪd.ər/
strike /straɪk/ (**struck, struck**)
superheat /ˈsuː.pəˌhiːt/
surface /ˈsɜː.fɪs/
sustain /səˈsteɪn/
swelling /ˈswelɪŋ/
tag /tæg/
tender /ˈten.dər/
tertiary /ˈtɜː.ʃər.i/
thermal /ˈθɜː.məl/
thready /ˈθred.i/
throughout /θruːˈaʊt/
throw /θrəʊ/ (**threw, thrown**)
tissue /ˈtɪʃ.uː/, /ˈtɪs.juː/
trench /trentʃ/
triage /ˈtraɪ.ɪdʒ/
tympanic /ˈtɪm.pə.nik/
membrane /mem.breɪn/
tympanic /ˈtɪm.pə.nik/
upper /ˈʌp.ər/
venous /ˈviː.nəs/
victim /ˈvɪk.tɪm/
voice /vɔɪs/
wave /weɪv/
withdraw /wɪðˈdrɔː/
withdrawal /wɪðˈdrɔː.əl/
witness /ˈwɪt.nəs/
zone /zəʊn/

Part 5 Gynaecology, obstetrics, paediatrics

Unit 1

Case study 1

Supine hypotension syndrome occurs from: reduction of cardiac output due to compression of the inferior vena cava. ◄

1_____ hypotension syndrome (or vena cava syndrome) occurs when the pregnant 2_____ compresses the 3_____ ____ ____ when the patient is in a supine position. This results in a 4_____ in blood return back to the heart and a reduction of 5_____ _____. This syndrome can occur as early as the third month of gestation.

a. Supine; b. cardiac output; c. inferior vena cava; d. decrease; e. uterus

Case study 2

You are caring for a female patient who is at 35 weeks gestation. She was involved in a car accident and complains of neck pain. You suspect spinal injury and fully immobilize her on a long spine board.

- You would then: carefully 1_____ the board on its left side 10 -15 degrees. ◄

The backboard must be tilted on its left side 10 -15 degrees to prevent supine 2_____ _____. Tilting the board will allow the 3_____ to displace to the left and prevent compression of the 4_____ vena cava.

a. hypotension syndrome; b. uterus; c. tilt; d. inferior

Case study 3

The major concern with a prolapsed cord is that it: will be compressed and reduce blood flow to the infant, resulting in 1_____. ◄

The major concern with a prolapsed cord is 2_____ of the cord by the head of the infant. This can result in a reduced 3_____ ____ to the infant and can lead to foetal hypoxia.

a. compression; b. blood flow; c. hypoxia

Case study 4

Abdominal pain in the region of the ovary during ovulation is known as: 1_____.

- Mittelschmerz is German for "2_____ pain" and is defined as abdominal pain in the region of the ovary during 3_____. ◀

> a. middle; b. ovulation; c. Mittelschmerz

Case study 5

In obstetrics, a woman's parity refers to her number of:
1_____ deliveries. ◀

This is common obstetric medical terminology. The term "gravida" means: number of 2_____.

3_____ or gravidity refers to the number of times a woman has been 4_____.

A multigravida and 5_____ pregnancy history includes: many pregnancies and no births

6_____ is when a woman has been pregnant more that once. Nullipara is a woman who has not yet delivered her first child.

> a. viable; b. pregnant; c. nullipara;
> d. Multigravida; e. Gravida; f. pregnancies

Case study 6

Your patient is 26 years old and 30 weeks pregnant. She complains of sudden severe tearing abdominal pain with some minor vaginal bleeding. Upon careful 1_____, her abdomen is very tender and her uterus seems to be tightly 2_____.

- You suspect: abruptio placenta. ◀

Abruptio placenta is premature separation of the placenta from the uterus. There are different 3_____ that can occur depending on the severity of the abruption.

Classic presentation includes a sudden, 4_____, tearing pain and the development of a 5_____ boardlike abdomen. Bleeding can be severe or not present depending on many factors.

> a. stiff; b. palpation; c. sharp;
> d. presentations; e. contracted

Case study 7

Placenta abruption is a
1_____ _____ caused by:

- 2_____ of the fertilized ovum in a fallopian tube
- the uterus covering the 3_____ opening
- premature separation of the placenta from the uterine wall. ◀
- spontaneous 4_____

It is a true medical emergency because it poses a life threat to the mother and 5_____.

> a. foetus; b. medical emergency; c. abortion;
> d. implantation; e. cervical

Case study 8

The normal 1_____ changes to vital signs during the second trimester of pregnancy include: blood pressure 2_____, 3_____ _____ rises. ◀

> a. physiological; b. pulse rate; c. falls

97

Case study 9

The next four questions are based on the following scenario:

You are called to the scene of a 26-year-old female patient who is 27 weeks pregnant and in active labour. The patient states "the baby is coming." You perform a visual examination of the perineum and notice a prolapsed cord.

You would immediately place the patient in which position?

- hips 1_____ as much as possible ◄
- knee-chest position ◄

Position the mother with the hips elevated as much as possible or in the knee-chest position in an attempt to 2_____ pressure on the cord.

You would instruct the patient to:

- push with each contraction
- pant with each contraction. ◄
- bear down
- hold her breath

You would instruct the patient to pant with each contraction to prevent 3_____ _____ and applying pressure on the cord.

With a gloved hand, placing two fingers into the vagina to elevate the presenting part to relieve pressure on the cord. Provide oxygen and rapid transport to a hospital that can perform a 4_____ _____.

- Additional treatment would include: with a gloved hand, placing two fingers into the vagina to raise the foetus off the cord, providing oxygen and transport ◄

Care for the prolapsed cord would include:

- application of a sterile dressing ◄
- attempting to reposition the cord
- packing in ice to prevent it from drying

Applying a sterile 5_____ to the exposed cord will minimize 6_____ change. If the cord is exposed to room temperature, the temperature of blood 7_____ to the infant will decrease. This can cause hypothermia.

Additionally, a temperature change of the blood may cause the umbilical vessels to 8_____ resulting in 9_____ blood flow to the infant.

a. relieve; b. caesarean delivery; c. elevated; d. bearing down; e. raise; f. spasm; g. dressing; h. flowing; i. decreased; h. temperature

Case study 10

The hormone secreted by the 1_____ _____ that stimulates the uterus to produce stronger 2_____ is: oxytocin ◄

The medication (oxytocin) is used to induce labour or control 3_____ haemorrhage.

> a. postpartum; b. pituitary gland;
> c. contractions

Case study 11

The most common sexually
1_____ disease is:

- chlamydia ◄
- gonorrhoea
- syphilis
- herpes

Gonorrhoea, syphilis,
and 2_____ are also
3_____ transmitted diseases.

> a. herpesvirus; b. sexually; c. transmitted

Case study 12

You are treating a 20-year-old
female complaining of abdominal
pain that becomes more intense
when walking. She states that if
she shuffles her feet when she
walks, the pain isn't as intense.

Other signs and symptoms
include fever, 1_____, and
nausea. This patient is most
likely 2_____ ____:

- endometritis
- pelvic inflammatory
  disease ◄
- ruptured ovarian cyst
- mittelschmerz
- cystitis

Pelvic inflammatory disease
is often accompanied by increased
pain when 3_____.

The patient will bend forward
and take short, slow steps.

4_____ of the abdomen and
nausea are also common with PID.

> a. chills; b. Guarding; c. suffering from;
> d. walking

Case study 13

The next three questions are
based on the following scenario:

You are called to a 32-year-
old female who is in her twenty-
eighth week of pregnancy. She
complains of dizziness, blurred
vision, and a feeling that she
is going to pass out. She is
emotionally 1_____ and crying.
At her doctor's 2_____
last week, her doctor scolded her
for gaining too much of weight.

Her hands and ankles are
oedematous and her face is
puffy.Vitals are BP 178/108,
pulse 104, respirations 24.

You suspect that this patient:

- is emotionally upset
- has preeclampsia ◄
- has borderline hypotension
- has postpartum depression

3_____ signs and symptoms
of preeclampsia include headache,
dizziness, 4_____, blurred
vision, nausea, vomiting, proteinuria,
hypertension, and oedema.

Treatment for this
patient would include:

- rapid transport with
  lights and siren

- administering nitroglycerin to lower the blood pressure
- transporting for psychiatric evaluation
- keeping the patient calm, and transporting without lights and siren ◄

If you suspect preeclampsia, you should 5_____ _____ to prevent seizures, which include keeping the patient calm and transporting without lights and sirens.

You are enroute to hospital when the patient has a 6_____ ___ _____.

- Treatment for this patient includes: maintaining an airway, administering oxygen, administering magnesium sulphate 2-5 g, monitoring vital signs. ◄

Treatment of seizure activity in eclampsia includes placing the patient in the left lateral 7_____ position, maintaining the airway, administering high-flow oxygen, 8_____ IV access, and the administration of 2-5 grams of magnesium sulphate IV. If seizures cannot be controlled, sedatives may be required.

a. establishing; b. common; c. upset;
d. confusion; e. take precautions;
f. recumbent; g. grand mal seizure;
h. appointment

Case study 14

The next two questions are based on the following scenario:

Your patient is a 38-year-old 1_____ in her thirtieth week of gestation. She presents with bright red vaginal bleeding but 2_____ abdominal pain. Her 3_____ is soft and feels "out of place." Her problem began following sexual intercourse. You suspect:

- a uterine rupture
- placenta praevia ◄
- an ectopic pregnancy
- abruptio placenta

Placenta praevia is usually in a multigravida in her third trimester of pregnancy. A recent history of 4_____ _____ or vaginal examination just before the onset of vaginal bleeding is not uncommon. The onset of painless bright red vaginal bleeding or spotting is considered the 5_____ _____ of placenta praevia.

- Management of this patient includes: IV fluids, high-flow oxygen, transport for evaluation. ◄

A vaginal exam should not be attempted when placenta praevia is suspected. The exam may 6_____ the placenta and cause a severe haemorrhage.

a. puncture; b. sexual intercourse; c. hallmark sign; d. denies; e. multigravida; f. uterus

Case study 15

APGAR assessment of a newborn should be performed: at 1_____ _____ _____ minutes after birth.◄

It is important to wait one full minute to perform the first 2_____ assessment. A second APGAR should be 3_____ at five minutes.

a. APGAR; b. one and five; c. performed

Case study 16

If the amniotic sac has not ruptured and the baby's head 1_____, you should: use your fingers to 2_____ and puncture the sac, then push the sac away from the nose and mouth. ◄

If the 3_____ ___ is present around the baby's head, use your fingers to pinch the sac, and then 4____ __ ____ from the nose and mouth. Using a scalpel or scissors is not recommended.

a. amniotic sac; b. push it away; c. emerges; d. pinch

Case study 17

1_____ _____ should be performed on any newborn with a heart rate less than 2__ _____ per minute. ◄

If a newborn's heart rate is 60-80 and does not increase despite 3_____ and 4_____, it is necessary to start chest compressions.

a. 60 beats; b. stimulation; c. ventilation; d. Chest compressions

Case study 18

Your 26-year-old female patient complains of nausea, dizziness, sudden onset of sharp left lower quadrant pain, and shoulder pain. You suspect:

- a ruptured appendix
- an ectopic pregnancy ◄
- cholecystitis
- kidney stones

An ectopic pregnancy should be suspected when 1_____ _____ is present in women of childbearing age who are sexually active. An ectopic pregnancy can be difficult to 2_____ from other conditions. The classic 3_____ of symptoms includes abdominal pain, 4_____ bleeding, and amenorrhoea.

Other symptoms include 5_____ pain to the shoulder, nausea, vomiting, or syncope. Signs of shock may be present if the 6_____ ruptures.

a. distinguish; b. vaginal; c. abdominal pain; d. referred; e. triad; f. ectopic

Case study 19

The function of the placenta includes all of the following:

- the transfer of antibodies ◄
- the transfer of 1_____ ___ _____ ◄
- the excretion of CO_2 and waste products ◄

The placenta has many functions including the transport of oxygen, nutrients, and other substances to the foetus and the 2_____ of CO_2 and other 3_____ products.

a. excretion; b. waste; c. oxygen and nutrients

Case study 20

What is the most appropriate care for a suspected 1_____-_____ patient? – Perform a limited 2_____ _____ and care for injuries requiring immediate treatment. ◄

EMS providers should limit the patient's history to the elements necessary to provide care. Patient contact should be 3____-_____ and supportive.

a. non-judgemental; b. sexual assault;
c. physical examination

Vocabulary 1

abortion /əˈbɔː.ʃən/
abruptio placentae /
æbˈrʌp.ʃi.əʊ.pləˈsen.tiː/
abruption /əˈbrʌp.ʃən/
amenorrhoea /ˌeɪ.men.əˈriː.ə/
amniotic /ˌæm.niˈɒt.ɪk/ **sac** /sæk/
antibody /ˈæn.tiˌbɒd.i/
appendix /əˈpen.dɪks/
apply /əˈplaɪ/
appointment /əˈpɔɪnt.mənt/
bear /beər/ **down** /daʊn/
bend /bend/ (**bent, bent**)
blurred /blɜːd/
boardlike /bɔːd.laɪk/
borderline /ˈbɔː.də.laɪn/
breath /breθ/
caesarean section /sɪˌzeə.ri.ənˈsek.ʃən/
care /keə/ **for** /fɔː/
careful /ˈkeə.fəl/
cervical /səˈvaɪ.kəl/

childbearing /ˈtʃaɪldˌbeə.rɪŋ/
chill /tʃɪl/
chlamydia /kləm.iˈde.ə/
cholecystitis /ˌkəʊ.lɪ.sɪˈstaɪ.tɪs/
compress /kəmˈpres/
condition /kənˈdɪʃ.ən/
contract /kənˈtrækt/
cord /kɔːd/
cyst /sɪst/
cystitis /sɪˈstaɪ.tɪs/
decrease /dɪˈkriːs/
delivery /dɪˈlɪv.ər.i/
distinguish /dɪˈstɪŋ.gwɪʃ/
eclampsia /ɪˈklæmp.si.ə/
ectopic pregnancy /
ekˌtɒp.ɪkˈpreg.nən.si/
emerge /ɪˈmɜːdʒ/
emotionally /ɪˈməʊ.ʃən.əl.i/
endometritis /ˌen.də.miˈtraɪ.tɪs/
establish /ɪˈstæb.lɪʃ/
evaluation /ɪˌvæl.juˈeɪ.ʃən/
excretion /ɪkˈskriː.ʃən/
exposed /ɪkˈspəʊzd/
fallopian tube /fəˌləʊ.pi.ənˈtjuːb/
fertilize /ˈfɜː.tɪ.laɪz/
flowing /ˈfləʊ.ɪŋ/
foetal /ˈfiː.təl/
forward /ˈfɔː.wəd/
gonorrhoea /ˌgɒn.əˈriː.ə/
gravida /ˌgræv.ɪ.də/
gravidity /grævˈɪd.ɪ.ti/
gynaecology /ˌgaɪ.nəˈkɒl.ə.dʒi/
hallmark /ˈhɔːl.mɑːk/
herpes /ˈhɜː.piːz/ **zoster** /zɒ.stər/
herpes /ˈhɜː.piːz/
herpes /ˈhɜː.piːz/ **simplex** /ˈsɪm.pleks/
herpes-virus /ˈhɜː.piːzˈvaɪ.rəs/
hip /hɪp/
hold /həʊld/
implantation /ˌɪm.plænˈteɪ.ʃən/
instruct /ɪnˈstrʌkt/
kidney /ˈkɪd.ni/ **stones** /stəʊnz/
knee /niː/ **-chest** /tʃest/
position /pəˈzɪʃ.ən/
labour /ˈleɪ.bər/

light /laɪt/
magnesium /mæg'niː.zi.əm/
sulphate /'sʌl.feɪt/
minimise /'mɪn.ɪ.maɪz/
minor /'maɪ.nə/
mittelschmerz /mɪtl.ʃmərθ/
multigravida /mʌl.ti'græv.ɪ.də/
newborn /'njuː.bɔːn/
non-judgemental /ˌnɒn.dʒʌdʒ'men.təl/
nullipara /nʌ'lɪp.ər.ə/
nutrient /'njuː.tri.ənt/
obstetrics /ɒb'stetrɪks/
oedematous /ɪ'diː.mə.təs/
ovarian /əʊ'veə.ri.ən/
ovary /'əʊ.vər.i/
ovum /'əʊ.vəm/ pl **ova**
oxytocin /ˌɒk.sɪ'təʊ.sɪn/
pack /pæk/
packing /'pæk.ɪŋ/
paediatrics /ˌpiː.di:'æt.rɪks/
pant /pænt/
parity /'pærɪti/
pass /pɑːs/ **out** /aʊt/
pelvic /'pel.vɪk/ **inflammatory** /
ɪn'flæm.ə.tər.i/ **disease** /dɪ'ziːz/
perform /pə'fɔːm/
perineum /ˌper.ɪ'niː.əm/
pituitary gland /pɪ'tjuː.ɪ.tər.iˌglænd/
placenta /plə'sen.tə/ **praevia**/ priː.vi.ə/
postpartum /ˌpəʊst'pɑː.təm/
precaution /prɪ'kɔː.ʃən/
preeclampsia /ˌpri.ɪ'klæmp.si.ə/
premature /'prem.ə.tʃər/
presenting /prɪ'zent.ɪŋ/ **part** /pɑːt/
product /'prɒd.ʌkt/
prolapsed /prəʊ'læpst/
proteinuria /'prəʊ.ti:n.jʊə'ri:.ə/
puffy /'pʌf.i/
puncture /'pʌŋk.tʃə/
push /pʊʃ/
recumbent /rɪ'kʌm.bənt/
reposition /ˌriː.pə'zɪʃən/
scalpel /'skæl.pəl/
scissors /'sɪz.əz/
scold /skəʊld/

separation /ˌsepə'reɪʃən/
severity /sɪ'ver.ɪ.ti/
sexual /'sek.sjʊəl/
intercourse /'ɪn.tə.kɔːs/
shuffle /'ʃʌf.l̩/
siren /'saɪərən/
spot /spɒt/
spotting /spɒt.ɪŋ/
state /steɪt/
stiff /stɪf/
supportive /sə'pɔː.tɪv/
suspected /sə'spek.tɪd/
syphilis /'sɪf.ɪ.lɪs/
tender /'ten.dər/
tightly /'taɪt.li/
umbilical /ʌm'bɪl.ɪ.kəl/
upset /ʌp'set/
uterine /'juː.tər.aɪn/ **wall** /wɔːl/
viable /'vaɪ.ə.bl̩/
vision /'vɪʒ.ən/
waste /weɪst/ **product** /'prɒdʌkt/
weight /weɪt/

Unit 2
Case study 1

The next two questions are based on the following scenario:

You arrive on the scene of a 25-year-old female who states she is 9 months pregnant and is in 1_____ labour. The patient states she is gravida 3, para 2. She states that her "2_____ _____" about 15 minutes ago and the baby is coming. Vital signs are BP 152/86, pulse 96, respirations 24.

- The term gravida means: number of pregnancies ◄

Upon 3_____ examination, you notice that crowning is present.

- You should: prepare for
  4_____ because
  the birth of the baby
  is imminent.◄

a. apparent; b. delivery; c. water broke;
d. visual

Case study 2

The next two questions are
based on the following scenario:

You arrive on the scene of a
motor vehicle crash and notice that a
car has struck a telephone pole. There
is extensive damage to the vehicle.

You find a confused female in
her mid-twenties complaining of
neck, chest, and abdominal pain.
She keeps asking if her baby is
going to be okay. You find out that
she is eight months pregnant.

Assessment reveals a large
laceration to the forehead with
active bleeding. BP 96/54,
pulse 142, with pale cool skin,
respirations 24 and shallow.

- Treatment includes:
  administering 100% oxygen,
  rapid 1_____
  from the vehicle with
  c-spine immobilization
  onto a backboard, placing
  her on a 2_____
  on the left side, starting
  two large-bore IVs while
  enroute to the hospital.

During transport, she suddenly
goes into cardiac arrest. The patient
is apnoeic and 3_____

and the cardiac monitor shows
ventricular fibrillation.

- What should be your next
  action? – Defibrillate,
  4_____ ____, and intubate,
  administer epinephrine
  1 mg IVP. ◄

Treatment for a pregnant
patient in cardiac arrest would
include defibrillation, CPR,
intubation, and administration of
appropriate 5_____.

a. medications; b. extrication; c. backboard;
d. begin CPR; e. pulseless

Case study 3

You are treating a 22-year-old
female 1_____ __ severe
abdominal pain and left shoulder
pain. Vital signs are BP 88/64,
pulse 128 and regular, respirations
of 22, skin cool and wet. She states
that she has a small amount of pink
vaginal 2_____. This patient
is most likely experiencing:

- a ruptured ectopic
  pregnancy ◄
- endometriosis
- pelvic inflammatory disease
- amenorrhoea

An ectopic pregnancy should 3__
_____ when abdominal pain
is present in women of childbearing
age who are 4_____ active.
An ectopic pregnancy can be
difficult to distinguish from other
5_____. The classic triad of

symptoms includes abdominal pain, vaginal bleeding, and 6_____.

from the nose and mouth to help to prevent 7_____.

a. conditions; b. discharge; c. be suspected;
d. complaining of; e. amenorrhoea; f. sexually

a. aspiration; b. positioning; c. same;
d. drainage; e. newborn; f. lower; g. is clamped

Case study 4

You are providing positive-pressure 1_____ to a newborn.

- Regarding oxygen administration to a newborn this statement is correct: Never 2_____ a newborn of oxygen for fear of oxygen toxicity. ◄

If central cyanosis is present, or you are unsure about the 3_____ of ventilation, the administration of 4_____ oxygen is necessary.

a. deprive; b. supplemental; c. ventilation;
d. adequacy

Case study 5

To prevent over- or undertransfusion of blood from the umbilical cord to the 1_____, correct 2_____ of the newborn until the umbilical cord 3__ _____ should be: at the level of vagina. ◄

Keep the newborn at the 4____ level of the vagina with the head slightly 5_____ than the rest of the body.

This will prevent over- or undertransfusion of blood from the umbilical cord to the newborn and facilitate 6_____ of secretions

Case study 6

The umbilical vein: carries oxygenated blood from the placenta to the foetus.

- The umbilical cord consists of one 1____ and two 2_____. ◄

The umbilical vein carries oxygenated blood from the 3_____ to the foetus. The umbilical arteries transport 4_____ products from the foetus to the placenta.

a. waste; b. arteries; c. vein; d. placenta

Case study 7

Contraction intervals are correctly 1_____: from the beginning of one contraction to the 2_____ of the next.◄

Many health care providers 3_____ measure intervals from the end of one contraction to the beginning of the next.

- Contraction length is correctly measured: from the beginning of one contraction to 4____ ____ of that contraction. ◄

a. beginning; b. measured; c. incorrectly;
d. the end

Case study 8

You have a female patient at 39 weeks' gestation. She has 1_____ contractions 2_____ 45-60 seconds at one to two-minute intervals and is crowning.

- Treatment for this patient should include: preparing for delivery. ◄

Regular contractions lasting 45-60 seconds at one to two-minute intervals and 3_____ indicate delivery is imminent.

```
a. regular; b. crowning; c. lasting
```

Case study 9

Four assessment manoeuvres used to 1_____ foetal position is called: the Leopold manoeuvre. ◄

The Leopold manoeuvre is 2_____ of the abdomen in four different assessment steps. This is used to identify the 3_____ of foetuses, the foetal presentation, presenting 4_____, degree of descent, point of maximum intensity of foetal heart tones, and internal 5_____ of the foetus.

```
a. palpation; b. determine; c. part; d. number;
e. rotation
```

Case study 10

You are delivering a child when you observe the umbilical cord 1_____ around the neck.

- Your first action should be: to gently 2_____ the cord from around the neck. ◄

Initial care for 3_____ _____ (cord around the neck) is to first try to gently remove the cord from around the neck. If this is not successful and the cord is so tight that it is 4_____ labour, it will be necessary 5__ _____ the cord in two places and 6____ between the clamps.

```
a. wrapped; b. to clamp; c. nuchal cord;
d. remove; e. inhibiting; f. cut
```

Case study 11

You are delivering a child in a breech presentation. You have delivered the feet and chest. You note that the 1_____ of the child is moving and suspect the child is attempting to breathe.

- You should: insert two fingers in the vagina to form an airway around the infant's 2_____ ____ _____. ◄

If the infant starts to breathe with its face pressed against the vaginal wall, it is necessary 3__ _____ two fingers in the vagina to form 4__ _____ around the infant's nose and mouth.

```
a. an airway; b. nose and mouth; c. chest,
d. to insert
```

Case study 12

- Applying gentle 1_____ to the infant's head to prevent explosive delivery is essential because: this will allow the 2_____ to stretch and reduce the chance of tearing. ◄

Applying gentle countertraction to the infant's head to prevent 3_____ delivery is essential to decrease the likelihood of tearing of the perineum and decreases the potential for rapid 4_____ of the baby's skull through the birth canal, which may cause 5_____ injury.

a. countertraction; b. intracranial;
c. expulsion; d. explosive; e. perineum

Case study 13

Meconium-stained 1_____ _____ indicates: a foetal hypoxic incident. ◄

Hypoxia causes an increase in 2_____ activity along with the relaxation of the 3____ _____, which allows meconium to pass into the amniotic fluid.

a. digestive; b. anal sphincter; c. amniotic
fluid

Case study 14

The next two questions are based on the following scenario:

You are sent to private residence for a 13 months-old child with a barky cough. He is awake, slow to respond, and visibly uncomfortable. The 1_____ cough is audible without a stethoscope but lung sounds reveal inspiratory stridor at rest. There is use of 2_____ muscles and you note nasal flaring.

You would suspect the child to be suffering from:

- epiglottitis
- croup ◄
- bronchiolitis
- a common cold

3_____ is a viral infection of the upper airway that causes inflammation of the 4_____ region that can lead to airway 5_____. Inspiratory stridor is often present. Other assessment findings include nasal flaring, tracheal tugging or retractions. The vital signs of this patient are compensatory to the airway obstruction.

This child can be categorized as a child who is experiencing:

- respiratory arrest
- respiratory insuffiency
- prerespiratory arrest
- respiratory failure ◄

Respiratory failure is 6_____ for the following reasons: tachypnoea, tachycardia, nasal flaring, 7_____, audible airway noises (stridor/ barky) cough, and slowness to respond, which indicates a decreased level of 8_____.

a. barky; b. Croup; c. retractions;
d. accessory; e. obstruction; f. evident;
g. subglottic; h. consciousness

Case study 15

You have been called to treat a five-year-old child previously diagnosed with and upper respiratory infection. She now presents with increased work of breathing, fever, and increased cough. The child appears pale, is lying on the couch, and slow 1__ _____. She has obvious nasal flaring with a respiratory rate of eight per minute.

- This child is most likely in: respiratory distress with 2_____ respiratory failure. ◄

Respiratory distress is defined as the inability to maintain 3_____ _____ sufficient to meet the needs of the body. Evidence of abnormal respirations (tachypnoea or bradypnoea) or increased work of breathing, use of accessory muscles, nasal flaring, 4_____, and decreased 5_____ can also signal respiratory distress in the paediatric patient.

a. to respond; b. gaseous exchange; c. mentation; d. grunting; e. impending

Case study 16

Signs and symptoms associated with shaken baby syndrome might include: an intracranial haemorrhage, resulting from 1____ _____ between the brain and skull in children under the age of 24 months. ◄

The result of 2_____ _____ in a baby less than 24 months old may include damage to nerve tissues deep 3_____ ____ _____ and torn veins between the brain and the skull, which can cause severe bleeding.

a. violent shaking; b. within the brain; c. torn veins

Case study 17

You respond to a call for a two-month-old female who is reported by the mother to be seizing. Upon arrival, you find the infant lying in a crib motionless, no 1_____ _____ is evident. The mother reports that the episode began approximately 10 minutes ago. Your assessment reveals a flaccid infant with slow respiration of 10 per minute, bulging anterior fontanelle, and several areas of bruising on the extremities 2__ _____ _____ of healing.

- From the information given and the general appearance of the infant, you suspect: child abuse, most probably shaken baby syndrome ◄

You may suspect 3_____ _____ _____ based on 4_____ __ the anterior fontanelle without fever or overhydration as a cause. In addition, the multiple areas of bruising provide information that may indicate 5_____ _____.

a. in various stages; b. shaken baby syndrome; c. child abuse; d. bulging of; e. seizure activity

Case study 18

Intraosseous access allows for the administration of fluids, medications, and blood products into the 1_____ _____.

- Possible complications of intraosseous infusion include all of the following: osteomyelitis, fractures, compartment syndrome. ◄

IO infusions will generally improve the patient's condition or improve his or her vascular volume, thereby increasing the BP and cardiac output.

2_____ can occur if the needle is left in place for longer than 24 hours.

3_____ can occur when the extremity is not well stabilized or an attempt was made at an improper site where the bone is weaker.

4_____

_____ occurs when extravasation is not detected.

a. Fractures; b. bone marrow; c. Compartment syndrome; d. Osteomyelitis

Case study 19

The MOST appropriate 1_____ manoeuvre for an infant in SVT involves: holding ice packs firmly to the face. ◄

Applying ice to the 2_____ of the infant, being careful not to obstruct the nose and mouth. If the child is old enough to follow 3_____, have the child hold his/her 4_____ and blow into an occluded straw or 5_____ the child to bear down.

a. encourage; b. face; c. breath; d. directions; e. vagal

Case study 20

You are dispatched to a private residence for an eight-year-old boy complaining of trouble breathing. On arrival, you find the patient 1_____, with blue lips and rapid laboured respirations. He is able to answer questions with only one- or two-word 2_____.

Physical examination reveals a respiratory rate of 50 per minute, diminished breath sounds and 3_____ are heard over the right lung field with dullness to percussion. He also has a temperature of 104° F (40° C).

- Based on your assessment, this patient may be experiencing: respiratory 4_____, most probably due to pneumonia. ◄

The patient may be experiencing respiratory failure, most probably due to 5_____ based on tachypnoea, increased work of breathing, diminished breath sounds, dullness to 6_____, and elevated temperature.

a. pneumonia; b. sentences; c. percussion; d. crackles; e. lethargic; f. failure

Case study 21

Answer the next four questions on the basis of the following information.

You respond to the residence of a 4-year-old male who was

109

found in his backyard, head down in a 5 gallon (19 L) bucket of water. The child, according to the mother, was in the water 1_____ four minutes.

The child is cyanotic, pulseless, and apnoeic. The ECG shows he is in asystole. The child weights approximately 40 pounds (18 kg).

A physician at the scene of an accident instructs you to provide care for a patient that you know to be inappropriate given the patient's present condition.

- Your best course of action will be to: contact the medical control physician and ask him to speak with the on-scene physician.◄

The medical control physician should be able to engage with the on-scene physician in discussion with the patient's condition, the level of care that will be provided by the EMS 2_____, and the transportation destination decision.

- What would be the most reliable method for determining the proper medication dosing for this paediatric patient? – Use the Broselow Tape or another length-weight 3_____ system. ◄
- All of the following medications can be given through the endotracheal tube to paediatric

patient: lidocaine, epinephrine, atropine ◄

Valium is usually given orally or rectally

- After endotracheal intubation of this patient, what step should be done first? – Confirm the ETT placement ◄

Your first step following placement of the ET tube is to confirm its placement in the trachea. After 4_____ of placement, secure the tube with tape or using a commercial device to help 5_____ dislodging of the tube. Pay especially close 6_____ to these tubes as they are easily displaced, even when secured.

Depending upon which size tube you use, it may or may not be a cuffed tube. Medication administration will follow after confirmation of 7_____ and securing the tube.

a. attention; b. placement; c. prevent; d. approximately; e. personnel; f. measuring; g. confirmation

Vocabulary 2

accessory /ək'ses.ər.i/
activity /æk'tɪv.ɪ.ti/
adequacy /'æd.ə.kwə.si/
amenorrhoea /ˌeɪ.men.ə'riː.ə/
anal /'eɪ.nəl/
apnoeic /æp'niː.ɪk/
apparent /ə'pær.ənt/
asystole /ə.sɪs.tə.lɪ/
at /ət/ **rest** /rest/
attempt /ə'temp t/

audible /'ɔ:.dɪ.bl̩/
backyard /ˌbæk'jɑ:d/
barky /'bɑ:.ki/
bear /beər/ down /daʊn/
birth /'bɜ:θ/ canal /kə'næl/
bone /bəʊn/ marrow /'mær.əʊ/
break /breɪk/ (broke broken)
breech /bri:tʃ/ presentation /
ˌprez.ən'teɪ.ʃən/
bucket /bʌkɪt/
bulge / bʌldʒ/〜
clamp /klæmp/
cold /kəʊld/
commercial /kə'mɜ:ʃəl/
compartment /kəm'pɑ:t.mənt/
syndrome /'sɪn.drəʊm/
confirmation /ˌkɒn.fə'meɪ.ʃən/
contraction /kən'træk.ʃən/
countertraction /ˌkaʊn.tər'træk.ʃən/
course /kɔ:s/
crackle /'kræk.l̩/
crash /kræʃ/
crib /krɪb/
croup /kru:p/
crowning /'kraʊ.nɪŋ/
defibrillate /ˌdi:'fɪb.rɪ.leɪt/
deprive /dɪ'praɪv/
descent /dɪ'sent/
destination /ˌdes.tɪ'neɪ.ʃən/
detect /dɪ'tekt/
discharge /dɪs'tʃɑ:dʒ/
dislodge /dɪ'slɒdʒ/
distinguish /dɪ'stɪŋ.gwɪʃ/
drainage /'dreɪ.nɪdʒ/
dullness /'dʌl.nəs/
endometriosis /ˌen.dəʊˌmi:.tri'əʊ.sɪs/
engage /ɪn'geɪdʒ/
epiglottitis /ˌep.ɪ.glə'taɪ.tɪs/
essential /ɪ'sen.tʃəl/
explosive /ɪk'spləʊ.sɪv/
delivery /dɪ'lɪv.ər.i/
expulsion /ɪk'spʌl.ʃən/
extravasation /eksˌtræ.və'seɪ.ʃən/
facilitate /fə'sɪl.ɪ.teɪt/
fear /fɪə/

flaccid /'flæksɪd/
fontanelle /ˌfɒn.tə'nel/
gallon /'gæl.ən/
gaseous /'geɪ.si.əs/
gently /'dʒent.li/
grunt /grʌnt/
heal /hi:l/
ice /aɪs/ pack /pæk/
imminent /'ɪm.ɪ.nənt/
impending /ɪm'pen.dɪŋ/
improper /ɪm'prɒp.ər/
improve /ɪm'pru:v/
inability /ˌɪn.ə'bɪl.ɪ.ti/
incident /'ɪnt.sɪ.dənt/
indicate /'ɪn.dɪ.keɪt/
infusion /ɪn'fju:.ʒən/
inhibit /ɪn'hɪb.ɪt/
insuffiency /ˌɪn.sə'fɪʃ.ənt.si/
intraosseous /ˌɪn.trə'ɒs.i.əs/
intubate /ɪn'tju:.beɪt/
likelihood /'laɪ.kli.hʊd/
measure /'meʒ.ər/
meconium /mɪ'kəʊ.nɪ.əm/
mentation /men'teɪ.ʃən/
motionless /'məʊ.ʃən.ləs/
nuchal /nu:.kəl/
osteomyelitis /ˌɒs.ti.əʊ.maɪ.əl'aɪ.tɪs/
overhydration /ˌəʊvə.haɪ'dreɪ.ʃən/
pain /peɪn/
pelvic /'pel.vɪk/ inflammatory /
ɪn'flæm.ə.tər.i/ disease /dɪ'zi:z/
potential /pə'ten.ʃəl/
prerespiratory /ˌpri:'res.pər.əˌtɔr.i/
presentation /ˌprez.ən'teɪ.ʃən/
regarding /rɪ'gɑ:.dɪŋ/
relaxation /ˌri:.læk'seɪ.ʃən/
remove /rɪ'mu:v/
residence /'rez.ɪ.dəns/
retraction /rɪ'træk.ʃən/
rotation /rəʊ'teɪ.ʃən/
seize /si:z/
seizure / 'si:.ʒə/
sentence /'sen.təns/
shake /ʃeɪk/ (shook, shaken)

shaken /ˈʃeɪkən/ **baby** /ˈbeɪ. bi/ **syndrome** /ˈsɪn.drəʊm/
sphincter /ˈsfɪŋk.tər/
stage /steɪdʒ/
stethoscope /ˈsteθ.ə.skəʊp/
subglottic /sʌbˈglɒt.ɪk/
suddenly /ˈsʌd.ən.li/
thereby /ˌðeəˈbaɪ/
tight /taɪt/
torn /tɔːn/
tracheal / trəˈkiː.əl/
tug /tʌg/
umbilical cord /ʌmˈbɪl.ɪ.kəlˌkɔːd/
uncomfortable /ʌnˈkʌmp f.tə.bl̩/
unsure /ʌnˈʃɔːr/
ventricular /venˈtrɪk.jə.lər/
fibrillation /ˌfaɪ.brɪˈleɪ. ʃən/, /ˌfɪb.rɪˈleɪˌʃən/
violent /ˈvaɪələnt/
wrap /ræp/

Unit 3

Case study 1

Defibrillation in an infant or child: is 1_____ every 2 minutes as indicated ◄

After 5 cycles of CPR (2 minutes), 2_____ the rhythm and pulse and defibrillate again if a 3_____ rhythm is present.

a. shockable; b. reassess; c. repeated

Case study 2

You have just delivered a 1_____-_____ baby in your ambulance. The initial APGAR score is 5.

Treatment should consist of: effective ventilation.◄

Most newborn infants respond quite favourably to 2_____, drying, suctioning, and 3_____. Occasionally, administration of oxygen with assisted ventilations may be necessary. Vascular access and 4____ are utilized only after the infant fails to 5_____ effectively to ventilatory assistance.

a. stimulation; b. full-term; c. warming; d. respond; e. CPR

Case study 3

Which of the following clinical 1_____ is MOST consistent with 2_____ ingestion in a child?

- diaphoresis, miosis, tachycardia, and bronchospasm
- hypertension, tachycardia, diaphoresis, and mydriasis.◄
- miosis, bradycardia, hypoventilation, and hypotension
- mydriasis, diarrhoea, hypothermia, and hallucinations

Hypertension, tachycardia, diaphoresis, and 3_____ (dilated pupils) are consistent with cocaine or 4_____ use.

a. Presentations; b. amphetamine; c. mydriasis; d. cocaine

Case study 4

Which of the following assessment finding would indicate that a paediatric patient

is progressing from respiratory
distress to respiratory failure?

- nasal flaring
- 1_____ rate over 32
- poor muscle tone ◄
- grunting/head bobbing

Nasal 2_____, elevated
respiratory rate, grunting and head
bobbing all indicate respiratory
distress. The development of poor
3_____ _____ indicates the patient
is tiring and is an 4_____
sign of respiratory failure.

a. respiratory; b. muscle tone; c. flaring;
d. ominous

Case study 5

While enjoying an "off" day
from work, you hear your neighbour
screaming. You rush outside to see
her 1_____ her four-year-old
child from the swimming pool.

- The child is limp, blue,
  and 2____ _____
  to any stimulus. What
  should you do? – Send the
  mother to call 112, open
  an airway and initiate
  3_____ _____. ◄

The 4____ rescuer
should initially provide rescue
breathing to the child while
someone is sent to call 112.

a. pulling; b. lone; c. rescue breathing; d. not
responsive

Case study 6

Identify the anatomical
differences in the paediatric airway
compared to the 1_____ _____.
– The airway diameter is smaller,
the larynx is more anterior, the
tongue is proportionally larger. ◄
The airway 2_____
in children is smaller than an
adult airway, the larynx is more
3_____ making visualization
difficult the 4_____ is
proportionally larger to the jaw.

a. anterior; b. tongue; c. diameter; d. adult
airway

Case study 7

Beta blocker ingestion in small
children would 1____ likely cause:

- acute hypoglycaemia ◄
- agitation or irritability
- marked hypertension
- ventricular fibrillation

Ingestion of beta blockers,
ethanol or other 2_____,
3_____, or oral hypoglycaemic
agent can lead to hypoglycaemia.

a. insulin; b. MOST; c. alcohols

Case study 8

It is important to compare central
and 1_____ pulses in the
paediatric patient to determine:

- the presence of shock ◄
- skin colour
- mental status
- airway patency

The presence or absence of shock may be indicated by a difference between the 2_____ and peripheral pulses. Pulse 3_____ or deficit may be a sign of poor peripheral 4_____.

a. perfusion; b. central; c. peripheral; d. differences

Case study 9

A child wearing a helmet strikes a large rock on his bicycle and flies over the 1_____. The patient would MOST likely suffer:

- associated head injury
- stretching or tearing injuries to the kidneys
- open or closed fractures to the lower extremities
- compression injuries to the intraabdominal organs ◄

Injury from bicycle handlebars typically includes 2_____ injuries to the intraabdominal organs and 3_____ injuries. Upper 4_____ injuries are also common.

a. pancreatic; b. extremity; c. compression; d. handlebars

Case study 10

You have administered lidocaine to an eight-year-old. 1_____, decreased mental status, muscle twitching, and seizures are side effects that may result from its administration. ◄

Lidocaine has central nervous system properties that cause drowsiness, decreased 2_____ _____, muscle 3_____, and the possibility of 4_____.

a. Drowsiness; b. seizures; c. twitching; d. mental status

Case study 11

Of the following 1_____ below, which is most likely to 2_____ _____ shaken baby syndrome?

- hypoglycaemia
- abdominal bruising
- subdural haematoma ◄
- lower extremity fracture

3___ _____ (including the possibility of a subdural haematoma) is a 4_____ _____ in shaken baby syndrome.

a. common finding; b. Head injury; c. choices; d. result from

Case study 12

Your squad is dispatched to the scene of a six-year-old child with an elevated temperature. The mother tells you that the child was fine last night and got up this morning complaining of a sore throat and trouble swallowing.

The initial assessment reveals a sick-looking child who is leaning forward in the 1_____ _____. He is obviously drooling. From this information you suspect:

- bronhciolitis
- croup
- epiglottitis ◄
- meningitis

2_____ is a bacterial infection causing the acute 3_____ of the epiglottis and the soft tissues above the glottic opening. Clinical findings include but are not limited to sudden onset high fever 102-104°F (38-40°C), pain on 4_____, typically sitting in tripod position, and 5_____.

```
a. Epiglottitis; b. swallowing; c. drooling;
d. tripod position; e. swelling
```

Case study 13

During transport of a child with epiglottitis, he becomes 1_____ and apnoeic. You are still able to 2_____ a weak pulse at a rate of 64 per minute.

- Your immediate action should be: position the child's head and provide bag-valve mask ventilation with 100% oxygen.◄

Any external 3_____ of the epiglottis (i.e., intubation or OPA 4_____) can cause complete airway obstruction in the child with epiglottitis. Carefully 5_____ the child's head and provide positive pressure ventilation with 100% oxygen.

```
a. palpate; b. unresponsive; c. manipulation;
d. position; e. insertion
```

Case study 14

Your patient is an ill-appearing four-months-old lying in his mother's arms. The mother tells you that the infant won't take a bottle and cries whenever she moves.

Your exam reveals a lethargic infant, warm to touch, with fine pinpoint 1_____ on the abdomen, chest, and face. The infant's 2_____ appears to be bulging.

- The information gained on exam should lead you to suspect: meningitis.◄

Recognize the syndrome of fever and petechia as a medical emergency. Inflammation of the 3_____ will cause the fontanelle 4__ _____ and appear full. 5_____ should be suspected in this patient.

```
a. to bulge; b. petechia; c. meninges;
d. fontanelle; e. Meningitis
```

Case study 15

This statement correctly relates to paediatric seizures: febrile seizures correlate to the speed in which the temperature rises, not to the 1_____ of the fever. ◄

How fast the 2_____ of the child rises will increase a child's risk for developing a 3_____.

```
a. seizure, b. degree, c. temperature
```

Case study 16

The next two questions are based on the following scenario:

You are dispatched to a local department store when a concerned customer notices an infant left unattended in a car. It is bitterly cold outside.

Once you gain entry into the car, you find the infant to be dusky in colour with no activity or 1_____. The respiratory rate is 12 per minute and irregular with 2_____ and short sighs.

The heart rate is 64 per minute with weak central pulses. The infant's hands are cold to touch. Capillary refill is 5 seconds.

- Your immediate action should be: ventilate with a bag-valve mask device and 100% oxygen. ◄

Recognize that the infant has inadequate oxygenation (3_____ colour) and immediately begin bag-valve mask ventilation with 100% oxygen.

After obtaining 4_____ _____ and delivering the pharmacological intervention, the patient's heart rate increases to 130 per minute with strong central pulses but no peripheral pulses.

- To further stabilize the infant, the next course of action should be to: begin rewarming the patient.◄

Considering the 5_____ temperature to be very cold, hypothermia is a significant cause of the patient's presentation. Begin 6_____ the patient.

a. movement; b. ambient; c. rewarming; d. venous access; e. dusky; f. grunting

Case study 17

A seven-year-old child has been 1_____ by a car and is lying 2_____ in the street. He has 3_____ head trauma.

- Identify the signs of Cushing's triad: increased BP, bradycardia, abnormal respirations. ◄

4_____ _____ (sometimes referred to as Cushing's reflex or response) characteristically presents with and 5_____ blood pressure, bradycardia, and abnormal (usually 6____) respirations.

a. elevated; b. slow; c. struck; d. motionless; e. obvious; f. Cushing's triad

Case study 18

Seizurelike activity triggered by stimuli other than cerebral electrical discharges, such as major mood disorders or severe environmental stress is defined as:

- partial seizure
- partial complex seizure
- generalized seizure
- pseudoseizure ◄

1_____ _____ (neurogenic) is a distributive shock producing hypotension relative to an increase in the vascular space in the absence of a loss of body fluids.

A 2_____ _____ injury results in a "lack of communication" between the 3_____ and the 4____ so there is no response to catecholamine release resulting in bradycardia and hypotension.

> a. spinal cord; b. Spinal shock; c. brain; d. body

Case study 19

To ensure that an infant's head is in a neutral position during 1_____ _____, you should:

- provide slight flexion of the head
- place padding under the infant's shoulders ◄
- 2_____ a towel roll behind the infant's neck
- use 3_____ rolls for lateral head stabilization

An infant has a large head in comparison to the rest of the body. To maintain the infant's head in a neutral position, place padding under the infant's 4_____.

> a. shoulders; b. spinal immobilization; c. place, d. towel

Case study 20

You respond to a MVC involving a young child. The child is found apnoeic, but still has a 1_____ pulse. You immediately begin positive pressure ventilation with a bag-valve mask device.

You note that the left side of the chest moves, but the right does not. 2____ _____ are absent on the right side and the 3_____ is deviated to the left.

- Your immediate action is to: perform a needle decompression on the right side. ◄

The signs and symptoms are consistent with a 4_____ _____ (absent breath sounds, tracheal 5_____, no or little chest movement on the affected side). Immediate needle decompression is warranted.

> a. tension pneumothorax; b. trachea; c. palpable; d. Lung sounds; e. deviation

Case study 21

Your patient is a 5-year-old girl who presents with breathing difficulty of rapid 1_____. She is sitting upright and 2_____. Her temperature is 104.6° F (40.3° C).

- What should you suspect? – Epiglotitis. ◄
- What does appropriate management of a child with 3_____ consist of? – Airway maintenance and administration of humidified oxygen. ◄

Management of epiglottitis consists of airway 4_____, oxygen, and prompt transport.

> a. drooling, b. maintenance, c. epiglottitis, d. onset

Vocabulary 3

agitation /ˌædʒ.ɪˈteɪʃən/
ambient /ˈæm.bi.ənt/
bitterly /ˈbɪt.ə.li/

bob /bɒb/
catecholamine /kat.ə.kəl.am.in/
compare /kəmˈpeər/
comparison /kəmˈpærɪsən/
complex /kɒm.pleks/
correlate /ˈkɒrɪˌleɪt/
deviate /ˈdiː.vi.eɪt/
discharge /dɪsˈtʃɑːdʒ/
dispatch /dɪˈspætʃ/
drool /druːl/
drowsiness /ˈdraʊ.zɪ.nəs/
dusky /ˈdʌs.ki/
favourably /ˈfeɪ.vər.ə.blˌi/
fly /flaɪ/ (flew, flown)
full-term (infant) /fʊlˈtɜːm/
generalized /ˈdʒen.ə rə.laɪzd/
handlebar /ˌhæn.dlˌ.bɑː/
humidified /hjuːˈmɪd.ɪ.faɪd/
identify /aɪˈden.tɪ.faɪ/
ingestion /ɪnˈdʒes.tʃən/
intraabdominal /ɪn.trə.æbˈdɒm.ɪ.nəl/
irritability /ˌɪr.ɪ.təˈbɪl.ɪ.ti/
kidney ˈkɪd.ni/
lean /liːn/ forward /ˈfɔː.wəd/
limp /lɪmp/
lone /ləʊn/
maintenance /ˈmeɪntɪnəns/
miosis /maɪˈəʊ.sɪs/
mood /muːd/ disorder /dɪˈsɔːˌdər/
muscle /ˈmʌsəl/ tone /təʊn/
mydriasis /maɪˈdraɪ.ə.sɪs/
occasionally /əˈkeɪ.ʒən/
ominous /ˈɒmɪnəs/
onset /ˈɒnˌset/
padding /ˈpæd.ɪŋ/
pancreatic /ˌpæŋ.krɪˈæ.tɪk/
partial /ˈpɑːˌʃəl/
patency /ˈpeɪ.tənt.si/
perfuse /pəˈfjuːz/
petechia /piˈtiːˌki.ə/ pl petechiae
pin-point, pinpoint / ˈpɪn.pɔɪnt/
prompt /prɒmp t/
property /ˈprɒp.ə.ti/
proportionally /prəˈpɔːˌʃən.əli/
pseudoseizure /ˈsjuːˌdəʊˈsiːˌʒər/

pull /pʊl/
reassess /ˌriːˈə'ses/
responsive /rɪˈspɒnt.sɪv/
result /rɪˈzʌlt/
rewarm /ˌriːˌwɔːm/
rock /rɒk/
roll /rəʊl/
rush /rʌʃ/
sick-looking /sɪkˈlʊk.ɪŋ/
sigh /saɪ/
slight /slaɪt/
sore /sɔː/ throat /θrəʊt/
spinal /ˈspaɪ.nəl/ cord /kɔːd/
squad /skwɒd/
stretch /stretʃ/
swallow /ˈswɒl.əʊ/
tiring /ˈtaɪə.rɪŋ/
towel /taʊəl/
trigger /ˈtrɪg.ər/
tripod /ˈtraɪ.pɒd/
twitch /twɪtʃ/
unattended /ˌʌn.əˈten.dɪd/
warrant /ˈwɒr.ənt/

Unit 4
Case study 1

Your assessment of an unresponsive 7-year-old child reveals that he is 1_____ and 2_____. After performing a 2-minute period of 3____ you assess his cardiac rhythm, which reveals 4_____ _____.

• You should: defibrillate and immediately resume CPR.◄

a. ventricular fibrillation; b. CPR; c. apnoeic; d. puseless

Case study 2

A small child has fallen through the ice while skating. After 30 minutes, the child is pulled from the icy water apnoeic and pulseless.

- Your first action in the management of this child should be to: secure the child's airway and control the cervical spine. ◄

Since it is unknown if there are any c-spine injuries from the 1____ through the ice, you must 2____ ____ ____ and control the cervical spine during 3_____.

a. secure the airway; b. fall; c. resuscitation

Case study 3

You have intubated a six-week-old infant found in respiratory arrest. While performing ventilation, the child becomes blue and the pulse rate drops into the lower 50s.

- Your next step should be to: auscultate the chest. ◄

1_____ of the chest for proper endotracheal tube 2_____ is necessary. If lung sounds are diminished or absent, it may be necessary to 3_____, ventilate, 4_____, and then reintubate.

a. extubate; b. placement; c. reassess; d. Auscultation

Case study 4

A child has suffered multisystem trauma and IV access cannot be obtained. You determine the best 1_____ of action would be establish an IO.

- A 2_____ for intraosseous insertion is: 3_ _____ of the lower extremity. ◄

a. a fracture; b. course; c. contraindication

Case study 5

An injury to which abdominal organ is most likely to cause death in the paediatric patient?

- pancreas
- liver ◄
- spleen
- kidney

The liver is a 1_____, vascular organ in the right upper quadrant. 2_____ or 3_____ of the liver can cause severe 4_____. Injury to the liver is the most common abdominal injury that leads to death in paediatric.

a. haemorrhage; b. solid; c. laceration; d. Rupture

Case study 6

You have performed a 1_____ ____ ____ on a child and are prepared to transport. In which situation is it appropriate to perform the detailed exam enroute to the hospital?

- fracture of the humerus
- amputated thumb
- mottled skin with tachycardia ◄
- fractured tibia with numbness in the foot

A sign of poor perfusion includes 2_____ _____ and tachycardia. This is indicative of 3_____ and a detailed exam should be performed enroute to the hospital. Other indicators of shock include weak peripheral pulses and prolonged 4_____ _____ time.

a. shock; b. capillary refill; c. mottled skin; d. Rapid Trauma Survey

Case study 7

You are treating a child with a tension pneumothorax. Needle decompression is needed.

- The correct site for insertion of needle is: top of the third rib in the midclavicular line. ◄

1_____ the needle over (on top of) the second or third rib avoids 2_____ puncturing or laceration of the adjoining 3_____ and 4_____ located at the inferior border of the ribs.

a. Inserting; b. inadvertent; c. nerves; d. vessels

Case study 8

Concerning paediatric airway management this statement is true: bradycardia can result from suctioning a child. ◄

1_____ may result in bradycardia from stimulation of the 2_____ _____, particularly in children less than six months old. Do not use 3_____ suction attempts.

a. Suctioning; b. prolonged; c. vagus nerve

Case study 9

Which of the following is most likely to cause shock in a child?

- laceration to the face
- a fractured radius
- cerebral oedema
- a splenic injury. ◄

The 1_____ is a blood-filled organ located in the left upper quadrant. 2_____ _____ can cause injury to the spleen resulting in 3_____ _____ and shock. The spleen is the most injured organ resulting in shock, while the 4_____ is the most injured organ resulting in death of a paediatric patient.

a. Blunt trauma; b. spleen; c. liver; d. blood loss

Case study 10

Which action is most important when 1_____ an unresponsive child?

- performing chest compression
- checking for a pulse
- administering supplemental oxygen

- manually opening
  the airway ◄

Establishing a 2_____
_____ is the most important
treatment 3_____ in providing care
for an 4_____ patient.

> a. unresponsive; b. patent airway; c. treating;
> d. step

Case study 11
You respond to the local high
school football practice field for a
sports injury. The coach tells you
that the patient made a tackle and
after the play did not 1____ __. Your
patient is 2_____ on the ground
with all of his equipment on. He is
3_____ but slow to answer questions.

- You should remove the
  football 4_____ if:
  you do not have an easy
  access to the airway. ◄

Unless special circumstances
exist such as respiratory distress or
airway 5_____, the helmet
should not be 6_____ by EMS.

> a. get up; b. awake; c. compromise; d. supine;
> e. helmet; f. removed

Case study 12
Cuffed endotracheal tubes
are usually not 1_____ in
children: under the age of eight. ◄
In a child less than eight, the
normal anatomic 2_____
at the level of the 3_____
_____ provides a "functional
cuff" and eliminates the need

for a cuffed tracheal tube under
most 4_____.

> a. narrowing; b. circumstances; c. cricoid
> cartilage; d. indicated

Case study 13
Suctioning of the infant's mouth
and nose should be performed after:

- 1___ ____ is
  clamped and cut
- the infant 2_____ to cry
- the chest 3___ ____
  _____
- the head has been
  delivered ◄

> a. begins; b. the cord; c. has been delivered

Case study 14
You are assessing a newborn
infant who presents with respiratory
distress. Physical 1_____ reveal
that the patient has a low birth weight,
a small head, and small eye openings.
Besides the obvious respiratory
distress, you might suspect the
infant to be suffering from:

- a heroin 2_____
- crack cocaine ingestion
- foetal alcohol syndrome ◄
- apnoea of 3_____

Characteristics of a newborn
with foetal 4_____ _____
include low birth weight, a small
head, and small eye openings.

> a. alcohol syndrome; b. overdose; c. infancy;
> d. findings

Case study 15

You are assessing an 18-month-old male who presents with obvious 1_____ _____. Inspiratory stridor is heard with evident use of all 2_____ _____. The trouble breathing is worse at night. No other significant findings are visible. The child is on no medications and has otherwise been well. You suspect:

- epiglottitis
- asthma
- bronchiolitis
- croup ◄

3_____ _____, absence of drooling, trouble swallowing, and symptoms persistently worse at night leads to the conclusion of 4___ _____.

a. the croup; b. Inspiratory stridor; c. breathing difficulty; d. accessory muscles

Case study 16

External signs that may indicate an intraabdominal injury in a paediatric patient may include:

- pale skin, abdominal contusion, seat belt abrasions across the abdomen ◄
- dilated pupils, bradycardia, poor peripheral pulses
- tracheal deviation, JVD

1____ _____, abdominal contusion, 2____ ____ abrasions, or unexplained 3_____ may suggest the possibility of intraabdominal injury with a probability of abdominal 4_____.

a. haemorrhage; b. seat belt; c. Pale skin; d. shock

Case study 17

From the following list, identify an example of distributive shock:

- hypovolemic shock
- anaphylactic shock ◄
- cardiogenic shock
- psychogenic shock

1_____ _____ is a shock state that exists when there is no lost of 2____ _____, but the fluid distribution is altered from an increase in the vascular space or leaking of fluid from the 3_____ _____. This results in an 4_____ of fluid relative to the vascular space. Types of distributive shock include anaphylactic, septic, and neurogenic.

a. vascular space; b. insufficiency; c. body fluid; d. Distributive shock

Case study 18

You are 1_____ ___ a child with respiratory distress. You note a 2_____ high-pitched sound with each breath. You suspect this is indicative of:

- stridor ◄
- wheezing
- crackles
- rhonchi

3_____ is a harsh high or low-pitched sound caused by

breathing through a partially blocked airway; wheezing is a high or low-pitched 4_____ sound; crackles/rhonchi represent 5_____ in the larger bronchial airways.

a. Stridor; b. fluid; c. whistling; d. caring for; e. harsh

Case study 19

A priority in evaluating a two-year-old with diarrhoea and vomiting includes determining:

- temperature 1_____
- a viral infection
- a respiratory 2_____
- adequate hydration ◄

Of the choices listed, evaluating the patient for adequate hydration is the 3___ _____. Evaluating the patient's 4_____ and the presence of infection are necessary but secondary to determining adequate hydration.

a. top priority; b. temperature; c. elevation; d. infection

Case study 20

You have initiated an IO line in a paediatric patient suffering from severe 1_____. What is the most reliable indicator of successful placement of the IO needle?

- take an X-ray
- the ability to draw arterial blood through the IO
- aspiration of bone marrow ◄
- no evidence of fractures after insertion

One of the ways to determine 2_____ _____ of the IO needle is by aspiration of the 3___ _____. Additionally, an unobstructed infusion of fluid without evidence of infiltration can also be used. _-4____ are not needed to confirm placement. You should not be able to aspirate 5_____ _____ from a properly placed IO needle.

a. arterial blood; b. bone marrow; c. successful placement; d. X-rays; e. dehydration

Case study 21

Answer the next five questions on the basis of the following information.

You arrive to find a 6-year-old on the floor of his classroom, unconscious, incontinent, and responsive to pain only.

The school nurse states that the child shook 1_____ for approximately two minutes and has been 2_____ ever since. She knows that he takes phenobarbital because she gave him one at lunch, but she is unable to provide further medical history.

- This child most likely suffers from: seizure disorder.◄

The clinical presentation is one of seizures that could occur for a variety of 3_____, including diabetes. However, the use of the drug phenobarbiral is commonly associated with 4_____ _____.

- Phenobarbital is an
  example of: sedative
  or anticonvulsant.◄
- If this child is on medication,
  why did he have this episode
  at school? – Medications
  only limit the number
  of seizures a person
  has; they do not always
  eliminate the seizures.◄

Anticonvulsants serve to
limit the number of seizures a
patient has, but they do not stop
them from occurring altogether.

- Treatment for this patient
  should include: oxygen
  and monitoring.◄
- This patient should be
  transported to a hospital
  because: medication levels
  need to be determined by
  laboratory analysis.◄

This patient needs to be
5_____ to a hospital because
medication levels should be assessed
by laboratory methods. Seizures
may or may not continue to occur.

a. reasons; b. transported; c. unconscious;
d. seizure disorders; e. violently

Vocabulary 4

abrasion /əˈbreɪ.ʒən/
adjoining /əˈdʒɔɪ.nɪŋ/
alter /ˈɒl.tər/
amputate /ˈæm.pjʊ.teɪt/
anticonvulsant /ˌæn.tɪ.kənˈvʌl.sənt/
aspirate /ˈæs.pɪ.rət/
blood /blʌd/ loss /lɒs/

bone /bəʊn/ marrow /ˈmær.əʊ/
border /ˈbɔː.dər/
cardiogenic /ˈkɑː.di.ə.ˈdʒen.ɪk/ shock /ʃɒk/
coach /kəʊtʃ/
compromise /ˈkɒm.prəˌmaɪz/
conclusion /kənˈkluː.ʒən/
crack /kræk/
cricoid /ˈkraɪ.kɔɪd/
cartilage /ˈkɑː.təl.ɪdʒ/
croup /kruːp/
cuff /kʌf/
distributive /dɪˈstrɪbjʊtɪv/
draw /drɔː/
equipment /ɪˈkwɪp.mənt/
foetal /ˈfiː.təl/
get up /get.ʌp/
harsh /hɑːʃ/
helmet /ˈhel.mət/
humerus pl -ri /ˈhjuː.mə.rəs/
hydration /haɪˈdreɪ.ʃən/
inadvertent /ˌɪn.ədˈvɜː.tənt/
incontinent /ɪnˈkɒn.tɪ.nənt/
indicator /ˈɪn.dɪ.keɪ.tər/
infancy /ˈɪn.fənt.si/
inferior /ɪnˈfɪə.ri.ər/
infiltration /ˌɪn.fɪlˈtreɪ.ʃən/
laceration /ˌlæsəˈreɪʃən/
leaking /liː.k.ɪŋ/
list /lɪst/
liver /ˈlɪv.ər/
mottled /ˈmɒt.ḷd/
narrow /ˈnær.əʊ/
numbness /ˈnʌm.nəs/
nurse /nɜːs/
obvious /ˈɒb.vi.əs/
overdose /ˈəʊ.və.dəʊs/
pancreas /ˈpæŋ.kri.əs/
partially /ˈpɑː.ʃəl.i/
patent /ˈpeɪ.tənt/
pitch /pɪtʃ/
priority /praɪˈɒr.ɪ.ti/
psychogenic /ˌsaɪ.kəʊˈdʒe.nɪk/
puncture /ˈpʌŋk.tʃər/
radius /ˈreɪ.di.əs/

responsive /rɪˈspɒnt.sɪv/
resume /rɪˈzjuːm/
seat /siːt/ **belt** /belt/
sedative /ˈsed.ə.tɪv/
seizure / ˈsiː.ʒər/ **disorder** /dɪˌsɔː.dər/
skate /ˈskeɪt/
space /speɪs/
spleen /spliːn/
splenic /spliːn.ɪk/
survey /ˈsɜː.veɪ/
tackle /ˈtæk.l̩/
thumb /θʌm/
tibia /ˈtɪb.i.ə/ pl -ae
vagus /vəɪ.gəs/ pl -gi
weight /weɪt/
whistle /ˈwɪs.l̩/
X-ray /ˈeks.reɪ/

Unit 5

Case study 1

You are performing 1_____
_____ with a bag-mask
device for an 2_____ child.

- How often should you
  3_____ rescue breaths?
  - Once every 6 seconds ◄

a. provide; b. apnoeic; c. rescue breathing

Case study 2

A small child has been struck
by a car travelling approximately
25 1___. The child is unresponsive.
The airway maneuver of
choice for this patient is:

- jaw-thrust with c-spine
  stabilization ◄
- head-tilt/chin-lift
- 2_____
  with jaw-thrust

- hyperflexion of the head to
  the "3_____" position

With the probability of
significant trauma and c-spine
injury, the child's airway should
be assessed using a 4___-_____
maneuvre while stabilizing the
5_____ _____. Head-tilt/chin-
lift hyperextension and hyperflexion
cause manipulation of the cervical
spine and are not indicated when
cervical spine injury is suspected.

a. jaw-thrust; b. cervical spine; c. sniffing;
d. MPH; e. hyperextension

Case study 3

Which of the following
findings or factors would make
you 1___ ___ immediate transport
of a pregnant woman rather than
2_____ delivery in the field?

a) the mother's urge to push
b) the presence of crowning
c) meconium-stained
   amniotic fluid ◄
d) multiparity with
   explosive births

Because meconium staining
in the amniotic fluid can indicate
3_____ _____, it may
mean that the best thing to do is to
transport the mother immediately.
Choices a), b), and d) suggest that
birth is imminent and transport is
4___ _____. If you must deliver
the infant when 5_____ staining
is present, you should be prepared to
provide immediate 6_____
of the trachea and to 7_____

the child prior to stimulation,
drying, warming, or positioning.

a. not advisable; b. meconium; c. foetal
distress; d. intubate; e. attempt; f. suctioning;
g. opt for

Case study 4

During delivery you notice
that the 1_____ _____ is
discoloured and has a foul odour.

• What should you do
first? – Suction the
upper airway using a
meconium aspirator. ◄

Suction the newborn before
stimulating it to 2_____.
Endotracheal suctioning may be
3_____ if meconium is
noted in the 4_____ _____.

a. breathe; b. amniotic fluid; c. upper airway;
d. warranted

Case study 5

How should you 1_____
bleeding after the normal
2_____ of an infant? –
Perform fundal massage. ◄
Massaging the top of the
uterus 3_____ it to contract
and 4_____ control of
normal postpartum bleeding.

a. promotes; b. control; c. stimulates;
d. delivery

Case study 6

In prehospital management of
a very ill neonate: Interventions
should be reassessed at
30-second intervals.◄

Interventions during a neonatal
1_____ should be
assessed often, so that 2_____
are noted as soon as they 3_____.

a. changes; b. occur; c. resuscitation

Case study 7

You must perform chest
compressions on a newborn
infant if, after oxygenation and
ventilation, the heart rate persists
in being less than: 80/min ◄
The threshold for
1_____ in a newborn
infant is 80 beats per minute, and
the range where you would consider
the 2____ ____ compressions
along with other 3_____
is between 60 and 80 BPM.
Any infant with a heart rate less
than 60 BPM should immediately
receive 4_____, but if the
rate remains between 60-80 and is
not rapidly increasing despite positive
pressure 5_____ with
100% oxygen, you should perform
chest compressions for 30 seconds,
reassess, and repeat as needed.

a. ventilation; b. bradycardia; c. treatments;
d. need for; e. compressions

Case study 8

Which is the correct method
to stimulate 1_____
in a neonate?

• Hold it by the feet while
you slap the buttocks.
• Slap the soles of the feet
and rub the back.◄

- Let the cool air cause
it to shiver a little.
- Rub the head but avoid
touching the fontanelle.

Stimulate a neonate by slapping
the soles of the feet and rubbing
the back. The infant should not be
allowed to lose any 2_____ ___,
and you should avoid 3_____
the head to keep from putting any
pressure on the 4_____.

a. fontanelle; b. body heat; c. touching;
d. respirations

Case study 9

How should you control bleeding
after the normal delivery of an infant?

- Pack the vagina with
1_____ _____.
- Apply 2_____ pressure
the the genitalia
- 3_____ the pelvis.
- Perform fundal massage ◀

Massaging the top of the
4_____ stimulates it to contract,
and promotes control of normal
5_____ bleeding.

a. Elevate; b. direct; c. uterus; d. postpartum;
e. sterile gauze

Case study 10

The minimum size bag-
valve mask device used for
neonates, infants, and children
should be: 450 ml.◀
Although it is likely that the
1___-_____ ____ will not deliver
450 ml of volume, it is important

to have a device 2_____ __
delivering excessive volumes because,
as the bag 3__ _____,
there is dead space, from which
air cannot be 4_____ expelled.

a. is compressed; b. fully; c. bag-valve mask;
d. capable of

Case study 11

An isotonic solution is one
that: has an electrolyte composition
like that of blood plasma ◀
1_____ _____ such as
Ringer's lactate or normal 2_____
have electrolyte compositions
similar to that of 3_____ _____
although they lack the large protein
molecules found within blood.

a. blood plasma; b. Isotonic solutions;
c. saline

Case study 12

One way to determine the size
of the endotracheal tube to use in a
child is to use the following equation:
16+ the child's age divided by 4.

- Another consideration
is the size of the child's:
Cricoid ring. ◀

1__ _____ to the child's
age, the size of the 2_____
____ should be based on the size
of the cricoid ring, which is 3___
_____ part of a child's airway.

a. the narrowest; b. endotracheal tube; c. in
addition

Case study 13

Cardiac arrest in young children is most commonly associated with: respiratory problems or diseases.◄

Most 1_____ cardiac arrests are the result of 2_____ accidents that result in respiratory 3_____.

a. preventable; b. compromise; c. childhood

Case study 14

A late sign of 1_____ in children is: bradycardia ◄

Bradycardia in a child is an 2_____ sign of a 3_____ brain.

a. hypoxic; b. ominous; c. hypoxia

Case study 15

Why is 1_____ of the paediatric patient with a bag-valve mask more difficult than ventilation of an adult? – It is more difficult to create a 2____ ____ in an infant.◄

The bridge of the nose in a paediatric patient may make a mask seal more difficult to 3_____. Additionally, the mask size needed to fit in paediatric patient's face may not be available.

a. achieve; b. good seal; c. ventilation

Case study 16

Which of the following statements regarding 1_____ _____ in the paediatric patient is correct?

- The curved 2_____ is preferred in infants and children.

- The narrowest 3_____ of the airway in infants and children is just below the glottic opening ◄

- Cuffed 4_____ tubes should be used in children under the age of eight years.

Straight laryngoscope blades are preferred in children. Uncuffed tubes are needed in order to be firmly seated at the narrowing of the 5_____.

a. trachea; b. airway management; c. blade; d. diameter; e. endotracheal

Case study 17

An 18-month-old female presents with lethargy. The parent states that the patient began looking 1_____ a few hours ago and has become increasingly 2_____ to arouse. The patient had exhibited 3_____ feeding and vomited once prior to your arrival.

She presents with 4_____, cool skin, a pulse rate of 200, and a respiratory rate of 40. She responds to 5_____ stimuli with a weak cry. The EKG shows a rapid narrow complex tachydysrhythmia.

- What is the patient's primary problem? – Dysrhythmia ◄

The relatively 6_____ _____ of this condition and lack of dehydration history points to a primary dysrhythmia as the 7_____ _____ of her presentation.

> a. underlying cause; b. difficult; c. poor;
> d. pale; e. painful; f. irritable; g. sudden onset

Case study 18

Answer the next three questions on the basis of the following information.

You respond to the home of a 2-year-old girl who is experiencing 1_____ and difficult breathing.

The child's mother states that she has had a cold for the past several days and a seal-like bark for the past 20 minutes.

Physical exam reveals she has a fever of 102° F (38.9° C) and 2____ ____ skin. Inspiratory 3_____ is heard upon of lung sounds. Vital signs are blood pressure 100/70, pulse rate of 100, and respiratory rate of 40 that is laboured and with sternal retractions noted.

- This patient is most likely 4_____ ____: croup ◄

This patient is exhibiting the classic signs and symptoms of croup.

- What is the 5_____ treatment for this child? – Saline given by nebulizer treatment and oxygen.◄

A 6_____ saline mist is the appropriate treatment of croup. Do not interfere with the airway in case there is any tissue swelling present.

- A related disease or condition that can result

in rapid and total airway obstruction is: epiglottitis.◄

Epiglottitis, a condition whereby the patient's airway can become 7_____ obstructed, is related to croup.

> a. stridor; b. suffering from; c. appropriate;
> d. laboured; e. nebulized; f. totally; g. hot dry

Case study 19

Your patient is 2 years old.

- How can you reassure her before listening to her chest with your stethoscope? – Gain her trust by letting her listen to your chest first. ◄

1_____ can often be reassured by being allowed to handle 2_____ objects. They will not understand detailed 3_____ and should not be 4_____ to disassemble equipment.

> a. Toddlers; b. allowed; c. explanations;
> d. unfamiliar

Case study 20

You respond to a 2-year-old female who is postictal following seizure activity. The patient's parents report that the child was sleeping when she began to shake and turn blue. She has had a runny nose, but she has had no medications lately. There is no history of seizures.

- This patient is most likely suffering from which condition? – A febrile seizure. ◄

Fever-induced 1_____ are common in young children with only minor illnesses. Once a child has a febrile seizure, he or she is 2_____ __ repeat episodes, which can occur at 3_____ temperatures than the first seizure.

- What vital signs would you expect this patient to have? – Increased body temperature, tachycardia, and tachypnoea. ◄

4_____ body temperature, tachycardia, and tachypnoea are common in a child who is recently postictal from febrile seizures.

- What would be appropriate treatment if this patient continues in a prolonged 5_____ state? – Remove the child's excess clothing, administer oxygen and an IV, and transport. ◄

Oxygen, an IV, and transport is an appropriate treatment for this patient. Remove excess clothing from the patient to passively cool him or her, but do not allow the patient to get chilled. 6_____ the child with room-temperature water if the temperature is excessively high.

Never use 7_____ on the skin as a cooling agent. Alcohol can be absorbed directly through the skin.

```
a. alcohol; b. prone to; c. Increased;
d. postictal; e. lower; f. seizures; g. Sponge
```

Case study 21

Your patient is 10 months old. He has tachypnoea and wheezing and a fever of 100.6°F (38.1°C).

- What do you suspect is wrong with your patient? – Bronchiolitis ◄

1_____ and tachypnoea in a child younger that age 1 is most often due to bronchiolitis brought on by the RSV virus. Asthma in children this young often presents as 2_____.

Epiglottitis will often have a fever 3_____ _____ 100.6°F (38.1°C), and the epiglottitis patient will be drooling as respiratory distress 4_____.

Croup will present with junky-sounding airways and the classic 5_____-_____ cough.

```
a. worsens; b. seal-barking; c. higher than;
d. Wheezing; e. Coughing
```

Vocabulary 5

absorb /əbˈzɔːb/
achieve /əˈtʃiːv/
advisable /ədˈvaɪ.zə.bl̩/
amniotic fluid /ˌæm.ni.ɒt.ɪkˈfluː.ɪd/
arouse /əˈraʊz/
aspirator /æs.pə.reɪ.tər/
bark /bɑːk/
buttock /ˈbʌt.ək/
chill /tʃɪl/
chin /tʃɪn/
composition /ˌkɒm.pə'zɪʃ.ən/
cooling /ˈkuː.lɪŋ/
cuff /kʌf/
curved /kɜːvd/
disassemble /ˌdɪs.əˈsem.bl̩/
equation /ɪˈkweɪ.ʒən/
expel /ɪkˈspel/

febrile /ˈfiː.braɪl/
feeding /ˌfiː.dɪŋ/
firmly /ˈfɜːm.li/
fit /fɪt/
foul /faʊl/
fundall /ˈfʌn.dəl/
fundus /ˈfʌn.dəs/ pl. **-di**
handle /ˈhæn.dl̩/
hyperflexion /ˌhaɪ.pəˈflæk.ʃən/
irritable /ˈɪr.ɪ.tə.bl̩/
isotonic /aɪ.səʊ ˈtɒn.ɪk/
jaw /dʒɔː/
junky- /ˈdʒʌŋ.ki/ **sounding** /ˈsaʊndɪŋ/
keep from /kiːp/ **(kept, kept)**
lack /læk/
lactate /lækˈteɪt/
lift /lɪft/
massage /ˈmæs.ɑːʒ/
mist /mɪst/ mlha, aerosol
MPH, Miles /maɪlz/ **Per** /
pə/ **Hour** /aʊə/
multiparity /mʌl.tiˈpær.ɪt.ɪ/
need /niːd/
neonate /ˌniː.əʊˈneɪ.t/
odour /ˈəʊ.dər/
opt /ɒpt/
oxygenation /ˈɒk.sɪ.dʒə.neɪ.ʃən/
point /pɔɪnt/ **to** /tʊ/
postictal /ˈpəʊstˈɪkt.əl/
preventable /prɪˈven.tə.bl̩/
prior /ˈpraɪə/ **to** /tʊ/
put /pʊt/ **pressure** /ˈpreʃ.ər/
range /reɪndʒ/
reassure /ˌriː.əˈʃɔːr/
retraction /rɪˈtræk.ʃən/
room /ruːm/
RSV, Human /hjuːmən/ **Respiratory**
/rɪˈspɪr.ə.tər.i/ **Syncytial** /
sɪnˈsɪ.ʃɪ.əl/ **Virus** /ˈvaɪrəs/
rub /rʌb/
runny /ˈrʌn.i/
seal /siːl/
seated /ˈsiː.tɪd/
shiver /ˈʃɪv.ər/
slap /slæp/

sniffing /snɪf.ɪŋ/
sole /səʊl/
solution /səˈluː.ʃən/
sponge /spʌndʒ/
stain /steɪn/
straight /streɪt/
swelling /ˈswelɪŋ/
tachydysrhythmia /ˌtæk.ɪ.dɪsˈriθ.mɪə/
threshold /ˈθreʃ.h əʊld/
thrust /θrʌst/
tilt /tɪlt/
toddler /ˈtɒd.lər/
turn /tɜːn/ **blue** /bluː/
underlying /ˌʌndəˈlaɪ.ɪŋ/
unfamiliar /ʌn.fəˈmɪl.i.ər/
urge /ɜːdʒ/
ventilation /ˌven.tɪˈleɪ.ʃən/

Part 6
Operations

Scene safety; legal considerations; vehicle operations; communications; documentation; infection controlling; quality improvement; DNR; basic patient assessment; basic physiology; hazardous materials; mass casualty incidents; scene management

Unit 1
Case study 1

You arrive on the scene of a two-car MVC. The driver of the first vehicle is 1_____.
Consent for this patient is said to be:

- informed
- implied ◄
- expressed
- involuntary

2_____ is assumed from any patient requiring emergency 3_____ who is physically, mentally, or emotionally unable to provide expressed consent.

a. Intervention; b. Consent; c. unconscious

Case study 2

A properly written 1_____ _____ _____ (PCR) is important because: the PCR may be the only 2_____ for pertinent information for receiving 3_____ _____ as well as other people interested in the event. ◄

a. healthcare professionals; b. patient care report; c. source

Case study 3

Which of the following patients would 1_____ most from the application of the PASG/MAST?

- a 10-year-old male, suspected spinal 2_____, no blood loss
- 72-year-old female, suspected 3_____ shock, no blood loss
- 40-year-old male, suspected lower extremity fracture, low blood pressure ◄
- 67-year-old female, suspected 4_____ sprain, high blood pressure

Indications for use of the PASG are to control bleeding, stabilize fractures, and 5_____ blood pressure.

a. raise; b. benefit; c. cardiogenic; d. fracture; e. ankle

Case study 4

The PCR is a legal document making it necessary to record accurate: incident times. ◄

All 1_____ _____ are to be recorded accurately for legal purposes including time of 2____, time of 3_____, time of arrival, time of medication 4_____, etc.

> a. administration; b. incident times; c. dispatch; d. call

Case study 5

Findings that require no 1_____ _____, but require documentation as evidence of a thorough history and exam are termed: pertinent negatives. ◄

2_____ _____ are findings that require no medical treatment but help to show the completeness of the paramedic's 3_____ ___ _____ on the PCR.

> a. Pertinent negatives; b. history and exam; c. medical intervention

Case study 6

The proper way to correct a written error on the PCR is to: draw a single line through the error, initial, and date the area. ◄

To 1_____ an error on a PCR, 2_ _____ _____ should be struck through the error, with the EMT-Paramedic's 3_____ next to the error and dated.

> a. a single line; b. initials; c. correct

Case study 7

An incomplete or 1_____ patient care report: may cause subsequent caregivers to provide inappropriate treatment based on the report. ◄

The 2_____ and completeness of the patient care report may have a significant 3_____ on ongoing care and treatment of the patient.

> a. accuracy; b. illegible; c. impact

Case study 8

Revisions to the original patient care report: are done on a separate 1_____ _____ and then attached to the original. ◄

Revisions are acceptable and must be done on a 2_____ report form and then 3_____ to the original document.

> a. attached, b. separate, c. report form

Case study 9

Appropriate 1_____ language on a PCR includes:

- medical terminology ◄
- slang
- personal opinion
- personally acceptable abbreviations

Medical 2_____ is an integral part of good 3_____ on a PCR.

> a. documentation; b. terminology; c. professional

Case study 10

A telephone is an example of:

- simplex
- a duplex ◀
- multiplex
- trunked

A duplex communication system allows the user to both 1_____ ____ _____ at the same time. A 2_____ _____ allows a person to listen or speak at one time. A multiplex system allows a person to listen and speak, as well as 3_____ ____. A trunked system pools all frequencies and routes transmissions to the next available frequency.

> a. listen and speak; b. transmit data;
> c. simplex system

Case study 11

For communication to be effective, the 1_____ must give appropriate:

- ideas
- encodings
- decodings
- feedback to the sender ◀

2_____ is a vital part of communication, allowing the sender to know that the receiver understands the 3_____.

> a. feedback; b. message; c. receiver

Case study 12

When communicating medical information, using 1_____ _____

can: shorten transmission and provide an 2_____ form of communication. ◀

Proper terminology helps to make communication clear, 3_____, and unambiguous.

> a. concise; b. unambiguous; c. proper terminology

Case study 13

Disadvantages of a simplex system may include that: the process is slower and more formal.◀

In a simplex system the user is able 1_____ to listen or speak. The major 2_____ include the fact that the process is slower, more formal, and 3___ _____ discussion.

> a. not facilitating; b. disadvantages; c. only

Case study 14

Disadvantages of using a cellular telephone for EMS communications include that: geography can 1_____ ___ the system or signs. ◀

An advantage of 2_____ _____ includes promoting a less formal, 3_____ discussion of EMS events. Disadvantages include 4_____ __ _____ signals due to geographical area or cell sites.

> a. shorter; b. lost or broken; c. cellular telephones; d. interfere with

Case study 15

Functions of an EMS dispatcher include all of the following:

- call taking ◄
- alerting and directing the EMS response ◄
- giving prearrival instructions to the caller ◄

EMS 1_____ serve by receiving the call, taking information regarding the 2_____ of the event, and providing prearrival 3_____ to assist prior to the EMS Unit's arrival.

a. nature; b. instructions; c. dispatchers

Case study 16

Communication from the EMS dispatcher that provides the caller with 1_____ _____, may be life sustaining to the patient during a critical event, provides immediate 2_____ to the caller as well as ongoing information to responding Units is:

- incident data collection
- predispatch education
- prearrival instructions ◄
- incident referral data

3_____ instructions provide immediate instructions and assistance to patients prior to arrival of EMS Units.

a. Prearrival; b. emotional support; c. assistance

Case study 17

Bacteria, viruses, and fungi are 1_____ of:

- pathogenic hosts

- nonspecific inflammatory 2_____
- disease processes
- infectious agents ◄

3_____ _____ have the potential of causing an infection.

a. infectious agents; b. examples; c. agents

Case study 18

The body's first line of 1_____ against infection is:

- the skin ◄
- the 2_____ system
- the gastrointestinal 3_____
- humoral response

The skin is the body's first line of defense against 4_____ _____.

a. infectious agents; b. system; c. defense; d. respiratory

Case study 19

You respond to the home of a patient with an unknown illness for two days. You approach the call suspecting an infectious or 1_____ disease. What action is not appropriate for the patient's care?

- gloves and protective eye goggles are worn ◄
- a full history and detailed physical exam is obtained ◄
- make the patient a "load and go" due to the potential for paramedic exposure

pertinent /'pɜːtɪnənt/
pool /puːl/
prearrival /ˌpriː.ə'raɪ.vəl/
promote /prə'məʊt/
protection /prə'tekʃən/
quantity /'kwɒn.tɪ.ti/
record /'rekɔːd/
referral /rɪ'fɜː.rəl/
report /rɪ'pɔːt/
revision /rɪ'vɪʒ.ən/
sender /'sen.dər/
separate /'sep.ər.ət/
shorten /'ʃɔː.tən/
simplex /'sɪm.pleks/
single /'sɪŋɡəl/
slang /slæŋ/
sprain /spreɪn/
subsequent /'sʌb.sɪ.kwənt/
take /teɪk/ care /keər/
task /tɑːsk/ úkol,
trunking /'trʌŋkɪŋ/
unambiguous /ˌʌnæm'bɪgjʊəs/

Unit 2
Case study 1
Which of the following
1_____ groups is NOT
transmitted via 2_____?

- Hepatitis A ◄
- Hepatitis B
- Hepatitis C
- Hepatitis D

Hepatitis A is transmitted
via the 3____/_____ route.

a. blood; b. oral/faecal; c. hepatitis

Case study 2
The next two questions are
based on the following scenario:

You are called to a local
1_____ _____ for a
gentleman with complaint of a cough
for two or three weeks, night sweats,
and weight loss. You suspect:

- hepatitis A
- HIV
- TB (tuberculosis) ◄
- meningitis

2_____ presents with
a chronic cough 3_____ for
two to three weeks, low-grade fever,
and night sweats. Certain populations
are at a higher risk of developing TB
including children less than 3 years
old and 4_____ patients.

You diagnose the above
illness and know the disease
is spread through:

- exposure to blood
- exposure through
  airborne droplets ◄
- exposure to body fluids
- direct physical contact

a. Tuberculosis; b. geriatric; c. homeless
shelter; d. persistent

Case study 3
You respond to a home of a
patient with complaint of sudden
onset of fever/chills, joint pain,
neck stiffness, and severe headache.
Upon examination the medics note
a petechial rash. You suspect:

- rabies
- influenza
- hepatitis A

- meningitis ◄

Meningitis signs and symptoms include a 1_____ _____, vomiting, fever, and 2_____ of sudden onset. The patient may have a petechial rash and usually has 3_____ _____.

> a. muscle rigidity; b. chills; c. severe headache

Case study 4
The causative organism of 1_____ ___ is the varicella zoster virus, which is a member of the:

- varicella virus group
- zoster virus group
- herpesvirus group ◄
- rubivirus group

The 2_____ group also contains a virus responsible for genital herpes and the common 3____ _____.

> a. chicken pox; b. cold sore; c. herpesvirus

Case study 5
Reportable infectious/ communicable disease exposures 1_____:

- contact of infectious materials with eye, mouth, or mucous membrane ◄
- working with a partner with a URI
- contact with blood and body fluids on intact gloves

- spill of infectious material in the EMS Unit with no contact

2_____ includes contact of infectious material with eyes, mouth, exposed mucous membrane, or 3_____ skin.

> a. include; b. nonintact; c. Exposure

Case study 6
Exercising the degree of care, skill, and judgement that would be expected under like or similar 1_____ by a similarly trained, reasonable paramedic in a similar 2_____or location is the 3_____ __:

- duty to act
- standard of care ◄
- malfeasance
- proximate cause

> a. community; b. definition of; c. circumstances

Case study 7
The four 1_____ of a negligence claim include:

- the duty 2__ ___ ◄
- breach of duty ◄
- proximate cause ◄
- 3_____ damages ◄

> a. elements; b. to act; c. actual

Case study 8
You arrive on the scene of a two-car MVC (motor vehicle collision). The driver of the first

vehicle is 1_____. Consent
for this patient is said to be:

- informed
- implied ◄
- expressed
- involuntary

Consent is assumed 2_____
from any patient requiring emergency
intervention who is physically,
mentally, or emotionally unable to
provide expressed 3_____.

a. implied; b. unconscious; c. consent

Case study 9

You and your partner are
treating a 16-year-old female with
lower abdominal pain. The patient's
husband arrives and informs you
his wife may be 1_____.

- You can treat this
  patient without parental
  consent based on: an
  emancipated minor is
  considered an adult. ◄

Care for this patient would
not require 2_____ _____
because the patient is married and
therefore an 3_____ minor.

a. pregnant; b. emancipated; c. parental
consent

Case study 10

You are called to the middle
of a bridge to transport a violent
patient who is suicidal. Per local
police, the patient threatened to
jump from the bridge and needs a

psychiatric evaluation. The patient
refuses transport threatening to
sue anyone who touches him.

- You transport this patient
  against his 1____ based on:
  involuntary consent. ◄

This patient can be treated
and transported against his
will under 2_____
_____. Law enforcement
personnel can direct transport and
treatment of a patient who is 3_
_____ to himself or others.

a. involuntary consent; b. a threat; c. will

Case study 11

You and your partner are
treating a patient who needs to be
transported to the hospital for chest
pain. You have established an IV,
placed the patient on the monitor,
administered oxygen and aspirin.
Your partner checks his watch and
notes that his 1_____ __ ____. You
remove the monitor and politely
tell the patient the oncoming crew
will come and 2_____ him
to the hospital shortly. Leaving
this patient is an example of:

- false imprisonment
- assault
- battery
- abandonment ◄

3_____ is the
termination of the paramedic-
patient relationship without ensuring
appropriate 4____ ___ the patient.

139

a. Abandonment; b. care for; c. shift is over; d. transport

Case study 12

Unlawful 1_____ of an individual without his or her consent could lead the paramedic open to 2_____ __: battery ◄

Battery is an unlawful touching of someone without his or her 3_____.

a. Consent; b. touching; c. allegations of

Case study 13

1_____ directives are documents that express the patient's wishes in the event that he or she is 2_____ or otherwise unable to 3_____ his or her choice for care.

* These include living wills, do not resuscitate orders, and: durable power of attorney for health care ◄

Durable power of attorney for 4_____ _____ or health care proxy once signed and witnessed are effective until the patient revolves them.

a. health care; b. express; c. unconscious; d. Advance

Case study 14

The paramedic's primary responsibility at a crime scene or 1_____ scene is:

* quality patient care
* 2_____ documentation

* thorough knowledge of the event
* to protect self and other EMS personnel ◄

The primary responsibility of the paramedic at all scenes is the 3_____ of himself or herself and other 4____ _____.

a. EMS personnel; b. protection; c. accident; d. quality

Case study 15

Laws that protect a paramedic if he or she acts 1__ _____ _____, is not negligent, acts within his or her scope of 2_____, and does not accept 3_____ for service constitutes the: Good Samaritan laws. ◄

a. payment; b. in good faith; c. practice

Case study 16

You and your partner are overheard in the elevator discussing a patient's injuries from a motor vehicle crash. Your conversation included pertinent personal and medical information about the patient.

* A call was placed to your 1_____ because: you failed to keep patient confidentiality.◄

Breach of 2_____ - any medical or personal information about a patient should not be discussed 3__ _____ or released without the patient's consent.

a. in public; b. confidentiality; c. supervisor

Case study 17

Commonly mandated injuries that are reportable to local authorities include all of the following:

- child abuse or neglect ◄
- animal bites ◄
- gunshot/stab wounds ◄

Injuries reportable to local authorities include spousal abuse, child 1_____ __ _____, elder abuse, sexual 2_____, gunshot/stab wounds, animal bites, and 3_____ diseases.

a. assault; b. communicable; c. abuse or neglect

Case study 18

Intentional false communication that injures another person's 1_____ or good name is a definition of:

- invasion of privacy
- breach of confidentiality
- informed slander
- defamation ◄

Defamation includes 2_____, which is verbal, and libel, which is 3_____.

a. slander; b. written; c. reputation

Case study 19

Personal protective equipment used to operate safely in the rescue environment includes all of the following:

- head 1_____ ◄
- eye protection ◄

- 2____ protection ◄
- personal flotation devices ◄
- 3_____ protection ◄
- high visibility clothing ◄
- specialized 4_____ ◄

a. protection; b. footwear; c. thermal, d. hand

Case study 20

It is generally considered 1_____ to walk in fast-moving water:

- ankle
- knee deep ◄
- waist
- chest

Walking in fast-moving water places the person at risk of having an 2_____ pinned and then being pulled under by 3___ _____.

a. extremity; b. the current; c. unsafe

Vocabulary 2

abuse /ə'bjuːz/
act /ækt/
airborne /'eə͵bɔːn/
allegation /͵æl.ə'geɪʃən/
assault /ə'sɒlt/
authority /ɔː'θɒr.ɪ.ti/
battery /'bæt.ər.i/
be /biː/ **over** /'əʊ.vər/
bite /baɪt/
breach /briːtʃ/
causative /'kɔː.zə.tɪv/
chickenpox /'tʃɪk.ɪn.pɒks/
claim /kleɪm/
cold /kəʊld/ **sore** /sɔːr/
confidentiality /͵kɒn.fɪ.den.tʃi'æl.ɪ.ti/
consent /kən'sent/
constitute /'kɒn.stɪ.tjuːt/

141

crew /kruː/
crime /kraɪm/
current /ˈkʌr.ənt/
damage /ˈdæm.ɪdʒ/
defamation /ˌdefəˈmeɪʃən/
directive /daɪˈrek.tɪv/
Do Not Resuscitate /
rɪˈsʌs.ɪ.teɪt/ order /ˈɔː.dər/
droplet /ˈdrɒp.lət/
durable /ˈdjʊərəbəl/
duty /ˈdjuː.tɪ/
elder /ˈeldə/
element /ˈelɪmənt/
emancipated /ɪˈmæn.sɪ.peɪ.tɪd/
enforcement /ɪnˈfɔː.smənt/
expressed /ɪkˈspresd/
faecal /ˈfiː.kəl/
faith /feɪθ/
false /fɒls/ imprisonment /
ɪmˈprɪz.ən.mənt/
fast-moving /fɑːstˈmuː.vɪŋ/
flotation /fləʊˈteɪ.ʃən/
equipment /ɪˈkwɪp.mənt/
footwear /ˈfʊt.weər/
genital /ˈdʒen.ɪ.təl/
grade /greɪd/
gunshot /ˈgʌn.ʃɒt/
hepatitis /ˌhep.əˈtaɪ.tɪs/
herpes-virus /ˈhɜː.piːzˈvaɪ.rəs/
homeless /ˈhəʊm.ləs/
implied /ɪmˈplaɪd/
influenza /ˌɪn.fluˈen.zə/
informed /ɪnˈfɔːmd/
intentional /ɪnˈtenʃənəl/
invasion /ɪnˈveɪ.ʒən/
involuntary /ɪnˈvɒləntərɪ/
judgment /ˈdʒʌdʒ.mənt/
law /lɔː/
libel /ˈlaɪ.bəl/
living /ˈlɪvɪŋ/ will /wɪl/
malfeasance /mælˈfiː.zəns/
mandate /ˈmæn.deɪt/
minor /ˈmaɪ.nə/
mucous membrane /
ˌmjuː.kəsˈmem.breɪn/

neglect /nɪˈglekt/
negligence /ˈneglɪdʒəns/
negligent /ˈneg.lɪ.dʒənt/
nonintact /ˌnɒn.ɪnˈtækt/
oncoming /ˈɒnˌkʌmɪŋ/
overhear /ˌəʊvəˈhɪə/
parental /pəˈren.təl/
personnel /ˌpɜːsəˈnel/
petechial /piˈtiː.ki.əl/
pin /pɪn/
polite /pəˈlaɪt/
power /paʊər/ of attorney /əˈtɜː.ni/
privacy /ˈpraɪvəsɪ/
proximate /ˈprɒk.sɪ.mət/
proxy /ˈprɒk.sɪ/
rabies /ˈreɪ.biːz/
reportable /rɪˈpɔːtˈebəl/
responsibility /rɪˌspɒn.səˈbɪ.lɪ.tɪ/
resuscitate /rɪˈsʌs.ɪ.teɪt/
revolve /rɪˈvɒlv/
rigidity /rɪˈdʒɪd.ɪ.ti/
rubivirus /ruːbɪˈvaɪ.rəs/
scope /skəʊp/
shelter /ˈʃel.tər/
shift /ʃɪft/
sign /saɪn/
skill /skɪl/
slander /ˈslɑːndə/
spousal /ˈspaʊzəl/
standard /ˈstæn.dəd/
stiffness /ˈstɪf.nəs/
sue /sjuː/
supervisor /ˈsuː.pə.vaɪ.zər/
sweat /swet/
termination /ˌtɜː.mɪˈneɪ.ʃən/
thorough /ˈθʌr.ə/
threat /θret/
threaten /ˈθret.ən/
touch /tʌtʃ/
transmit /trænzˈmɪt/
treat /triːt/
unlawful /ʌnˈlɔː.fʊl/
unsafe /ʌnˈseɪf/
varicella /ˌvær.ɪˈsel.ə/
visibility /ˌvɪz.ɪˈbɪl.ɪ.ti/

waist /weɪst/
will /wɪl/
wish /wɪʃ/
witness /ˈwɪt.nəs/
zoster /zɒ.stər/

Unit 3

Case study 1

Low-head dams are considered "drowning machines" due to: recirculating currents created by water moving over a uniform obstruction. ◄

Low-head dams create a recirculating current, which can repeatedly 1_____ the victim under the water, making 2_____ difficult. These dams also make 3_____ _____ hazardous.

a. rescue operations; b. escape; c. pull

Case study 2

The body responds to cold water by rapidly losing heat. Protective measures exist within the body, which stimulates a parasympathetic response, decreasing heart rate, causing peripheral vasoconstriction, and shunting blood to the core.

- This cold protective response is known as the: mammalian dive reflex. ◄

The 1_____ ____ _____ is a protective physiologic response, which increases 2_____ by shunting blood to the core, 3_____ heart rate, and dropping 4_____ _____.

These factors are affected by the person's age and 5_____ _____ and the water temperature.

a. decreasing; b. survivability; c. health status; d. mammalian dive reflex; e. blood pressure

Case study 3

The following are considered oxygen-deficient environments or 1_____ spaces:

- storage tanks ◄
- grain bins or 2_____ ◄
- 3_____ vaults ◄
- wells ◄
- manholes ◄

a. confined; b. underground; c. silos

Case study 4

You are the first Unit on the scene of a multiple-vehicle crash. Upon arrival, each of the following actions would be appropriate:

- to establish scene command ◄
- the scene sizeup ◄
- control scene hazards ◄

The first Unit to arrive on the scene should begin the scene sizeup, which includes 1_____ _____, calling for back-up Units, controlling any 2_____, and locating any 3_____ _____. It would be not appropriate for the primary Unit to locate and transport the 4_____ _____ injured patient.

a. hazards; b. most critically; c. establishing command; d. triage patients

Case study 5

Which of the following definitions best describes a disaster?

- motor vehicle collision with two to three patients
- an everyday incident that generates three or more patients
- a bus or train collision with 25-30 injured
- an incident that overwhelms resources and may damage the infrastructure of a region ◄

1_ _____ is an incident that may generate hundreds of patients, 2___ _____ the existing resources, and may damage the 3_____ of the region shutting down railroads, hospitals, and other normal operations.

a. may overwhelm; b. A disaster; c. infrastructure

Case study 6

You are assigned the duties of safety officer under the incident command of a local mass casualty 1_____. You understand the 2_____ of this position to:

- monitor all on-scene actions to ensure no potentially harmful situations are created

- coordinate all operations of this incident that involve outside agencies
- collect data regarding the incident and relay information to the press or media
- act as an officer who supervises a specific safety Unit or area ◄

The safety officer monitors all on-scene actions to ensure that no potentially 3_____ _____ are created.

a. harmful situations; b. responsibilities; c. incident

Case study 7

The "S" in the acronym START is for:

- suitable
- simple ◄
- salvageable
- sorting

1_____ stands for simple triage and rapid transport. This system focuses on four easily identifiable 2_____: (1) ability to walk, (2) respiratory 3_____, (3) pulses/perfusion, (4) 4_____ status.

a. findings; b. START; c. effort; d. neurological

Case study 8

You are the 1_____ _____ at a car versus bus collision. Your first victim is approximately 30 years old, awake, alert and oriented.

He is the driver of the car that collided with the bus head on. He complains of lower abdominal pain and has obvious 2_____ to both femurs. Respirations 24, pulse 140, BP 80/ palpated, capillary refill > 2 sec. How would you triage the following patient?

- green
- yellow
- red ◄
- black

This patient should be tagged Red with immediate life threats including the possibility of bilateral 3_____ _____ and intraabdominal bleeding.

a. femur fractures; b. triage officer; c. deformity

Case study 9

You are treating a patient with diabetic ketoacidosis. The patient is tachycardic and has deep, rapid respirations.

- The most likely cause for the 1_____, 2_____ respirations is that: the body is compensating for a low pH by increasing respirations. ◄

The 3_____ recognizes a decrease in pH or excess of H+ ions and attempts to compensate by 4_____ the respiratory effort.

a. brain; b. increasing; c. deep; d. rapid

Case study 10

You are treating a patient with hyperventilation syndrome due to an anxiety attack.

- What acid-base derangement will hyperventilation produce? – Respiratory alkalosis. ◄

1_____ _____ results from an 2_____ in respirations and an excessive 3_____ of CO_2.

a. Respiratory alkalosis; b. elimination; c. increase

Case study 11

Hyperventilation resulting from pure anxiety leads to:

- 1_____ acidosis
- respiratory alkalosis ◄
- a decreasing blood pH
- hepatic failure

2_____ can result in an excess elimination of 3_____ _____ leading to respiratory alkalosis.

a. Hyperventilation; b. respiratory; c. carbon dioxide

Case study 12

Parenteral routes of drug administration include all of the following:

- intravenous ◄
- intramuscular ◄
- topical ◄

1_____ _____ for delivery of medication include all those areas 2_____ the gastrointestinal tract. Parenteral routes include 3_____, 4_____, intramuscular, subcutaneous, topical, and 5_____. The sublingual route administers the drug through the enteral route, or through the gastrointestinal tract.

a. intravenous; b. inhalations; c. Parenteral routes; d. outside; e. endotracheal

Case study 13

The six rights of medication administration include:

- right 1_____ ◄
- right dose ◄
- right time ◄
- right 2_____ ◄
- right patient ◄
- right 3_____ ◄

a. medication; b. route; c. documentation

Case study 14

A 53-year-old female who is being treated for chronic pain with morphine sulphate continues to complain of pain despite taking her medications 1__ _____. The patient is most likely experiencing what 2_____ to this medication?

- 3_____ reaction
- tolerance ◄
- dependence
- antagonism

Tolerance is a decreased response to the 4____ _____ of a drug after taking the drug over a period of time.

a. as prescribed; b. response; c. same amount; d. allergic

Case study 15

At the scene of a MVC your ambulance should 1__ _____ at least 100 feet (30.5 metres) from the accident, uphill and upwind to ensure:

- 2___ _____ of the vehicle
- the safety of your crew ◄
- that the crime scene is not violated
- clear distance for secondary Units to arrive

The number one 3_____ of every EMS call is assurance of your personal safety.

a. priority; b. the safety; c. be parked

Case study 16

The following statements regarding scene safety with regard to helicopter and air medical transport are all true:

- Generally a helicopter requires a 1_____ ____ of approximately 100 feet (30.5 metres) by 100 feet (30.5 metres). ◄
- Ensure that the landing zone is 2_____ __ wires, loose debris, towers or vehicles. ◄
- Mark the landing zone with a single flare and do

not shine lights directly into the pilot's eyes. ◄

The helicopter should 3_____ be approached in a crouched position away from the tail rotor. Approach a helicopter that is on a slight incline from the 4_____ side.

a. downhill; b. landing zone; c. cautiously; d. clear of

Case study 17

Promptly recognizing the need for 1_____ management, assessing the scene for 2_____, contacting Dispatch to mobilize other Units for care and 3_____ of the patient, establishing rapport with the patient and other paramedics on the scene represent the paramedic's:

• ethical responsibility
• roles ◄
• triage criteria
• care responsibility

Recognizing an emergency exists, assessing the situation, managing the emergency care, 4_____ efforts of your team as well as other agencies involved in the care and transportation of the patient, and establishing 5_____ with the patient and other EMS crew are all examples of a paramedic's roles.

a. transportation; b. coordinating; c. rapport; d. danger; e. emergency

Case study 18

In the 1_____ C-FLOP, when describing the practices of the Incident Management System the "O" 2_____ ___:

• operations ◄
• ongoing assessments
• order of command
• officer in charge

The mnemonic C-FLOP stands for: C – command, F – 3_____/ administration, L – logistics, O – operations, P – planning.

a. stands for; b. finance; c. mnemonic

Case study 19

The next questions are based on the following scenario:
You are assigned to triage patients at the scene of an explosion in a park. You are using the METTAG system of triage.

The first victim you come in contact with has no palpable pulse and no respiratory effort. The patient has a major laceration on the scalp with an open skull fracture.

• You would tag this person as: Black. ◄

The designation of this patient would be 1_____ due to the 2_____ of signs of life and injuries that were possibly 3_____ with life. The morgue area should be a triage area away from other treatment areas.

The next patient with whom you come into contact is a 34-year-old female who is wandering around the incident looking for her three-year-old daughter. The patient has multiple abrasions to her face and arms.

- You would most likely triage this patient: Green. ◄

This patient can be triaged to the 4_____ treatment area. The green treatment area is the area where patients require 5_____ __ __ care in preparation for transport.

The third patient you find is awake, alert, and oriented. The patient has tachypnoea with shallow respirations. Your assessment reveals a sucking chest wound on the right side of the chest, a fracture of the right femur, and a large laceration on the forehead.

- You will most likely 6_____ this patient: Red.◄

This patient has 7_____ injuries that require immediate attention. The 8___ treatment area has the equipment and skilled providers to best care for, stabilize, and transport this patient.

a. incompatible; b. absence; c. little or no; d. green; e. Critical; f. triage; g. red; h. black

Case study 20

You and your partner are the first EMS Unit to arrive on the scene of a single-car MVC, car versus pole. Electrical lines are down across the car. One victim is trapped inside the vehicle.

- What action would be most correct? – Contact Dispatch and have the 1_____ _____ turn the power off to the lines prior to attempting rescue of this patient. *

The rescuer's 2___ _____ is the safety of himself or herself and other rescuers. Attempting any rescue prior to cutting power to the downed lines would 3_____ the safety of rescuers and the patient.

a. power company; b. jeopardize; c. top priority

Vocabulary 3

antagonism /ænˈtæg.ə.nɪ.zəm/
assign /əˈsaɪn/
assurance /əˈʃɔː.rəns/
back-up /ˈbæk.ʌp/
be /biː/ **in charge** /tʃɑːdʒ/ **of**
bin /bɪn/
carbon /ˈkɑː.bən/ **dioxide** / daɪˈɒk.saɪd/
cautiously /ˈkɔː.ʃəs.li/
command /kəˈmɑːnd/
company /ˈkʌm.pə.ni/
confined /kənˈfaɪnd/
core /kɔːr/
crouch /kraʊtʃ/
dam /dæm/
dependence /dɪˈpen.dənt s/
derangement /dɪˈreɪndʒd.mənt/
diabetic /ˌdaɪəˈbet.ɪk/
disaster /dɪˈzɑː.stər/
distance /ˈdɪs.tənt s/
dive /daɪv/

down /daʊn/
downhill /ˌdaʊnˈhɪl/
drop /drɒp/
electrical /ɪˈlek.trɪ.kəl/ line /laɪn/
elimination /ɪˌlɪm.ɪˈneɪ.ʃən/
escape /ɪˈskeɪp/
flare /fleər/
forehead /ˈfɒrɪd/, /ˈfɔːˌhed/
generate /ˈdʒen.ər.eɪt/
grain /greɪn/
harmful /ˈhɑːm.fəl/
hazard /ˈhæz.əd/
head-on /ˌhed.ˈɒn/
health /helθ/ status /ˈsteɪ.təs/
identifiable /aɪˈden.tɪ.faɪ.ə.bl̩/
incline /ɪnˈklaɪn/
incompatible /ˌɪn.kəmˈpæt.ɪ.bl̩/
infrastructure /ˈɪn.frəˌstrʌk.tʃər/
intramuscular /ˌɪn.trəˈmʌs.kjʊ.lər/
intravenous /ˌɪn.trəˈviː.nəs/
jeopardize /ˈdʒep.ə.daɪz/
landing /ˈlændɪŋ/ zone /zəʊn/
locate /ləʊˈkeɪt/
loose /luːs/
mammalian /məˈmeɪ.li.ən/
manhole/ ˈmænˌhəʊl/
morgue /mɔːg/
operation /ˌɒp.ərˈeɪ.ʃən/
order /ˈɔːdə/
overwhelm /ˌəʊ.vəˈwelm/
parenteral /pəˈren.tə.rəl/
peripheral /pəˈrɪf.ər.əl/
power /paʊər/
prescribe /prɪˈskraɪb/
press /pres/
promptly /ˈprɒmptlɪ/
railroad /ˈreɪl.rəʊd/
rapport /ræˈpɔːr/
recirculate /riːˈsɜː.kjʊ.leɪt/
relay /ˈriːleɪ/
repeatedly /rɪˈpiː.tɪd.li/
rotor /ˈrəʊtə/
safety /ˈseɪftɪ/
salvageable /ˈsæl.vɪdʒə.bl̩/
scalp /skælp/

shine /ʃaɪn/
silo /ˈsaɪ.ləʊ/
simple /ˈsɪm.pl̩/
sorting /sɔː.tɪŋ/
stand /stænd/ for /fə/
storage /ˈstɔː.rɪdʒ/
sublingual /sʌbˈlɪŋ.gwəl/
suitable /ˈsjuː.tə.bl̩/
supervise /ˈsuː.pəˌvaɪz/
survivability /səˈvaɪv.ə.bɪl.ə.ti/
tail /teɪl/
tank /tæŋk/
tolerance /ˈtɒl.ər.əns/
topical /ˈtɒp.ɪ.kəl/
underground /ˌʌn.dəˈgraʊnd/
uphill /ˌʌpˈhɪl/
upwind /ˌʌpˈwɪnd/
vault /vɔːlt/
violate /ˈvaɪəˌleɪt/
wander /ˈwɒn.dər/
well /wel/
wire /waɪər/

Unit 4

Case study 1

You are the paramedic in charge of a single patient entrapped in a vehicle that was involved in a head-on crash. The extrication of this patient will require a lengthy period of time.

- Your 1_____ during the time of disentanglement will be that: management of this patient will remain the same as for other emergency patients. Initiation of assessment and care should be started as soon as possible. ◄

Keep in mind that rapid 2_____ ___ _____ may not be possible. Management of this patient should remain the same as similar emergency patients. You must 3_____ assessment and care as soon as possible.

a. initiate, b. extrication and transport, c. responsibility

Case study 2

You are transporting a patient who has been exposed to a hazardous material. You have come into contact with this patient with level D hazmat protection equipment on.

- You have most likely experienced: a secondary exposure. ◄

For a secondary contamination level D 1_____ protection equipment is the lowest level of protection. Level D equipment consists of structural fire-fighting, or turn-out gear. 2_____ _____ occurs when an uncontaminated person comes 3____ _____ with a contaminated person.

a. into contact; b. Secondary contamination; c. hazmat

Case study 3

The paramedic faces many stress-inducing situations. All of the following are phases of the stress response:

- alarm reaction ◄

- resistance ◄
- exhaustion ◄

The three phases of the body's 1_____ to stress are alarm reactions (of the 2_____ ___ _____ response), resistance, and as the body sustains increasing stress, the level of resistance to stress rises, and higher levels of stress must occur for the 3_____ _____ to occur. 4_____ follows as stress continues and coping mechanisms begin to fail.

a. fight or flight; b. alarm reaction; c. response; d. Exhaustion

Case study 4

While eating lunch at a local eatery, you and your partner are 1_____ a call you had just completed. The patient's relative who is sitting at the next table 2_____ your partner talking about the patient's condition. Your partner has violated the patient's

- right to consent
- right to confidentiality ◄
- 3_____ of refusal of treatment
- character by defamation

Information related to the patient's condition or treatment is considered 4_____ information.

a. confidential; b. overhears; c. discussing; d. right

Case study 5

While assessing a patient complaining of abdominal pain, you should first:

- palpate/auscultate
- inspect/percuss
- inspect then auscultate the abdomen.◀
- palpate/percuss

Inspection is the visual assessment of the patient. Inspection can reveal many important aspects of the patient. 1_____ of abdominal sounds should 2_____ palpation and 3_____.

a. auscultation; b. precede; c. percussion

Case study 6

A 50-year-old male is experiencing an acute 1_____ of asthma. Your partner establishes an IV and you prepare to administer albuterol via a hand-held 2_____. Your actions are in direct accordance with your local protocol.

- This type of standing order is considered: off-line medical direction.◀

3__-____ medical direction includes the authority of a medical director or advisory group to establish treatment protocols or standing orders.

a. nebulizer; b. exacerbation; c. Off-line

Case study 7

You and your partner respond to the home of an elderly gentleman who is unresponsive. Your assessment reveals no respiratory effort, skin that is cool and mottled with obvious pooling, and no palpable pulse. The patient's wife presents a valid Do Not Resuscitate order. All of the actions below would be correct:

- address the wife using gentle eye contact and choosing appropriate words ◀
- explain to the wife that her loved one has died, do not use terms that can be misinterpreted ◀
- offer assistance to the survivor(s) if necessary ◀

This patient has a valid 1___ (Do Not Resuscitate) order and no obvious 2_____ __ ____. The correct actions would be to address the survivor in terms that leave no doubt about the outcome of the 3_____. Use gentle reassuring eye contact and offer any 4_____ that may be needed to the survivor.

a. assistance; b. DNR; c. signs of life; d. deceased

Case study 8

You are one of the many EMS workers who just completed working the scene of a 1_____ plane crash that left several hundred people 2_____ __ _____. You and your crew are called in for CISD (Critical Incident Stress Debriefing). You understand this to be:

- a technique for reducing stress on scene that includes fluid replacement, food services, and change of assignments
- a formal, structured, planned intervention done by a trained team within 24-72 hours of a posttraumatic event. 3____ ____ includes mental health workers and peers.◄
- a spontaneous post-call discussion of the events
- a short informal meeting that gives the crew a chance to vent and verbalize their feelings about this 4_____

a. incident; b. devastating; c. dead or injured; d. The team

Case study 9

Your crew is dispatched to the home of an obese woman who has fallen. The general rules for lifting and moving this patient include all of the following:

- Position the load as close to your body as possible. ◄
- Bend your knees, let the 1____ _____ of the legs do the work of lifting. ◄
- Take your time, do not hurry, and maintain a wide base of support. ◄

Proper 2_____ _____ should be utilized during all patient encounters. Ask for assistance if needed. Do not 3_____ the rescuer's or the patient's safety.

a. jeopardize; b. lifting techniques; c. large muscles

Case study 10

Documentation of a patient's 1_____ for care or transport should include all of the following:

- the paramedic's advice to the patient ◄
- online medical control's 2_____ ◄
- a complete narrative of the 3_____ ◄

a. advice; b. event; c. refusal

Case study 11

Legislation that governs the 1_____ of medicine and may prescribe a physician's ability to delegate authority to perform medical acts by the paramedic is:

- licensure
- 2_____ direction
- 3_____ of care
- medical practice act ◄

a. standard; b. medical; c. practice

Case study 12

You 1___ _____ the patient involved in a two-car MVC with severe blunt trauma to the abdomen. You suspect internal haemorrhage. The patient's BP is 100/52 with a pulse rate of 130. You know the 2_____ in the heart rate is the body's attempt to maintain:

- metabolism
- system integration
- homeostasis ◄
- end-organ damage

3_____ is the natural tendency of the body to maintain a steady state of 4_____within the body's internal envvironment.

a. Homeostasis; b. equilibrium; c. elevation; d. are assesing

Case study 13

The 1_____ of water across a cell membrane is known as:

- oncotic pressure
- osmosis ◄
- diffusion
- osmolarity

2_____ is the movement of any solvent (usually water) across a 3_____ _____.

a. Osmosis; b. cell membrane; c. movement

Case study 14

The set of 1_____ ____ _____ that a paramedic is permitted to perform during a medical situation is called:

- primary practice
- consent to 2_____
- scope of practice ◄
- regional practice

3_____ of practice is generally defined by state statute and defines what an EMS provider can 4_____.

a. Scope; b. duties and skills; c. perform; d. practice

Case study 15

When is use of "reasonable" force or use of restraints permissible for a patient?

- The patient is alert, cooperative, but 1_____.
- The patient has altered level of consciousness, caused by injury, substance abuse, or illness. ◄
- It is never appropriate to use any 2_____ on a patient.
- This is at the 3_____ of the paramedic or the crew's officer.

If the patient is altered and is placing himself or others in harm's way, the EMS provider should use any method within reason to 4_____ the patient's actions.

a. control; b. force; c. anxious; d. force

Case study 16

Drawing a patient's blood without her 1_____ may be an example of:

- battery ◄
- slander
- false imprisonment
- assault

In most situations, unpermitted 2_____ _____ is a form of battery. 3_____ is the threat of bodily harm.

a. physical contact; b. Assault; c. permission

Case study 17

In which of the following situations is an EMS provider required to make a report to law enforcement?

- suspected sexual assault ◄
- alcohol-related 1_____
- motor vehicle collision with 2_____
- illegal 3____ possession

Most states require the reporting of 4_____ or neglect of children, spouses, or older adults; 5____ and sexual assault; 6_____ and stab wounds; animal bites; and certain 7_____ diseases.

a. gunshot; b. communicable; c. trauma;
d. rape; e. abuse; f. entrapment; g. drug

Case study 18

A patient is in respiratory distress. She has a 1_____ DNR order.

- Which of the following treatments is correct? - 2_____ oxygen and a nebulized albuterol treatment. ◄

"Do Not Resuscitate" is not the same as "3__ ___ _____." Under these conditions, management of the condition is warranted.

a. valid; b. Provide; c. do not treat

Case study 19

The two primary goals of prehospital care of a sexual assault victim are to preserve the victim's privacy and dignity and to: preserve all physical evidence for the police ◄

In order to preserve 1_____ _____ of the assault, avoid cleaning wounds and do not allow the victim to bathe or 2_____ her clothing. If clothing is removed during 3_____ ____, it should be placed in a brown paper bag and 4_____ ____ to police officers. Maintain chain of custody carefully to 5_____ the evidence.

a. change; b. patient care; c. handed over;
d. physical evidence; e. preserve

Case study 20

You are dispatched to the home of a 1_____ patient who has signed a Do not Resuscitate order. What should you do?

- Contact medical control before providing any patient care. ◄

Contact 2_____ _____ about the specific situation before providing care; this will allow you to provide the type of care that is 3_____ only. Some states have specific 4_____ to follow with DNR patients and may even provide various levels of care in a variety of circumstances.

a. palliative; b. medical control; c. protocols;
d. dying

Case study 21

The term ethics refers to:

- professional
  1_____ of care
- rules, standards,
  and morals ◄
- upgrading standards
  2__ ____
- moral code of 3_____

4_____ refers to rules,
standards, and morals that govern
actions in a 5_____.

---

a. Ethics; b. profession; c. standards; d. of
care, e. conduct

Vocabulary 4

accordance /ə'kɔː.dənt s/
address /ə'dres/
advice /əd'vaɪs/
advisory /əd'vaɪ.zər.i/
alarm /ə'lɑːm/
appropriate /ə'prəʊ.pri.ət/
authority /ɔː'θɒr.ɪ.ti/
confidential /ˌkɒn.fɪ'den.t ʃəl/
confidentiality /ˌkɒn.fɪ.den.t ʃi'æl.ɪ.ti/
cope /kəʊp/ with /wɪð/
custody /'kʌs.tə.di/
debrief /ˌdiː'briːf/
debriefing /ˌdiː'briː.f.ɪŋ/
deceased /dɪ'siːst/
defamation /ˌdefə'meɪʃən/
delegate /'del.ɪ.gət/
devastating /'dev.ə.steɪ.tɪŋ/
dignity /'dɪg.nɪ.ti/
direction /da ɪ'rek.ʃən/
disentanglement /ˌdɪs.ɪn'tæŋ.gl̩.mənt/
drawing /'drɔː.ɪŋ/
eatery /'iː.təri/
encounter /ɪn'kaʊntə/
entrap /ɪn'træp/

entrapment /ɪn'træp.mənt/
equilibrium /ˌiːkwɪ'lɪbriəm/
ethics /'eθɪk/
evidence /'evɪdəns/
exacerbation /ɪgˌzæsə'beɪʃən/
exhaustion /ɪg'zɔːs.tʃən/
fight or flight /ˌfaɪt.ɔː.'flaɪt/
fire-fighting /'faɪəˌfaɪ.tɪŋ/
gear /gɪə/
govern /'gʌv.ən/
gunshot /'gʌn.ʃɒt/
hand /hænd/ over /'əʊ.vər/
hazmat /'hæz.mæt/
homeostasis /ˌhəʊ.mi.əʊ'steɪ.sɪs/
integration /ˌɪn.tɪ'greɪ.ʃən/
law /lɔː/ -enforcement /ɪn'fɔːs.
mənt/ agency /'eɪ.dʒən.si/
lengthy /'leŋ.θi/
licensure /'laɪ.sən.ʃər/
lifting /'lɪft.ɪŋ/
load /ləʊd/
misinterpret /ˌmɪs.ɪn'tɜː.prɪt/
moral /'mɒrəl/
narrative /'nærətɪv/
oncotic /ɒŋ.kɒ.tɪk/ pressure /'preʃ.ər/
online /'ɒn.laɪn/
osmolarity /ɒz.mə'lær.ə.ti/
osmosis /ɒz'məʊ.sɪs/
outcome /'aʊt.kʌm/
palliative /'pæl.i.ə.tɪv/
peers /pɪərz/
permissible /pə'mɪs.ə.bl̩/
permit /pə'mɪt/
pooling /puː.l.ɪŋ/
possession /pə'zeʃ.ən/
posttraumatic /ˌpəʊst.trɔːˌmæt.ɪk/
precede /prɪ'siːd/
preserve /prɪ'zɜːv/
rape /reɪp/
reasonable /'riː.zən.ə.bl̩/
refusal /rɪ'fjuː.zəl/
regional /'riː.dʒən.əl/
right /raɪt/
scope /skəʊp/
solvent /'sɒl.vənt/

spouse /spaʊs/
standing /stænd.ɪŋ/ **order** /ˈɔːdə/
statute /ˈstætjuːt/
steady /ˈsted.i/
survivor /səˈvaɪ.vər/
take /teɪk/ **time** /taɪm/
turn out /ˈtɜːnˌaʊt/
upgrade /ʌpˈgreɪd/
valid /ˈvælɪd/
vent /vent/

VOLUME 2

Unit 1
Case study 1

You are called for a 55-year-old man who "suddenly collapsed." He is 1_____ ___ _____.

- Initial management of this patient's airway should include. – Insertion of an oropharyngeal airway and ventilation with bag-valve mask.◄

An apnoeic and pulse less patient is unlikely to have an intact gag reflex, 2_____ an OPA to help control the 3_____ _____. A BVM will need at least 10 Lpm of oxygen flow in order to adequately 4_____the patient during ventilations.

a. oxygenate; b. apnoeic and pulse less; c. upper airway; d. necessitating

Case study 2

You respond to a college fraternity where you encounter a 19-year-old male with a partially obstructed airway. According to witnesses, he was eating pizza and drinking beer when he began to 1_____ ___ _____ his throat. The patient is able to speak in a 2_____ _____ only, and he has been coughing repeatedly for about 20 minutes.

- What is the best treatment for this patient? – Remove the 3_____ with forceps.◄

A conscious patient with a partial obstructed airway should be dealt with by 4_____ _____ and continuous monitoring of patient status. Interventions like Heimlich manoeuvre are considered counterproductive, as they may actually 5_____ the obstruction.

To perform a needle cricothyrotomy, you should place the patient: supine with head and neck hyperextended.◄

A 6_____ _____ will place the anatomical structure.

a. hoarse whisper; b. hyperextended position; c. worsen; d. obstruction; e. cough and grab; f. encouraging coughing

Case study 3

Your patient is a 26-year-old male with a midshaft 1_____ _____ and no other apparent injuries. The patient is 2_____ and oriented, and all vital signs are normal. The best way to 3_____ this fracture is to use:

- the PASG/MAST

- a long spine board
- a traction splint. ◄
- a softly padded board

In a stable patient, the PASG is unnecessary. The long board will not adequately immobilize this injury because the muscles of the leg will 4_____ and 5_____ the leg. A padded board may not provide adequate traction to prevent muscle spasms either, so the 6_____ _____ is the best choice.

a. shorten; b. immobilize; c. femur fracture; d. spasm; e. alert; f. transion splint

Case study 4

A 16-year-old male complains of a fever, sore neck, nausea, vomiting, and headache. During transport, he begins to have a 1_____. Which of the following would be your most likely field impression?

- 2_____ abscess
- cerebral 3_____
- meningitis ◄
- sepsis

While the other answers are possible, based upon the fever, vomiting, and headache complaints, this is most likely 4_____.

a. seizure; b. neoplasm; c. meningitis; d. brain

Case study 5

Your patient is a 24-year-old female who shows signs and symptoms of pelvic 1_____ _____.

- What is the goal of 2_____ _____ for this patient? – Make the patient as comfortable as possible and transport to the hospital. ◄

The goal of prehospital care for patients with PID is to 3_____ _____. There is no need to perform a 4_____ ____ or ask any questions regarding sexual contacts.

a. provide comfort; b. inflammatory disease; c. vaginal exam; d. prehospital care

Case study 6

You respond to a 22-year-old male who is complaining of 1_____ _____ of chest pain. The patient states that the pain 2__ _____ and sharp and that it started when he surfaced from a 3_____ ____ from 60 feet (18.2 metres) down. The patient's diving partner states that the patient 4_____ too rapidly.

- What is this patient most likely suffering from? – Pulmonary embolism. ◄

A too rapid ascent from a scuba dive may result in a pulmonary embolism due to lung 5_____.

- What does treatment for this patient consist of? – IV, high-flow oxygen, and rapid transport to a recompression chamber. ◄

An IV, 100% oxygen via a nonrebreather mask, and transport to a 6_____ _____ are essential for this patient.

- Due to his rapid ascent, this patient may also be suffering from another diving related emergency: decompression sickness.◄

Due to the 7_____ of the dive and the rapid ascent, this patient may also be suffering from 8_____ _____.

- What is an additional possible problem associated with this injury? – Nitrogen bubbles entering tissue spaces and smaller blood vessels. ◄

a. scuba dive; b. rapid onset; c. is tearing; d. decompression sickness; e. cyanotic; f. depth; g. surfaced; h. overinflation; i. recompression chamber

Case study 7

Your patient is a 28-year-old diver who has been using scuba equipment. His diving partner states that he was unconscious when he surfaced after 1_ ____.

- You should suspect: air embolism. ◄

2___ _____ presents as 3_____ _____ (including unconsciousness) during or after 4_____ from a dive, or as a sharp pain in the chest.

- Due to his rapid ascent, this patient may also be 5_____ ____ another diving related emergency: decompression sickness. ◄

Due to the depth of the dive and the rapid ascent, this patient may also be suffering from decompression sickness.

- What is an additional possible problem associated with this injury? – Nitrogen bubbles entering 6_____ _____ and smaller blood vessels.◄

In this patient, nitrogen 7___ _____ may have entered tissue spaces and blood vessels.

a. a dive; b. tissue spaces; c. Air embolism; d. ascent; e. suffering from; f. gas bubbles; g. neurological deficit

Case study 8

- This statement about care of a near-drowning 1_____ is correct: The patient should be admitted to the hospital for observation.◄

Due to the chance of post event pulmonary oedema, all 2___-_____ victims should be admitted to the hospital for 3_____.

a. victim; b. near-drowning; c. observation

Case study 9

Your patient is a 23-year-old man who complains of abdominal pain. The patient states that the pain began 1_____ and was originally located only in the area around the 2_____. Now, however, it has moved to the 3_____ _____ quadrant. The patient also complains of nausea and vomiting, and he has a fever of 102 °F (38.8 °C). Examination displays rebound 4_____.

- What would you suspect? – Apendicitis. ◄

a. tenderness; b. right lower; c. suddenly; d. umbilicus

Case study 10

A patient suspected of having an 1_____ aortic aneurysm will receive oxygen, an IV, ECG monitoring, and rapid transport as part of his or her treatment.

- What else should you do when treating such a patient? 2_____ the PASG/ MAST garment. ◄

Treat the patient for shock and transport rapidly. Do not 3_____ the abdomen. This is one of the few medical conditions that may still benefit from the use of PASG/MAST as the garment may tamponade any 4_____ that may be occuring. 5_____ which stimulate the cardiovascular system should be avoided.

a. Medications; b. bleeding; c. palpate; d. Apply; e. abdominal

Case study 11

A 42-year-old male complains of sudden, intense pain that is centered in his 1_____ _____. He is 2_____, 3_____, and diaphoretic, especially 4_____ the level of his umbilicus. He is tachycardic and hypotensive.

- What condition best describes the patient presentation? - Abdominal aortic aneurysm. ◄

The abdominal aorta is located in the 5_____-_____ space. A sudden 6_____ of pressure due to an aortic aneurysm will result in loss of perfusion below the site of injury.

a. lower back; b. below; c. pale; d. cool; e. retro-peritoneal; f. loss

Case study 12

You are called to the home of a 36-year-old man who is having a seizure. His wife reports that he has not taken his "1_____ _____" lately and that he has now had three seizures in a row without 2_____ _____. You have 3_____ the airway and are now ventilating with the 4_____ _____ _____.

- What should you do next? – Begin an IV, monitor cardiac rhythm, and administer diazepam. ◄

For a patient in 5_____ _____, treatment consists of establishing an IV, monitoring cardiac rhythm, and administering diazepam to stop the seizures.

> a. Status epilepticus; b. seizure pills;
> c. regaining consciousness; d. bag valve
> mask; e. secured

Case study 13

What is the primary reason that diazepam is given to a seizure patient?

- to suppress the spread of electrical activity in the brain and relax muscles. ◀

Although diazepam (Valium) does reduce 1_____, it is given to seizure patients to suppress the spread of 2_____ _____ through the brain as well as to 3_____ _____.

> a. anxiety; b. relax muscles; c. electrical
> activity

Case study 14

A 52-year-old male has been ejected from a car. He is apnoeic, with a slow pulse palpated at the 1_____ _____.

- What procedure would best manage this patient's airway? – Ventilate with the bag-valve mask and attach to high-flow oxygen. ◀

This patient needs immediate 2_____ ____ _____. Using a bag-valve mask will 3_____ this task most effectively.

> a. accomplish; b. oxygenation and ventilation;
> c. femoral artery

Case study 15

Your patient is a 27-year-old male who is found unconscious on a bathroom floor. He is not breathing, has 1_____ _____, and has a fresh 2_____ wound to his right forearm. He has 3_____ _____ that form a bluish streak over the veins on the backs on both hands. This patient is most likely suffering from which of the following?

- a seizure disorder
- multiple spider bites
- a narcotic overdose ◀
- anaphylactic shock

Common signs of a 4_____ _____ are described: Pinpoint pupils are characteristic of heroin and narcotic use, a fresh puncture wound over a vein indicates a recent 5_____ _____, and 6_____ _____ over the veins is consistent with the presence of track marks.

> a. bluish scarring; b. multiple scars;
> c. puncture; d. narcotic overdose; e. injection
> site; f. pinpoint pupils

Case study 16

A 24-year-old female is complaining of chest pain and difficulty breathing. She has been up for three days studying for finals and has been taking ephedrine supplements to help her 1_____

_____ and alert. She also admits to drinking twelve 2_____ soft drinks in the past day. Vitals are BP 80/40, P 180 carotid, and R 42. She is 3____ _____ and lethargic.

- The best treatment for this patient would include: cardioversion at 100 joules ◄

This patient presents in unstable supraventricular 4_____. Her condition may 5_____ quickly; therefore, immediate synchronized 6_____ is indicated.

a. cardioversion; b. caffeinated; c. stay awake; d. tachycardia; e. very pale; f. deteriorate

Case study 17

Your patient is a 19-year-old female who has been stung by a stingray while swimming.

- What should you do after 1_____ airway breathing and circulation are intact? – Apply heat or warm water to reduce pain and 2_____ the poison. ◄

Heat will cause the 3_____ to break down and 4_____ the harm to the patient.

a. detoxify; b. poison; c. ensuring; d. lessen

Case study 18

Your patient is a comatose 56-year-old male. His breath smells fruity and sweet and his respirations are very deep and rapid.

- After the initial assessment, you should provide the following treatments: Draw blood, start an IV of 0.9% NaCl, and give a 500 ml fluid bolus. ◄

This patient is showing signs and symptoms of diabetic 1_____. Avoid the use of 2_____ _____ if at all possible.

At the minimum, you should obtain a 3_____ _____ before administering any glucose containing solutions. The fluid bolus will help 4_____ the glucose contained within his blood.

a. glucose administration; b. glucometer reading; c. ketoacidosis; d. dilute

Case study 19

Your patient is a 30-year-old female who is complaining of a generalized rash and a dyspnoea after eating shellfish. The patient has small itchy, red welts all over her body and says her tongue feels like it is swollen. She complains of difficulty moving air in and difficulty 1_____ _ _____ _____. This patient's vital signs show a blood pressure of 110/60; a pulse of 100, strong and regular; and a respiratory rate of 36. Her breathing is somewhat shallow and 2_____.

- This patient is exhibiting the signs and symptoms of: an allergic reaction. ◄

This patient's blood pressure is still 3_____ ____ the allergic reaction; therefore, the patient is not in anaphylactic shock.

• This patient needs close monitoring because she could 4_____ ____: anaphylactic shock *

a. Compensating for; b. catching a full breath; c. progress into; d. laboured

Case study 20

You respond to a 17-year-old female found unconscious in her backyard by her parents. She has a newly developing skin rash on her right arm and is having difficulty breathing. You note that she is wheezing. Her parents state that she has no history of respiratory problems or other medical disorders.

Which of the following is a possible cause of her condition?

• Anaphylaxis ◄
• febrile seizures
• status asthmaticus
• epiglottitis

The environment she is in and previously unseen 1____, 2_____, difficulty breathing and negative past history are keys to this being a case of possible anaphylactic shock.

• What is the first step in managing this patient? – Aggressively manage the airway. ◄

You should aggressively manage the airway. It may be necessary to 3_____ _____ this patient, and you may get only one attempt. Once the tube contacts the larynx, the 4____ ____ can spasm and completely shut off the airway.

• The next step in treating this patient is to start a normal saline or Ringer's lactate IV and to give: epinephrine ◄

Epinephrine is a potent 5_____ and can reverse many of the effects of histamine 6_____. This patient is 7__ _____ and should first be treated with epinephrine. If respiratory 8_____ continues once the epinephrine has entered the patient's system, you may try using diphenhydramine (another antihistamine) or albuterol to bring about 9_____.

a. Antihistamine; b. distress; c. bronchodilation; d. carefully intubate; e. rash; f. vocal cords; g. in extremis; h. overload; i. wheezing

Vocabulary 1

abdominal /æbˈdɒm.ɪ.nəl/
thrust /θrʌst/
abscess /ˈæb.ses/
accomplish /əˈkʌm.plɪʃ/
admit /ədˈmɪt/
aggressively /əˈgres.ɪv.li/
air /ˈeər/ **embolism** /ˈem.bə.lɪ.zəm/
anaphylaxis /ˌæn.ə.fɪˈlæk.sɪs/
ascent /əˈsent/
bag /bæg/ **mask** /mɑːsk/
bolus /ˈbəʊ.ləs/

break /breɪk/ **down** /daʊn/
bring /brɪŋ/ **about** /əˈbaʊt/
bronchodilation /ˌbrɒn.kəʊ.ˈdɪleɪʃən/
caffeinated /ˈkæf.ɪ.neɪ.tɪd/
cardioversion /ˌkɑː.di.əˈvɜː.ʃən/
catching /ˈkætʃ.ɪŋ/
center /ˈsen.tər/
comfortable /ˈkʌmf.tər.bəl/
consciousness /ˈkɒn.ʃəs.nəs/
counterproductive /ˌkaʊn.tə.prəˈdʌk.tɪv/
cricothyreotomy /ˈkraɪ.kəˌθaɪəˈrɒ.tə.mɪ/
decompression /ˌdiː.kəmˈpreʃ.ən/ **sickness** /ˈsɪk.nəs/
deficit /ˈdef.ɪ.sɪt/
detoxify /diːˈtɒk.sɪ.faɪ/
dilute /daɪˈluːt/
diphenhydramine /di.fenˈhɪ.drə.miːn/
diving /ˈdaɪ.vɪŋ/ **reflex** /ˈriː.fleks/
drowning /ˈdraʊn.ɪŋ/
encourage /ɪnˈkʌr.ɪdʒ/
femoral /ˈfemərəl/
final /ˈfaɪ.nəl/
forceps /ˈfɔː.seps/
fraternity /frəˈtɜː.nə.ti/
fruity /ˈfruː.ti/
gag /gæg/ **reflex** /ˈriːfleks/
garment /ˈgɑːmənt/
glucose /ˈgluː.kəʊs/
goal /gəʊl/
grab /græb/
haemostasis /ˌhiː.məˈsteɪ.sɪs/
Heimlich maneuver /ˈhaɪm.lɪk.məˌnu.vər/
in extremis /ˌɪn.ɪkˈstriː.mɪs/
itchy /ˈɪtʃ.i/
MAST, Military Anti-Shock Trousers
mid /mɪd/
NaCl, sodium /ˈsəʊ.di.əm/ **chloride** /ˈklɔːraɪd/
near /nɪər/
necessitate /nəˈses.ɪ.teɪt/
neoplasm /ˌniː.əʊˈplæz.əm/

neurological /ˌnjʊə.rəˈlɒdʒ.ɪ.kəl/
nitrogen /ˈnaɪ.trə.dʒən/
nonrebreather /ˌnɒn.rəbrə.ðər/ **mask** /mɑːsk/
oropharyngeal /ˈɔː.rəˌfəˈrɪn.dʒi.əl/
overinflation /ˌəʊvə.ɪnˈfleɪʃ.ən/
overload /ˌəʊ.vəˈləʊd/
oxygenate /ˈɒk.sɪ.dʒə.neɪt/
padded /ˈpæd.ɪd/
PASG, Pneumatic /njʊˈmætɪk/ **Antishock** /ˈæn.tɪ.ʃɒk/ **Garment** /ˈgɑːmənt/
pneumatic /njʊˈmætɪk/
poison /ˈpɔɪ.zən/
pulseless /pʌls.ləs/
recompression /ˌriː.kəmˈpreʃ.ən/ **chamber** /ˈtʃeɪm.bər/
regain /rɪˈgeɪn/
retroperitoneal /ˌret.rəʊˌper.ɪ.təʊ.ˈniː.əl/
reverse /rɪˈvɜːs/
Ringer's lactate /ˈlækˈteɪt/
scar /skɑːr/
scuba diving /ˈskuː.bəˌdaɪ.vɪŋ/
shaft /ʃɑːft/
shellfish /ˈʃel.fɪʃ/
shut /ʃʌt/ **off** /ɒf/
softly /ˈsɒft.li/
sore /sɔːr/
spasm /ˈspæz.əm/
spider /ˈspaɪ.dər/
spine /spaɪn/ **board** /bɔːd/
splint /splɪnt/
status /ˈsteɪ.təs/
stingray /ˈstɪŋ.reɪ/
streak /striːk/
suddenly /ˈsʌd.ən.li/
suffering /ˈsʌf.ər.ɪŋ/
suit /sjuːt/
supplement /ˈsʌp.lɪ.mənt/
suppress /səˈpres/
track /træk/
traction /ˈtræk.ʃən/
tube /tjuːb/
umbilicus /ʌmˈbɪl.ɪ.kəs/

unconsciousness /ʌnˈkɒn.ʃəs.nəs/
unlikely /ʌnˈlaɪ.kli/
unseen /ʌnˈsiːn/
valve /vælv/
welt /welt/
whisper /ˈwɪs.pər/
worsen /ˈwɜː.sən/

Unit 2

Case study 1

What is the reason for giving 1_____ beta agonists to patients with severe allergic reactions?
- To reverse bronchospasm and relax airways ◄

2_____ _____ such as albuterol help in the treatment of severe allergic reactions by relaxing the 3_____ and thus relieving 4_____.

> a. Beta agonists; b. airway; c. bronchospasm; d. inhaled

Case study 2

Your patient is a 27-year-old male who has fallen from a 24-foot (7.3 m) ladder. As you are approaching and forming your general impression, you note that he is conscious and talking.

- What should you do first? – 1_____ stabilize his neck in a neutral position.◄

The 2_____ is always given first priority, but in this case, since the patient 3__ _____, the first step in his assessment and care would be to stabilize the

4_____ _____ as you begin your 5___ _____.

> a. ABC assessment; b. is talking; c. cervical spine; d. Manually; e. airway

Case study 3

When using the OPQRST 1_____ to assess a patient's pain, you would assess the R portion of the mnemonic by asking: "Does the pain move anywhere?" ◄

R stands 2_____. You should determine if the pain is radiating, 3_____, or causing any 4_____ _____. for

> a. radiation; b. referred; c. associated problem; d. mnemonic

Case study 4

The focused history and physical examination of a patient begins after you have: controlled immediate threats to the patient's life. ◄

The purpose of the focused history and physical examination is to detect additional problems after you have controlled 1_____ _____ to the patient's life.
The 2_____ _____ is typically performed during transport. 3_____ _____ may be consulted anytime during the call when you feel it is 4_____ or whenever your protocols and standing orders require it.

> a. Appropriate; b. Medical control; c. ongoing assessment; d. immediate threats

Case study 5

Using your sense of touch during a physical examination is called: palpation. ◄

The technique of 1_____ is using touch during a 2_____ _____ to gather information.

3_____ is listening with a stethoscope;

4_____ is using gentle tapping in order to identify the presence of air or fluid in body tissues.

> a. Percussion; b. Auscultation; c. physical examination; d. palpation

Case study 6

What are the components of the focused history and physical exam? – SAMPLE history and focused examination. ◄

The 1_____ _____ and physical exam, undertaken only after 2_____ _____ to life have been corrected, consists of ascertaining the nature of 3_____ __ _____, previous history (via SAMPLE), 4_____ _____, and focused exam.

> a. focused history; b. illness or injury; c. immediate threats; d. vital signs

Case study 7

What is the purpose of the OPQRST mnemonic? – To define the major complaint. ◄

The OPQRST mnemonic is used to define the 1_____ _____ associated with 2_____ _____ such as pain, dyspnoea, dizziness, and vague sensations.

It is not usually used in trauma or 3_____ _____.

> a. medical conditions; b. actual unconsciousness; c. chief complaint

Case study 8

What is a major concern when dealing with a patient with organophosphate poisoning? – Exposure of rescuers to the poison.◄

1_____ to organophosphate is a major concern. Proper 2_____ _____ are 3_____ to rescuer safety. 4_____ __ all patient clothing according to Environmental Protection Agency guidelines.

> a. Dispose of; b. Exposure; c. paramount; d. isolation procedures

Case study 9

Your patient is a farmer who has employed a crop cluster to spray his fields. The fields were sprayed earlier today and now the farmer has teary eyes, nausea and vomiting, diarrhoea, and excessive salivation.

- What was he most likely poisoned with? – Organophosphates. ◄

The symptoms of organophosphate 1_____ are described by the acronym SLUDGE (excessive 2_____, 3_____, 4_____, diarrhoea, gastrointestinal distress, 5_____).

a. salivation; b. absorption; c. emesis;
d. lacrimation; e. urination

Case study 10

What 1_____ is commonly used to treat patients who are the victims of organophosphate poisoning? - Atropine sulfate ◄

A large dose of atropine sulfate is used to 2_____ cholinergic poisoning from 3_____ and carbamates.

a. Counteract; b. organophosphates;
c. medication

Case study 11

A victim is unresponsive after possible exposure to 1_____ _____ in a closed garage. Which of the following procedures should you do first? –

- Wait for properly trained personnel to enter and evacuate the garage.◄
- 2____ the windows of the garage to ventilate the environment.
- 3_____ high-flow oxygen to the patient via positive pressure ventilations.
- 4_____ the patient from the environment.

Safety first! Of the three 5_____ options, 6_____ _____ and protected rescuers can remove the patient safely.

a. Extrication; b. Provide; c. carbon
monoxide; d. properly trained; e. Open;
f. Remove

Case study 12

Which finding is helpful 1__ _____ poisoning by spider venom from an acute abdominal condition?

- abdominal rigidity with no palpable tenderness ◄
- right-lower-quadrant pain in the absence of fever
- diaphoresis accompanied by 2_____ ___ _____
- the presence of multiple 3_____ _____ on the stomach

This finding is helpful in ruling out acute abdomen as the cause. 4_____ _____ generally always has pain associated with rigidity, whereas a 5_____ _____ may be painless initially due to the neurotoxicity of the 6_____. Spiders 7_____ bite more than once, ruling out the last choice as a realistic clue.

a. rarely; b. in distinguishing; c. spider bite;
d. bite marks; e. chills and fever; e. Acute
abdomen; f. venom

Case study 13

These are characteristic of a mild or moderate pit viper envenomation:

- 1_____ located around the wound site ◄
- 2_____ _____ like nausea or vomiting ◄
- Localised 3_____ at the wound site ◄

Pit viper 4_____ is generally very painful. Little or no

pain is characteristic of coral snake (5_____) envenomation.

> a. neurotoxic; b. Systemic effects; c. envenomation; d. Bruising; e. oedema

Case study 14

The physiological cause of the anxiety and restlessness that make up the classic 1_____ _____ of shock are a 2_____ _____ of what phenomena? – The release of catecholamines. ◄

The release of catecholamines that results from the initial drop in blood pressure causes the feelings of 3_____ ___ _____.

> a. early signs; b. anxiety and restlessness; c. direct result

Case study 15

A patient who experienced a seizure, rather than a period of syncope, usually reports that the episode: happened without any warning. ◄

1_____ unlike syncope, do not usually have 2_____ _____ such as a period of lightheadedness. Some seizures are 3_____ ___ a feeling or sensation of impending seizure called an aura.

> a. preceded by; b. Seizures; c. warning signs

Case study 16

During the initial phase of an acute stress reaction, what physiological response will occur? – Increased pulse rate and papillary dilatation. ◄

Both good stress (1_____) and bad stress (2_____) will initially cause symphatetic stimulation such as 3_____ heart and respiratory rate, bronchodilation, 4_____ _____, and increased blood flow to the 5_____ _____.

> a. skeletal muscles; b. distress; c. increased; d. dilated pupils; e. eustress

Case study 17

Continual reexperiencing of a traumatic event is a characteristic of which of the following?

- an 1_____ disorder
- stress and 2_____
- cumulative stress reaction
- delayed stress reaction ◄

3_____ _____ _____, or post-traumatic stress disorder, is characterized by reexperiencing of the traumatic event and diminished responsiveness to 4_____ ____, as well as physical and cognitive symptoms.

> a. burnout; b. anxiety; c. Delayed stress reaction; d. everyday life

Case study 18

What signs and symptoms are characteristic of a patient in compensated shock? – Lethargy; confusion; pulse and blood pressure normal to slightly elevated; skin cool; and capillary refill delayed.◄

The signs and symptoms given 1_____, 2_____, pulse and blood pressure normal to slightly elevated; skin cool; and 3_____ _____ delayed are characteristic of early, or compensated, shock. The single characteristic signalling the change from compensated to uncompensated shock is a drop in blood pressure that remains below normal despite 4_____ ___ _____. You 5_____ _____ wait to see a decrease in BP to decide if shock is present or not, since early 6_____ __ ___ _____ _____, sympathetic stimulation during compensation may result in a slight elevation of the diastolic blood pressure.

> a. intervention and treatment; b. lethargy;
> c. capillary refill; d. in the shock process;
> e. confusion; f. should never

Case study 19

What is the purpose of the body's 1_____ _____ to a stressor? – To prepare for the most efficient reaction. ◄

All the components of the stress reaction – 2_____ __ ACTH, relaxation of the young healthy adult, 3_____ _____, slowdown of 4_____, release of adrenaline – prepare the body to react to the 5_____ as efficiently as possible.

> a. stressor; b. bronchial tree; c. physiological
> response; d. release of; e. digestion

Case study 20

Why are vital signs changes not a good early indicator of shock in a young healthy adult? – The body attempts to compensate 1__ _____ normal vital signs. ◄

The body's physiological mechanism 2_____ ___ the insult that causes shock. Therefore, although changes in 3_____ _____ are ominous late signs in patients with poor tissue perfusion, they are unlikely to occur in a 4_____ _____ _____ who has just entered a state of shock.

> a. young healthy adult; b. by maintaining;
> c. compensate for; d. vital signs

Vocabulary 2

ACTH, Adrenocorticotropic /ə‚dri:.nəu‚kɔ:.tɪ.kəu'trɒf.ɪk/ **Hormone** /'hɔː.məun/
actual /'æk.tʃu.əl/
aldosterone /'ɔ:l.dəs.tər.əun/
ataxia /ə'tæk.si.ə/
atropine /'æt.rə.pɪn/ **sulfate** /'sʌl.feɪt/
aura /'ɔ:.rə/
beta-2 /'bi:tə.tu:/ **agonists** /'æg.ə.nɪsts/
burnout /'bɜ:naut/
carbamate /'kɑ:bə‚meɪt/
cervical /'sɜ:vɪkəl/ **spine** /spaɪn/
cholinergic /kɒ.lɪn.ə.dʒɪk/
cluster /'klʌs.tər/
cognitive /kɑg.nə.tɪv/
coral /'kɒr.əl/ **snake** /sneɪk/
counteract /‚kaun.tər'ækt/
crop /krɒp/
cumulative /'kju:.mju.lə.tɪv/
diarrhoea /‚daɪ.ə'ri:.ə/
digestion /daɪ'dʒes.tʃən/
dilatation /‚dɪl.ə'teɪ.ʃən/
disorder /dɪ‚sɔ:.dər/
efficiently /ɪ'fɪʃ.ənt.li/
emesis /e'mɪ.sɪs/
envenomation /ɪn‚ven.ə'meɪ.ʃən/
eustress /ju:.stres/

evacuate /ɪˈvæk.ju.eɪt/
event /ɪˈvent/
examination /ɪɡˌzæm.ɪˈneɪ.ʃən/
experienced /ɪkˈspɪə.ri.ənst/
general /ˈdʒen.ər.əl/
guideline /ˈɡaɪd.laɪn/
history /ˈhɪs.tər.i/
illness /ˈɪl.nəs/
in order to /ˈɔː.dər/
intake /ˈɪn.teɪk/
lacrimation /ˌlæk.riˈmeɪ.ʃən/
leading /ˈliː.dɪŋ/
lethargy /ˈleθ.ə.dʒi/
medical /ˈmed.ɪ.kəl/
mnemonic /nɪˈmɒn.ɪk/
moderate / ˈmɒd.ər.ət/
nature /ˈneɪ.tʃər/
neurotoxicity/ˌnjʊər.ə.tɒkˈsɪs.ɪ.ti/
onset /ˈɒnˌset/
OPQRST, Onset, Provocation,
Quality, Radiation, Severity, Time
oral /ˈɔː.rəl/
organophosphates /
ɔːˌɡæn.əʊˈfɒs.feɪts/
palpable /ˈpæl.pə.b̩l/
paramount /ˈpær.ə.maʊnt/
past /pɑːst/
phenomenon /fəˈnɒm.ɪ.nən/
pl phenomena
physiological /ˌfɪz.iˈɒl.ə.dʒi.kəl/
pit /pɪt/ viper /ˈvaɪ.pər/
portion /ˈpɔːˌʃən/
positive /ˈpɒz.ə.tɪv/
pressure /ˈpreʃ.ər/
previous /ˈpriː.vi.əs/
provocation /ˌprɒvəˈkeɪʃən/
quadrant /ˈkwɒd.rənt/
quality /kwɒlɪti/
radiation /ˌreɪ.diˈeɪ.ʃən/
reexperience /ˌriː.ɪkˈspɪə.ri.əns/
refill /ˈriː.fɪl/
responsiveness /rɪˈspɒn.sɪv.nəs/
restlessness /ˈrest.ləs.nəs/
salivation /ˈsæl.ɪ.veɪ.ʃən/

SAMPLE, Signs and Symptoms,
Allergies, Medications, Past
medical history, Last oral intake
severity / sɪˈver.ɪ.ti/
signal /ˈsɪɡ.nəl/
skeletal /ˈskel.ɪ.təl/
slowdown /ˈsləʊ.daʊn/
sludge /slʌdʒ/
SLUDGE, Salivation, Lacrimation,
Urination, Diarrhoea,
Gastrointestinal distress, Emesis
stressor /ˈstrɛs.ə/
symptom /ˈsɪmp.təm/
tap /tæp/
teary /ˈtɪə.r.i/
time /taɪm/
uncompensated /ʌnˈkɒmpənseɪtɪd/
unlike /ʌnˈlaɪk/
vague /veɪɡ/
venom /ˈvenəm/
warning /ˈwɔː.nɪŋ/
whereas /weərˈæz/

Unit 3
Case study 1

A patient presents with symptoms
of 1_____, 2_____, hives,
difficulty breathing, decreased
blood pressure, and dizziness.

- What should you suspect?
  – Anaphylaxis. ◀

3_____ accompanied by
difficulty breathing, strongly
4_____ anaphylaxis.

a. suggest; b. Hives; c. flushing; d. itching

Case study 2

While assessing a patient
complaining of difficulty

breathing, you note an 1_____
_____ _____, stridor, chest
tightness, and tachycardia.

- Based on these symptoms,
  you should suspect:
  anaphylaxis ◄

2_____ indicates an upper-
airway obstruction, in this case most
likely from an allergic reaction. A
patient with 3_____ would
exhibit difficulty breathing with
wheezing and rhonchi; a patient with
4_____ will exhibit wheezing
respirations; a patient suffering from
a CVA would have an altered mental
status but would not have stridor.

a. Asthma; b. Stridor; c. altered mental status; d. emphysema

Case study 3

What is the first sign of
1_____ _____ in a patient
2_____ _____ anaphylaxis?

- wheezing
- coughing
- hoarseness ◄
- dyspnoea

The first sign of laryngeal
oedema is usually a 3_____ _____.

a. hoarse voice; b. laryngeal oedema; c. suffering from

Case study 4

What are the two most common
causes of 1_____ anaphylaxis? –
Penicillin and insect bites/stings.◄
2_____ antigens are
likely to cause the most severe

reactions; penicillin and insect
stings are the two 3_____ _____
causes of severe anaphylaxis.

a. Injected; b. most common; c. severe

Case study 5

What is the 1_____ ____
for the management of acute
anaphylaxis? – Epinephrine.◄
To manage 2_____
_____ epinephrine is the
first medication used. Epinephrine
is a potent antihistamine and
immediately 3_____ the
physiological effects of the reaction
(vasodilation, bronchoconstriction,
and 4_____ _____).

a. airway swelling; b. primary drug; c. reverses; d. acute anaphylaxis

Case study 6

Epinephrine 1:1,000
may be indicated in:

- asthma ◄
- epiglottitis
- pertussis
- emphysema

As a 1_____,
epinephrine 1:1,000 is sometimes
2_____ in younger (<35
years old) 3_____ patients.

a. indicated; b. asthma; c. bronchodilator

Case study 7

An important disadvantage in
using both nasal- and oropharyngeal
airway adjuncts is that they:

are unable to protect the lower airway from aspiration ◄

Neither the nasopharyngeal nor the oropharyngeal airway is long enough to 1_____ the lower airway from 2_____ _____. Generally, the presence of 3_____ __ _____ in the airway does not affect their use, since suction is easily performed through and around these devices. The 4_____ come in a wide variety of sizes and styles. Use of the oropharyngeal airway is limited to patients who do not have a 5___ _____.

a. vomitus or blood; b. protect; c. gag reflex; d. devices; e. aspirated material

Case study 8

Your patient has suffered 1_____ trauma to the neck and is bleeding 2_____ from several large vessels.

- You should: apply an occlusive dressing then apply pressure. *

Apply an 3_____ _____ (a gloved hand can be used in the interim until the occlusive dressing is applied), then attempt to stop the bleeding with 4_____, _____ _____, but do not clamp neck vessels. Medical control may also direct 5_____ with a gloved finger.

a. profusely; b. tamponade; c. constant; direct pressure; d. occlusive dressing; e. penetrating

Case study 9

You are caring for a patient whose finger was just cut off in an accident.

- What should you do with the amputated finger? – Place the 1_____ finger in a plastic bag and 2_____ the bag in cold water. ◄

Do not allow the severed digit to 3___ ___ because tissues will begin to draw in the hypotonic fluid and 4_____ __, which may make reimplantation impossible. The 5____ _____ will help reduce 6_____ _____ by the cells of the severed digit and will help keep it 7_____ longer.

a. cold environment; b. get wet; c. severed; d. oxygen demand; e. swell up; f. immerse; g. alive

Case study 10

Assessment and care of a patient who is a victim of sexual assault should include the following: place sterile dressings on any wounds.◄

Do not 1_____ a vaginal exam, ask detailed questions about the 2_____ in the field, or 3_____ the patient to change clothes or bathe. You should not overly 4_____ any wounds you encounter, but instead wrap them up with dry 5_____ _____. Place any clothing or other evidence removed from a patient in a clean 6_____ ___ and take it with you to the hospital.

a. paper bag; b. assault; c. allow; d. sterile
dressings; e. perform; f. clean

Case study 11

Your patient is hypothermic with a body temperature of 93 °F (33.9 °C). The patient is likely 1__ _____ which of the following symptoms?

- severe shivering
- impaired judgement ◄
- respiratory depression
- bradycardia

This patient is experiencing early to moderate 2_____ and is likely to manifest 3_____ _____, 4_____ _____, normal blood pressure, and tachycardia. Severe 5_____ generally peaks around 95 °F and continues to decrease in intensity until 6____ _____ reaches the high 80s; it then stops altogether. Respiratory depression and bradycardia occur when the temperature 7_____ into the mid 80s.

a. shivering; b. impaired judgement;
c. hypothermia; d. to exhibit; e. slurred
speech; f. drops; g. body temperature

Case study 12

Shivering 1_____ in a hypothermic patient when the body temperature drops below: 86 °F (30 °Celsius).◄

2_____ is the body's attempt to 3_____ body temperature. Shivering continues until the body temperature reaches about 86 °F (30 °C). 4_____ __

shivering in a hypothermic patient indicates 5_____ _____.

a. Lack of; b. regulate; c. severe hypothermia;
d. Shivering; e. ceases

Case study 13

Which of the following patients shows signs and symptoms of heat exhaustion?

a) Male, age 34; severe 1_____ _____ in legs and abdomen; fatigue, and dizziness
b) Female, age 45; rapid; shallow respirations; weak pulse; cold, clammy skin; dizziness ◄
c) Male, age 42; deep respirations; 2_____ _____ pulse; dry, hot skin; loss of 3_____.
d) Female, age 70; shallow respirations; weak, rapid pulse; dilated pupils; 4_____.

Patients c) and d) show signs and symptoms of heat stroke, and patient a) shows signs of heat cramps.

a. consciousness; b. rapid, strong; c. muscle
cramps; d. seizures

Case study 14

Which of the following patient scenarios is the typical profile for a victim of classic 1___ _____?

- a healthy young adult who has been 2_____ in hot, humid weather

- someone 3_____ profusely and drinking large amounts of water without salt
- an elderly person with chronic illness who 4__ _____ to a hot room ◄
- 5__ _____ who is exposed to overly high ambient temperatures indoors

Although any of these individuals could suffer from heat stroke, the 6_____ _____ represents the typical profile of a victim of classic heat stroke.

a. is confined; b. sweating; c. elderly person; d. heat stroke; e. exercising; f. an infant

Case study 15

A patient begins to have a 1_____ _____ while running a marathon on a hot day. Which of the following procedures should you do first?

- Move the patient into the 2_____.
- 3_____ 5 mg diazepam intravenously.
- Establish an airway and ventilate the patient.◄
- Place 4____ _____ around the neck and under the arms.

While the other procedures are applicable to the treatment of a possible heat stroke victim, 5_____ the airway and 6_____ respirations should occur first.

a. Securing; b. ambulance; c. administer; d. cold packs; e. generalized seizure; f. ensuring

Case study 16

Which of the following patients is considered to be at 1____ ____ for a heat-related emergency?

- 29-year-old 2_____
- 48-year-old police officer
- 17-year-old athlete
- 78-year-old diabetic ◄

The very young, the very old, those undernourished, and those with chronic illness are all predisposed to 3____ _____ for a variety of reasons.

a. heat illness; b. high risk; c. amputee

Case study 17

You are called to the scene of a possible drowning at a local pool. Upon arrival, you discover that 1_____ have removed the patient from the pool and are performing 2_____ _____ since the patient is apnoeic with a pulse.

- 3_____ should consist of: defibrillation 200 joules. ◄

The patient presents in pulseless ventricular tachycardia, a 4_____ _____. Immediate defibrillation is indicated to terminate this event.

a. Management, b. lifeguards, c. lethal rhythm, d. rescue ventilations

Case study 18

What is the most important treatment consideration for a patient who is suffering from 1_____ _____? – Provide high-concentration oxygen with a nonrebreather mask. ◄

2_____ _____ at 100% concentration and intubate if the patient is not breathing 3_____.

> a. Provide oxygen, b. decompression sickness, c. spontaneously

Case study 19

What is the correct field treatment for a 1_____ body part? – Transport the patient to the hospital.◄

The correct treatment is 2_____ _____ in a water bath maintained between 100 ° F (37,8 ° C) and 106 °F (41°C), although this treatment should not be attempted 3__ ____ _____ because of the danger of 4_____. Pain management is essential because the procedure is 5_____ _____.

> a. in the field; b. gradual warming; c. extremely painful; d. refreezing; e. frostbitten

Case study 20

A patient presents with 1_____ _____ at a rate of six per minute.

- What should you do next? – 2_____

positive-pressure ventilation with a BVM ◄

The respiratory rate is too slow and must 3__ _____ immediately with 4_____ assistance.

> a. ventilatory; b. Administer; c. be corrected; d. shallow breaths

Vocabulary 3

accident /'æksɪdənt/
adjunct /'ædʒ.ʌŋkt/
alive /ə'laɪv/
amputee /ˌæm.pjʊ'tiː/
antigen /'æn.tɪ.dʒən/
applicable /ə'plɪk.ə.bl̩/
bathe /beɪð/
cease /siːs/
cerebrovascular /ˌser.ɪ.brə'væskjʊlə/
cut st off /kʌt/
CVA, Cerebrovascular/ˌser.ɪ.brə'væskjʊlə/
Accident /'æksɪdənt/
digit /'dɪdʒ.ɪt/
dilated /daɪ'leɪtɪd/
draw /drɔː/
exercise /'ek.sə.saɪz/
flush /flʌʃ/
frostbitten /'frɒstˌbɪt.ən/
gag /gæg/
gloved /glʌvd/
heat /hiːt/ **cramp** /kræmp/
heat /hiːt/ **exhaustion** /ɪg'zɔːs.tʃən/
heat /hiːt/ **stroke** /strəʊk/
hives /haɪvz/
humid /'hjuː.mɪd/
hypotonia /ˌhaɪpəʊ'təʊ.niə/
immerse /ɪ'mɜːs/
impaired /ɪm'peəd/
indoors /ˌɪn'dɔːz/
insect /'ɪn.sekt/
intensity /ɪn'ten.sɪ.ti/

interim /ˈɪn.tər.ɪm/
intravenously /ˌɪn.trəˈviː.nəs.li/
lifeguard /ˈlaɪf.gɑːd/
manifest /ˈmæn.ɪ.fest/
mental /ˈmen.təl/
mid /mɪd/
occlusive /ɒˈkluː.sɪv/
dressing /ˈdres.ɪŋ/
overly /ˈəʊ.vəl.i/
peak /piːk/
penetrate /ˈpen.ɪ.treɪt/
penetrating /ˈpen.ɪ.treɪ.tɪŋ/
pertussis /pəˈtʌ.sɪs/
pool /puːl/
rapid /ˈræp.ɪd/
refreeze /ˌriːˈfriː.z/
regulate /ˈregjʊˌleɪt/
sever /ˈsev.ər/
slurred /ˈslɜːd/
terminate /ˈtɜː.mɪ.neɪt/
tightness /ˈtaɪt.nəs/
undernourished /ˌʌn.dəˈnʌr.ɪʃt/
weak /wiːk/

Unit 4

Case study 1

Your patient is an adult female whom you suspect is unconscious as a result of an upper-airway obstruction. You use the head-tilt/chin-lift method 1__ ____ her airway and then attempt to give two 2_____, which are unsuccessful.

- What is the next thing you should do? – Reposition, and attempt to ventilate again. ◀

During the initial 3_____ _____, the next step after two unsuccessful attempts at ventilation for an unconscious adult patient is to 4_____ the head and try again. Once you have confirmed 5_____, you do not need to repeat this step (repositioning) again.

Perform the blind finger sweep following the 6_____ _____ before attempting ventilation each time. 7_____ _____ for relieving airway obstruction are reserved for very obese and pregnant adults.

a. Chest thrusts; b. obstruction; c. abdominal thrusts; d. resuscitation attempt; e. to open; f. reposition; g. ventilations

Case study 2

When 1_____ a patient, you should always: begin suctioning after the catheter is placed in the airway.◀

Attempts at suctioning should be limited to no more than 5-10 seconds (depending upon the level of 2_____). You should 3_____ the patient after each attempt, and you should not turn on the apparatus until the catheter is 4_____ _____.

In the case of a 5_____ _____ that has a hole in the system that allows you to control if suction is being applied or not by occluding the opening, you should only suction upon withdrawal.

This system may remain turned on at all times as long as you 6_____ _____ when suction is actually being applied to the patient.

a. placed properly; b. monitor closely; c. suction catheter; d. consciousness; e. suctioning; f. ventilate

Case study 3

You are called for a 54-year-old woman who is unconscious. Your assessment reveals the patient to be 1_____ ___ _____.

- Initial management of this patient's airway should include: insertion of an 2_____ airway and ventilation with a bag-valve 3_____. ◄

a. device; b. oropharyngeal; c. apnoeic and pulseless

Case study 4

Your patient has a partial airway obstruction but adequate air exchange.

- You should: monitor the patient closely while he or she continues trying to clear the airway him- or herself. ◄

If a patient has a 1_____ airway obstruction but adequate 2____ _____, allow her to continue her spontaneous efforts to clear the airway (3_____), but monitor her carefully. Your 4_____ may actually worsen the obstruction by making it 5_____.

If air exchange becomes inadequate, treat her as if the obstruction is total 6__ _____ the Heimlich, intubation, 7_____, or other efforts to relieve the 8_____.

a. by performing; b. interference; c. coughing; d. partial; e. air exchange; f. suction; g. obstruction; h. complete

Case study 5

After inserting a blind-insertion-airway device, what step should you take before inflating the balloon to ensure that the tube is properly positioned? – Look for chest rise and auscultate the lungs and abdomen. ◄

Regardless of which device you use, 1_____ of placement is generally advisable prior to 2_____ of any balloons on the device by looking for 3_____- ____ and fall and 4_____ ___ breath sounds in the chest and 5_____.

a. inflation; b. listening for; c. abdomen; d. chest rise; e. confirmation

Case study 6

What is the most definitive treatment of a patient with a flail chest injury? – Intubation and positive pressure ventilation. ◄

1_____ _____ ventilation of the patient with a 2_____ _____ _____ reverses the mechanism that causes the 3_____ chest wall movement, restores 4_____ _____, and 5_____ ____ of chest wall movement.

a. reduces pain; b. Positive pressure; c. paradoxical; d. tidal volume; e. flail chest injury

Case study 7

One breathing pattern is characterized by periods of apnoea followed by periods in which respirations first increase then decrease in both 1_____ ___ _____.

- This 2_____ is called: Cheyne-Stokes breathing.◄

Cheyne-Stokes respirations are characterized by periods of 3_____ lasting 10-60 seconds, followed by periods in which respirations gradually 4_____, then 5_____, in depth and rate.

a. decrease; b. apnoea; c. increase; d. pattern; e. depth and frequency

Case study 8

This statement regarding a 1_____ pneumothorax is true: It is usually limited to only 20% of the lung and is well tolerated by the patient.◄

A spontaneous pneumothorax occurs when a 2_____ (cystic lesion on the lobe of the lung) ruptures, allowing air to enter the 3_____ _____ from within the lung. It usually occurs in otherwise healthy individuals age 20 to 40. They are usually well 4_____ and occupy less than 20% of the lung.

a. pleural space; b. tolerated; c. spontaneous; d. bleb

Case study 9

The paper bag effect occurs when the occupant of a car takes deep breath just 1_____ _ _____, resulting in which of the following injuries?

- pneumothorax ◄
- pulmonary embolism
- shearing of the aorta
- lung laceration

The paper bag effect or the paper bag syndrome is thought to 2__ _____ for most pneumothoraces that result from car crashes. During this event the 3_____ _____ traps pressurized air in the 4_____. When compression occurs during the crash against the closed glottis, 5_____ _____ can occur to the hyperinflated 6_____ ___ _____, resulting in collapse.

a. chest; b. closed glottis; c. be responsible; d. alveoli and bronchioles; e. severe damage; f. before a collision

Case study 10

A patient is found lying supine on the floor with a 1_____ _____ to her right anterior chest, just below the breast. The patient is having 2_____ _____, with cool, clammy skin signs. No JVD is noted. Breath sounds are absent over the right side.

- This patient most likely is experiencing a: haemothorax. ◄

The lack of jugular venous 3_____ in the supine position is very telling; it suggests a 4_____ _____ of volume from the circulatory system.

a. difficulty breathing; b. stab wound; c. large loss; d. distension

Case study 11

A patient was hit several times in the left chest with the large end of a pool cue. The patient is in severe respiratory distress with tachycardia and tachypnoea. 1_____ can be felt over the left anterior fourth, fifth, sixth, and seventh rib area. Lung 2_____ are clear and equal, but diminished.

- What condition best describes the patient's presentation? – Flail chest segment. ◀

3_____ _____ is very possible in this case, due to the 4_____ of injury. The lack of other signs or symptoms such as jugular venous distension or unequal or absent breath sounds minimizes the possibilities of a 5_____ __ _____.

a. pneumothorax or tamponade; b. Flail segment; c. Crepitus; d. sounds; e. mechanism

Case study 12

This 1_____ in vital signs comprises Cushing's reflex, a sign of increasing 2_____ _____: respiratory rate increased, heart rate decreased, blood pressure increased ◀
Cushing's reflex is also sometimes called Cushing's triad or Cushing's 3_____.

a. response; b. intracranial pressure; c. change

Case study 13

The primary use of the Magill forceps in the field is to: directly 1_____ a visible foreign-body obstruction.◀
Magill forceps are used to remove an obstructing 2_____ _____ that is visible during laryngoscopy after 3_____ _____ have been unsuccessful.

a. remove; b. foreign body; c. abdominal thrusts

Case study 14

Progressively deeper, faster breathing 1_____ gradually with shallow, slower breathing is called: Cheyne-Stokes ◀
2_____-_____ respirations are 3_____ ___ ____. Biot's breathing is an irregular pattern.

a. alternating; b. regular and deep; c. Cheyne-Stokes

Case study 15

Which statements about deflation of the PASG/MAST in the field setting is correct?

- Deflation should be accomplished rapidly in the field.
- Deflate the legs first and then the 1_____ compartment.
- 2_____ the garment if the patient begins to experience dyspnoea.
- Deflation should not be attempted in the field without medical direction. ◀

IRENA BAUMRUKOVÁ

Because the PASG corrects a symptom and not the 3_____ _____, deflating should be 4_____ only in the hospital after the underlying 5_____is corrected.

a. attempted; b. underlying problem;
c. hypovolemia; d. abdominal; e. Deflate

Case study 16

The following conditions would result in an increase of a patient's PaO2: airway obstruction, hypoventilation, physical exertion.◄

PaO2 measures 1_____ _____ levels in the blood, which are influenced by 2_____ in CO_2 production or 3_____. Such levels would be increased by 4_____ _____ of muscles, by 5_____, or by an airway obstruction.

a. carbon dioxide; b. hypoventilation;
c. elimination; d. physical exertion;
e. alterations

Case study 17

Which of the following factors would normally cause a 1_____ in a patient's respiratory rate?

- anxiety
- sleep ◄
- fever
- hypoxia

A patient will breathe more slowly when 2_____ than when 3_____; all the other factors listed increase 4_____ _____.

a. awake; b. decrease; c. respiratory rate;
d. asleep

Case study 18

The volume of air normally inhaled and exhaled during each respiration is called the: tidal volume.◄

Tidal volume is the amount of air that moves into and out of the lungs during the 1_____ _____; minute volume is the total amount of air exchanged in the lungs in one 2_____; inspiratory 3_____ is the extra air that could be inspired in addition to the tidal volume; total 4____ _____ is the sum of the inspiratory reserve, tidal volume, expiratory reserve, and residual volume.

a. lung capacity; b. respiratory cycle;
c. reserve, d. minute

Case study 19

Which is the recommended method when measuring respiratory rate? – Count respirations while pretending to take a radial pulse.◄

Place your hand on the patient's wrist as if you were measuring his or her pulse and 1_____ ___ __ _____. This will prevent the patient from consciously 2_____ the respiratory rate. Placing the wrist and hand over the patient's 3_____ _____ is called the pledge of allegiance method.

a. chest wall; b. changing; c. count for 30 seconds

180

Case study 20

When using a peak flow meter to measure peak expiratory flow, the correct procedure is to: ask the patient to inhale deeply, then exhale once as quickly as possible, taking one reading. ◄

The correct procedure is to have the patient 1_____ _____ and 2_____ _____. Some meters ask you to repeat the procedure and 3_____ your findings, but you would still have the patient inhale deeply and quickly exhale with each 4_____.

a. average; b. inhale deeply; c. exhale quickly; d. reading

Vocabulary 4

allegiance /əˈliː.dʒəns/
alternating /ˈɒl.tə.neɪ.tɪŋ/
asleep /əˈsliːp/
average /ˈæv.ər.ɪdʒ/
balloon /bəˈluːn/
bleb /bleb/
confirmed /kənˈfɜːmd/
consciously /ˈkɒn.ʃəs.li/
count /kaʊnt/
cycle /ˈsaɪ.kl̩/
deflation /dɪˈfleɪ.ʃən/
exertion /ɪgˈzɜː.ʃən/
frequency /ˈfriː.kwən.si/
garment /ˈgɑː.mənt/
haemothorax /ˈhiː.məˈθɔː.ræks/
hole /hoʊl/
hypoventilation /ˌhaɪpoʊˌven.tɪˈleɪ.ʃən/
increase /ɪnˈkriːs/
inflation /ɪnˈfleɪ.ʃən/
interference /ˌɪn.tə'fɪə.rəns/
JVD, Jugular /ˈdʒʌg.jə.lər/ **Venous** / ˈviː.nəs/ **Distension** /dɪˈsten.t.ʃən/
lasting /ˈlɑː.stɪŋ/

method /ˈmeθ.əd/
otherwise /ˈʌð.ə.waɪz/
peak /piːk/ **flow** /floʊ/
place /pleɪs/
pledge /pledʒ/
pleural /ˈplʊə.rəl/
pool cue /kjuː/
pressurized /ˈpreʃ.ər.aɪzd/
pretend /prɪˈtend/
progressively /prəˈgres.ɪv.li/
rate /reɪt/
regular /ˈreg.jʊ.lər/
relieve /rɪˈliːv/
reserve /rɪˈzɜːv/
setting /ˈset.ɪŋ/
shear /ˈʃɪə.r/
sweep /swiːp/ **(swept, swept)**
take /teɪk/ **breath** /breθ/
tidal /ˈtaɪ.dəl/
total /ˈtoʊ.təl/
unequal /ʌnˈiː.kwəl/
visible /ˈvɪz.ɪ.bl̩/
wrist /rɪst/

Unit 5
Case study 1

What is an assessment finding of pulsus paradoxus associated with? – COPD ◄

1_____ _____, or a drop in 2_____ _____ with each respiratory cycle, is associated with chronic obstructive pulmonary disease (3____).

a. COPD; b. Pulsus paradoxus; c. blood pressure

Case study 2

What is bronchiolitis caused by? – The respiratory syncytial virus. ◄

The respiratory syncytial virus, which causes only 1_____ upper-respiratory infections in older persons, causes 2_____, a serious 3_____ _____ in infants and young children

> a. respiratory infection; b. mild;
> c. bronchiolitis

Case study 3

A disease that is associated with cigarette smoking and is related to, but distinct from, emphysema is: chronic bronchitis. ◄

In addition to emphysema, 1_____ _____ is associated with cigarette smoking. Either condition can lead to CHF. A 2_____ _____ can be caused by cigarette smoking, especially in young and thin males, but the disease process is unrelated to 3_____.

> a. emphysema; b. chronic bronchitis;
> c. simple pneumothorax

Case study 4

A dull sound heard during chest 1_____ may be associated with which condition? – Pneumonia. ◄

A 2____ _____ heard during chest percussion may be associated with pneumonia, 3_____, or 4_____ _____.

> a. Haemothorax; b. dull sound; c. pulmonary
> oedema; d. percussion

Case study 5

What condition best suggests respiratory failure? – Hyperextension of the neck. ◄

A patient in 1_____ _____ is compensating for the underlying condition, thereby preserving 2_____ to the brain. Once 3_____ _____ have collapsed, the loss of gas exchange at the brain will result in a change in 4_____ _____.

In a paediatric patient hypertension of the neck can complicate ventilation. Hyperextending the neck of a small child may result in an unintentional 5_____ of the airway, due to the softer 6_____ _____ supporting the trachea.

> a. Compensatory mechanisms; b. cartilage
> rings; c. respiratory distress; d. oxygenation;
> e. mental status; f. closure

Case study 6

These statements about airway obstruction caused by the tongue are correct:

- The tongue is the most common cause of 1_____ _____ in an unconscious patient. ◄
- Airway blockage does not depend on the 2_____ of the patient's head, neck, and jaw. ◄
- The 3_____ ____ _____ can contribute to

airway blockage in an unconscious patient. ◄

- Blockage of the airway by the 4_____ can occur when the patient is in any position. ◄

---
a. airway obstruction; b. oesophagus and epiglottis; c. position; d. tongue
---

Case study 7

The hypoxic drive is regulated by: low PaO2. ◄

COPD patients can no longer 1____ ____ normal regulatory mechanisms to control their 2_____. The hypoxic drive measures for low levels of oxygen in the 3____ _____ to increase respiratory rate.

---
a. rely upon; b. blood stream; c. respirations

Case study 8

What is the condition that is present when the pleural space expands because air enters from an interior wound? – A closed pneumothorax. ◄

1_____ _____ occurs when air enters the pleural space from an 2_____ _____. An open pneumothorax occurs when the chest wall is open so that air can enter directly into the chest from 3___ _____. A tension pneumothorax develops when a 4_____ _____ becomes large enough to cause pressure and structural changes within the chest.

---
a. Closed pneumothorax; b. the outside; c. simple pneumothorax; d. interior wound
---

Case study 9

What respiratory pattern is characteristic Kussmaul's respiration? – An 1_____ in both rate and depth.◄

Kussmaul's respirations, which are associated with 2_____ _____, are characterized by increased rate and depth of 3_____.

---
a. respirations; b. diabetic ketoacidosis; c. increase

Case study 10

What does the term stridor refer to? – A 1____-_____ sound upon inspiration from airway obstruction. ◄

Stridor is a sound made during 2_____ and is associated with croup and upper-airway 3_____. A harsh upper-airway sound that can be heard when the patient inhales and can usually be heard without a 4_____ and emanates from the area of the 5_____

---
a. throat; b. inspiration; c. obstruction; d. stethoscope; e. high-pitched
---

Case study 11

A whistling or musical sound heard on exhalation is referred to as what abnormal breath sound?

- snoring
- wheezing ◄
- stridor
- friction rub

1________, a whistling sound heard on 2___________, is generally associated with 3______. Snoring and stridor are 4_____-______ obstructions and a friction rub sounds like rubbing.

a. Wheezing; b. expiration; c. upper-airway; d. asthma

Case study 12

What condition is the pathophysiological result of near drowning in sea water? – Pulmonary oedema ◀

Because sea water is 1___________, fluid is drawn from the 2____________ into the 3________, causing pulmonary oedema. Because of this, all near-drowning patients should be hospitalized and monitored for a short time.

a. hypertonic; b. bloodstream; c. alveoli

Case study 13

Your patient is in respiratory distress. He is exhibiting jugular venous 1___________. Cracles are auscultated throughout his 2_____ _______. He is tachycardic, hypertensive, and tachypnoeic. What 3___ __ __________ is indicated for this patient's presentation?

- What are the correct 4_______ ___ _______ of the indicated medications? – Oxygen, intravenous line at 30 cc/hour, nitroglycerin sL, and 40 mg furosemide IV. ◀

This patient appears to be experiencing 5_____ pulmonary oedema.

a. distension; b. lung fields; c. choices and routes; d. set of treatment; e. acute

Case study 14

Which of the following factors increases the amount of energy necessary for the patient to expend for respiration?

- loss of pulmonary surfactant. ◀
- decrease in airway resistance
- increase in pulmonary compliance
- a decrease in body temperature

1_____ __ __________ __________, which can occur in pneumonia and other conditions, increases the tendency of the alveoli to 2________ and, thus, increases the work 3__________ ___ respiration.

a. necessary for; b. Loss of pulmonary surfactant; c. collapse

Case study 15

Signs and symptoms of traumatic asphyxia include: dyspnoea, bloodshot eyes, distended neck veins, and a cyanotic upper body. ◀

Traumatic asphyxia occurs when 1_______ ___ _______ pushes the chest wall inward, resulting in severe 2________________ and backflow of venous blood. Important signs and symptoms of

this include 3_____, bloodshot
eyes, distended neck veins, and
a 4_____ upper body.

a. dyspnoea; b. hypoventilation; c. cyanotic;
d. serious rib injury

Case study 16

You note snoring sounds
during your initial assessment of
a semiconscious trauma patient.

- What is your next step?
  – Perform the chin-lift/
  jaw-thrust manoeuvre.◀

1_____ indicates that the
airway is partially obstructed by
the patient's tongue. Clear the
airway first by positioning with the
2_____-____/___-_____ manoeuvre
or by inserting a nasopharyngeal
airway. An oropharyngeal airway
is 3___ _____ due to the
patient's LOC. Cervical stabilization
takes place prior to beginning
your ABC assessment and head
tilt/ chin lift is not advisable due
to the possibility of 4_-_____.

a. c-spine injury; b. not indicated; c. Snoring;
d. chin-lift/jaw-thrust

Case study 17

When administering IV fluids
to a trauma patient, it is critical
to continuously monitor which
1_____ ____? – Breath sounds. ◀
2_____ _____ are
particularly important to monitor
during IV fluid administration
because of the danger of 3_____

_____, which will initially
4_____ __ pulmonary oedema.

a. manifest as; b. fluid overload; c. vital sign;
d. breath sounds

Case study 18

A patient is found in a back
bedroom lying supine on the bed
with a hunting knife embedded in
her anterior chest, midline below
the right breast. The patient is in
obvious 1_____ _____.
She is cold, clammy, and diaphoretic
with flat neck veins. You hear no
breath sounds on the right side.

- This patient is most
  likely suffering from:
  haemothorax ◀

2____ ____ _____ while the
patient is supine indicate a lower
than normal pressure inside the
vasculature, most likely due to
3_____ ____. This would indicate a
haemothorax as the 4_____ _____
of the described signs and symptoms.

a. blood loss; b. Flat neck veins; c. primary
cause; d. respiratory distress

Case study 19

What is your first action for
an adult patient who is conscious
but who has a 1_____ _____
_____? – Deliver rapid
2_____ _____ until cleared
or unconsciousness results.◀
For the 3_____
patient, your first action would
be abdominal thrusts.

```
a. Abdominal thrusts; b. conscious;
c. complete airway obstruction
```

Case study 20

The most 1_____ cause
of upper-airway obstruction is:
relaxation of the tongue.◄

The loss of lingual control
during 2_____
occurs more commonly that
the other 3_____.

```
a. unconsciousness; b. conditions; c. common
```

Vocabulary 5

abbreviation /əˌbriːviˈeɪʃən/
abnormal /æbˈnɔː.məl/
asphyxia /æsˈfɪksɪə/
backflow /ˈbæk.fləʊ/
blockage /ˈblɒk.ɪdʒ/
bloodshot /ˈblʌd.ʃɒt/
bronchiolitis /ˈbrɒŋ.ki.ə'la.ɪ.tɪs/
cartilage /ˈkɑː.təl.ɪdʒ/ **ring** /rɪŋ/
consciousness /ˈkɒn.ʃəs.nəs/
COPD, Chronic /ˈkrɒnɪk/
Obstructive /əbˈstrʌk.tɪv/ **Pulmonary**
/ˈpʊl.mə.nə.ri/ **Disease** /dɪˈziːz/
danger /ˈdeɪn.dʒər/
deliver /dɪˈlɪv.ər/
diabetic /ˌdaɪəˈbet.ɪk/ **ketoacidosis**
/ˈkiːtəʊˌæs.ɪˈdəʊ.sɪs/
distinct /dɪˈstɪŋkt/
emanate /ˈem.ə.neɪt/
embedded /ɪmˈbed.ɪd/
exhalation /ˌeks.h ə'leɪ.ʃən/
expend /ɪkˈspend/
friction /ˈfrɪk.ʃən/
furosemide /fjʊr.ɒs'æm.aɪd/
harsh /hɑːʃ/
hyperextension /ˌhaɪ.pər'ɪk'stenʃən/
hypertonia /ˌhaɪ.pə'təʊ.nɪə/
hypoxic /haɪ'pɒk.sɪk/ **drive** /draɪv/
intravenous /ˌɪn.trə'viː.nəs/ **line** /laɪn/
lingual /ˈlɪŋgwəl/

LOC, Level /ˈlevəl/ **of**
consciousness /ˈkɒn.ʃəs.nɪs/
LOC, Loss /lɒs/ **of**
consciousness /ˈkɒn.ʃəs.nɪs/
obstructive /əbˈstrʌk.tɪv/
outside /ˌaʊtˈsaɪd/
PaCO₂, partial /ˈpɑːʃəl/ **pressure**
/ˈpreʃ.ər/ **of carbon** /ˈkɑː.bən/
dioxide /daɪˈɒk.saɪd/ **in arterial** /
ɑːˈtɪəriəl/ **blood** /blʌd/
particularly /pəˈtɪk.jʊ.lə.li/
primary /ˈpraɪ.mə.ri/
rely /rɪˈlaɪ/ **upon** /əˌpɒn/
semiconscious /ˌsem.iˈkɒn.ʃəs/
stabilization /ˌsteɪ.bɪ.laɪˈzeɪ.ʃən/
stream /striːm/
surfactant /sərfakˈtənt/
syncytial /sɪnˈsɪ.ʃi.əl/ **virus** /ˈvaɪrəs/
tendency /ˈten.dən.si/
traumatic /trɔːˈmæt.ɪk/
treatment /ˈtriːt.mənt/
unintentional /ˌʌn.ɪnˈten.ʃən.əl/
unrelated /ˌʌn.rɪˈleɪ.tɪd/
vasculature /ˈvæs.kjʊ.lə.tʃər/

Unit 6
Case study 1

These statements about
airway obstruction caused by
the tongue are correct:

- The tongue is the most
  common cause of 1_____
  _____ in an
  unconscious patient. ◄
- Airway blockage does not
  depend on the 2_____
  of the patient's head,
  neck, and jaw. ◄
- The 3_____
  ___ _____
  can contribute to

airway blockage in an
unconscious patient. ◄

Blockage of the airway by
the 4_____ can occur when
the patient is in any position.

> a. airway obstruction; b. oesophagus and
> epiglottis; c. position, d. tongue

Case study 2

An unconscious patient has
snoring respirations. When should
this condition be corrected?
– 1_____ _____
the respiratory status. ◄
2_____ respirations are
indicative of an airway issue and
should be 3_____ before
further assessment 4__ _____.

> a. is completed; b. corrected; c. Before
> evaluating; d. Snoring

Case study 3

A patient is short of breath after
impact with the 1_____ _____
in a motor vehicle crash. Breath
sounds are diminished on the left.

- What condition is most
  likely the cause of the
  patient's 2_____? –
  Simple pneumothorax. ◄

The question does not provide
any indication of a tension
pneumothorax. A pulmonary
3_____ or cardiac tamponade
should affect 4_____ _____.

> a. lung sounds; b. Complaint; c. contusion;
> d. steering wheel

Case study 4

Before using nitrous
oxide for a 1_____-_____
patient, you should exclude the
possibility that the patient has:

- cervical spine injury
- flail chest
- pericardial tamponade
- pneumothorax. ◄

Nitronox should not be used with
patients with head injury because
it can increase 2_____
_____. It should not be used with
patients who have 3_____
because the drug can move 4__
_____ to air spaces in the body.

> a. pneumothorax; b. by diffusion; c. chest-
> injury; d. intracranial pressure

Case study 5

Your trauma patient is
1_____ and apprehensive.
She is increasingly 2_____,
and breath sounds are rapidly
diminishing over her left lung. She
is exhibiting signs and symptoms
of 3_____. You should suspect

- haemothorax
- tension pneumothorax ◄
- cardiac 4_____
- flail chest

> a. agitated; b. shock; c. tamponade;
> d. cyanotic

Case study 6

Distended neck veins,
1_____ unilateral
breath sounds, and progressively

2_____ compliance
are indications of: tension
pneumothorax. ◄

Excessive pressure inside the
3_____ _____ due to the
tension pneumothorax will result
in all of the described symptoms.

> a. worsening; b. diminishing; c. thoracic
> cavity

Case study 7
The term tracheal tugging
refers to which of the following?

- the use of 1_____
_____ during respirations
- retraction if intercostal
muscles during inspiration
- cyanosis and 2_____
_____ with exhalation
- retraction of neck tissues
during respiration ◄

Tracheal tugging refers to
3_____ of neck tissues
during respiratory 4_____.

> a. effort; b. retraction; c. accessory muscles;
> d. nasal flaring

Case study 8
Your patient 1_____
cold, clammy skin; air hunger;
distended neck veins; 2_____
displacement; and 3_____
breath sounds on one side.

- You should suspect:
tension pneumothorax.◄

The signs and symptoms
of 4_____ _____,
the presence of air in the

5_____ _____ and
mediastinal shifting, are listed.

> a. tension pneumothorax; b. pleural space;
> c. tracheal; d. absent; e. exhibits

Case study 9
You can reduce gastric
distention during 1_____
_____ by: providing
ventilations deep enough to
cause 2_____ _____ only. ◄

Quickly 3_____ a BVM
may cause enough pressure to
4_____ ___ into the oesophagus.

> a. squeezing; b. chest rise; c. artificial
> ventilations; d. force air

Case study 10
Prehospital care of an
1_____ _____ includes:
occlusive dressing, high-flow
oxygen, and rapid transport. ◄

The steps involved in
management of this injury are
2_____ _____, high-
flow oxygen, and rapid transport.
3_____ is not necessary for
each patient. Needle decompression
is not necessary if tension
pneumothorax develops. If dyspnoea
4_____ open the dressing 5__
_____ some of the pressure that
is built up. An IV lifeline should be
6_____ but large volume
fluid resuscitation should be withheld.

> a. established; b. Intubation; c. open
> pneumothorax; d. worsens; e. to relieve;
> f. occlusive dressing

Case study 11

The following are signs and symptoms of acute pulmonary embolism: rapid, laboured breathing and tachycardia. ◄

The most common signs of a 1_____ _____ (rapid 2_____ breathing and tachycardia) are given; 3_____ is usually sudden, and there may be or may not be 4_____ _____.

> a. onset; b. chest pain; c. laboured; d. pulmonary embolism

Case study 12

Which of the following are signs and symptoms of air embolism?

a) Pruritus, skin 1_____ and cyanosis, pitting oedema in the ankles

b) chest pain, sharp with sudden onset, dyspnoea with coughing ◄

c) 2_____, auditory and vestibular disturbances, headache

d) Fatigue, pain in chest and 3_____ _____, nausea, and vomiting

All other options list signs and symptoms of 4_____ _____, only choice b) includes signs of 5___ _____ (sharp chest pain with sudden onset, dyspnoea with coughing).

> a. decompression sickness; b. pallor; c. lower abdomen; d. Dizziness; e. air embolism

Case study 13

After experiencing a sudden syncopal episode, a 41-year-old female is complaining of pleuritic chest pain and shortness of breath. Her vital signs are RR = 28, P = 126, and BP = 88/60. The pulse oximeter reads 89% on high-flow oxygen. Her breath sounds are clear.

Which of the following conditions best describes the patient's signs and symptoms?

- pulmonary embolism ◄
- pulmonary oedema
- chronic bronchitis
- acute asthma

The patient's presentation points to a 1_____ _____ as the likely cause. The other conditions are not normally associated with sudden 2_____, and adventitious lung sounds like 3_____ ___ _____ should be evident, unlike the patient's clear ones.

> a. crackles or wheezes; b. pulmonary embolism; c. syncope

Case study 14

What is the most commonly used drug in the 1_____ setting for patients with asthma? – Inhaled or nebulized albuterol. ◄

Albuterol, a 2_____, is frequently given via 3_____ ___ _____ in the field.

> a. inhaler or nebulizer; b. prehospital; c. bronchodilator

Case study 15

A patient presents with a sudden onset of 1_____ _____ _____
and respiratory distress. She has 2_____ lung sounds, a pulse rate of 110 and regular, BP of 112/76, and respirations of 28. Which of the following conditions best describes this patient presentations?

- Psychogenic hyperventilation
- Acute exacerbation of asthma
- Pulmonary embolism
- Pulmonary oedema

The lack of findings is almost as important as the reported ones. For example, 3____ _____ pedal oedema, crackles, or wheezes in the lung fields, or hypertension reduces the 4_____ of pulmonary oedema. The lack of medical history or wheezes 5_____ asthma as a possible cause.

a. not having; b. possibility; c. sharp chest pain; d. minimizes; e. clear

Case study 16

What does the disease process of emphysema cause within the 1____ _____? – A loss of elasticity in the alveoli due to 2_____ _____. ◄

Patients with emphysema have a loss of 3_____ in the alveoli due to prolonged insult. Bleb formation results in decreased ability of the 4_____ to expand and contract and an overall decreased 5_____ _____ of the lungs. Ruptured blebs do not result in lung "deflation".

a. alveoli; b. surface area; c. prolonged insult; d. lung tissues; e. elasticity

Case study 17

What is the primary treatment for a patient with chronic 1_____ who is NOT severely hypoxic? – Administering low-flow oxygen via 2_____. ◄

Patients with emphysema or 3_____ _____ benefit from 4_____ of low-flow oxygen and constant monitoring.

a. cannula; b. chronic bronchitis; c. emphysema; d. administration

Case study 18

What is the treatment for someone who is suffering an 1_____ of either emphysema or chronic bronchitis and is not too hypoxic? – Establish an 2_____, position the patient seated or 3_____-_____, administer low-flow oxygen, establish an IV lifeline, and transport. ◄

4___-____ _____ is appropriate for this patient if he or she is not too hypoxic. If a patient with emphysema or chronic bronchitis is 5_____, he or she needs more oxygen.

a. semi-seated; b. Low-flow oxygen; c. exacerbation; d. hypoxic; e. airway

Case study 19

Your patient, who has had a recent tracheostomy, tried to remove himself from the 1_____ and dislodged the trach cannula. Subcutaneous emphysema is now 2_____.

• What should you do next?
  –3_____ the tracheostomy tube and insert an
  4_____ ____. ◄

If the trach tube has been dislodged, it may not be easy to reinsert, so rest it in its 5_____ _____. Placing an endotracheal tube into the stoma and 6_____ ___ ____ will help rapidly establish a patient's airway.

```
a. original position; b. Remove; c. ventilator;
d. endotracheal tube; e. inflating the cuff;
f. evident
```

Case study 20

Which technique should you use to open the airway of a trauma patient? – The jaw thrust. ◄

The 1____ _____ is used to open the airway of patients with suspected 2____ _____ _____. Any trauma patient with questionable or unknown mechanism of injury should 3__ _____ to have a cervical spine injury until it is 4_____ ___.

```
a. jaw thrust; b. be assumed; c. ruled out;
d. cervical spine injury
```

Vocabulary 6

agitated /ˈædʒ.ɪ.teɪ.tɪd/
apprehensive /ˌæp.rɪˈhen.sɪv/
artificial /ˌɑː.tɪˈfɪʃ.əl/
ventilation /ˌven.tɪˈleɪ.ʃən/
ascites /æˈsaɪ.tɪːz/
BVM, Bag Valve Mask
cannula /ˈkæn.jʊl.ə/

displacement /dɪˈspleɪs.mənt/
evaluate /ɪˈvæl.ju.eɪt/
exclude /ɪkˈsklu:d/
inhaler /ɪnˈheɪ.lər/
mediastinal /ˌmiː.di.əsˈtaɪ.nəl/
nasal /ˈneɪ.zəl/ **flaring** /fleər.ɪŋ/
nebulizer /ˈneb.jə.laɪz.ər/
Nitronox /ˌnaɪ.trə.nɒks/
nitrous oxide /ˌnaɪ.trəsˈɒk.saɪd/
overall /ˌəʊ.vəˈrɔː.l/
pedal /ˈped.əl/
pitting /pɪt.ɪŋ/ **oedema** /ɪˈdiː.mə/
pruritus /prʊəˈraɪ.təs/
questionable /ˈkwes.tʃə.nə.bļ/
recent /ˈriː.sənt/
reinsert /ˌriː.ɪnˈsɜːt/
rest /rest/
semi /ˌsem.i/ **-seated** /ˈsiː.tɪd/
squeeze /skwiːz/
stoma /ˈstəʊ.mə/
thoracic /θɔːˈræs.ɪk/ **cavity** /ˈkæv.ɪ.ti/
tracheostomy /ˌtræk.iˈɒst.ə.mi/
tug /tʌg/
unilateral /ˌjuː.nɪˈlæt.ər.əl/
vestibular /vesˈtɪb.jə.lər/

Unit 7
Case study 1

An endotracheal tube that has been advanced 1____ ___ is prone to enter: right main bronchus. ◄

Because of 2_____ appearance of the distal trachea, it is most common for an ET tube that has been inserted too far to enter the 3_____ ____ _____, resulting in atelectasis and 4_____ of the left lung.

```
a. anatomical; b. insufficiency; c. right main
bronchus; d. too far
```

Case study 2

To ensure proper placement of the endotracheal tube, you should: confirm placement of the tube by two different methods.◄

To ensure proper placement always confirm 1__ ___ _____ _____: After watching the tube pass through the 2_____ _____, assess the chest for breath sounds in numerous locations and 3_____ _____, then check the proximal end of the tube for breath condensation. You may also use one of the several commercial 4_____ _____ that monitor end-tidal CO_2 or provide an audible whistling sound to confirm 5___ _____.

a. Confirmation devices; b. air movement; c. by two different methods; d. chest expansion; f. vocal cords

Case study 3

You are 1_____ the tracheal tube when you begin to hear the sound of the patient's breathing.

- Your next action would be to: wait for the patient to inhale and insert the tube farther.◄

As the tip of the nasotracheal tube reaches the glottic opening, you should hear the 2_____ _____ of the patient. Inserting of the tube past the vocal cords is timed to the 3_____ _____ in order to minimize 4_____ against the tube itself.

a. resistance; b. inhalation phase; c. respiratory effort; d. inserting

Case study 4

After placing an endotracheal tube, you note that breath sounds are much stronger on the right side of the chest than on the left.

- What does this suggest?
  – The ET has been inserted into the right mainstem bronchus ◄

If breath sounds are 1_____ on one side than on the other, or absent 2__ ___ _____, this suggests that the tube has been inserted 3___ ___ and is resting in one bronchus.

a. stronger; b. on one side; c. too far

Case study 5

After you orally intubate a patient, your partner 1_____ the patient with a bag-valve device. You 2_____ the lung sound to confirm placement. 3__ _____ are heard over the 4_____; breath sounds are present on the right side of chest and are decreased over the left.

- What should you do next?
  –Withdraw the tube slightly after deflating the cuff, reinflate the cuff, and reevaluate lung sounds. ◄

The original breath sounds indicated that the tube was placed in the trachea, but perhaps 5___ _____. Adjusting the depth of the tube so that the 6_____ ____ is sitting just above the carina will likely resolve this situation

> a. No sounds; b. epigastrium; c. distal end; d. ventilates; e. too deep; f. auscultate

Case study 6

Which of the following is a sign of oesophageal intubation?

a) air leak heard over the trachea
b) breath sounds absent on the left
c) bilateral chest wall expansion
d) abdominal movement with ventilation ◄

Right-side-only breath sounds are a sign of right 1_____ _____, ruling out choice b). Air leak over the trachea may be the sign of an 2_____ _____ ____, ruling out choice a). Bilateral chest wall expansion is a 3_____ _____, ruling out choice c). These findings point to the need to have a good baseline assessment of 4____ _____ and respiratory status prior to performing any 5_____.

> a. interventions; b. improperly inflated cuff; c. normal finding; d. lung sounds; e. mainstem intubation

Case study 7

You use end-tidal carbon dioxide 1_____ as a tool to determine if endotracheal intubation has been 2_____ obtained.

- The absence of 3_____ _____ in exhaled air after six ventilations indicates: that the endotracheal tube has been: placed in the oesophagus.◄

No carbon dioxide after six ventilations indicates either that the tube is in the 4_____ or that the patient has been 5_____ long enough that no carbon dioxide is being produced.

> a. oesophagus; b. dead; c. carbon dioxide; d. detector; e. correctly

Case study 8

While ventilating a patient with a bag-valve mask, you note decreasing compliance.

- How should you react to this finding? – Assess the cause of this finding and try to correct it. ◄

1_____ refers to how easily air flows 2_____ ____ ____ __ the lungs. If compliance is 3_____, look for the cause by first reassessing (with look, auscultate, and feel) the 4_____ and 5_____ _____ and then looking for signs that the patient is developing a tension pneumothorax; once you find the cause, try to correct it.

> a. decreasing; b. head position; c. Compliance; d. into and out of; e. airway

Case study 9

Ventilating a patient at
30 breaths per minute with a
1_____-_____ _____ and high-flow
oxygen may result in: alkalizing
the 2_____. ◄
    3_____ may
result in respiratory 4_____,
a harmful condition to the patient.

a. alkalosis; b. bag-valve mask; c. bloodstream; d. Hyperventilation

Case study 10

To adequately ventilate a patient
with a partial laryngectomy through
a stoma, you should: 1_____ the
nose and 2_____ the mouth. ◄
    A patient with a partial
3_____ has an ability to
exhale through the mouth and nose.
Therefore, you will have to close them
in order to 4_____ air into the lungs
while providing artificial ventilations.

a. direct; b. laryngectomy; c. pinch; d. close

Case study 11

Minute respiratory 1_____
is best described as: the 2_____
__ ___ moved in and out of the
3_____ during one minute.◄

a. lungs; b. volume; c. amount of air

Case study 12

Stroke volume can be
increased by all of the following:

- Increasing 1_____ _____
- Increasing 2_____
  _____
- Decreasing afterload ◄

Preload can be increased by
increasing venous return, increasing
the contractile force of the heart,
or by decreasing 3_____.

a. venous return;◄ b. afterload; c. contractile force ◄

Case study 13

- What is the 1_____
  treatment for patients
  with suspected 2_____
  _____ thrombosis? –
  Immobilization and elevation
  of the extremity. ◄

Prehospital treatment is limited to
3_____ ___ - _____
of the extremity and transportation.

a. elevation and immobilization; b. prehospital; c. deep venous

Case study 14

A patient with nonperfusing
1_____ _____
would receive the same
treatment as a patient with:
ventricular fibrillation. ◄
    Treatment for both conditions
consists of 2_____
defibrilation; 3_____
treatment includes 4____ and drugs.
5_____ therapy depends upon
whether a normal rhythm is initiated.

a. CPR; b. immediate; c. continued; d. Additional; e. ventricular tachycardia

Case study 15

You are managing a patient with
1_____ _____ and
multifocal PVCs. Suddenly, your

patient slumps 2_____
and goes into ventricular
fibrillation. You 3_____ that
your patient is pulseless.

- Your next action would be to:
  defibrillate at 200 joules ◄

Immediate defibrillation has been
proven to be effective in terminating
4_____ _____.
Even stopping for CPR in a witnessed
event such as this may be more
5_____ than 6_____.

> a. ventricular fibrillation; b. confirm;
> c. symptomatic bradycardia; d. harmful;
> e. unconscious; f. beneficial

Case study 16

How does the Valsalva
manoeuvre improve a 1____-_____
heartbeat? – It stimulates the vagus
nerve to slow the 2_____ _____. ◄
The Valsalva manoeuvre
(bearing down against a closed
glottis) stimulates the 3_____
_____, which innervates the heart.

> a. heart rate; b. vagus nerve; c. too-rapid

Case study 17

What rhythm might indicate
a 1_____ ___ cardioversion?
– Ventricular tachycardia
at a rate of 120.◄
If the tracheal tube has
been dislodged, it may not be
easy to reinsert, so rest it in its
2_____ _____. Placing
an endotracheal tube into the
3_____ and 4_____ ___

_____ will help rapidly establish
a patient's 5_____.

> a. inflating the cuff; b. airway; c. original
> position; d. stoma; e. need for

Case study 18

What is often the first sign of
the 1_____ of the development of a
potentially lethal dysrhythmia in an
MI patient? – Changing pulse rate. ◄
A change in the 2_____
_____ may be the first sign that a
3_____ is developing; this
is why recording baseline 4_____
_____ is particularly important.

> a. dysrhythmia; b. vital signs; c. pulse rate;
> d. onset

Case study 19

What is the purpose of
performing the Sellic's manoeuvre?

- to 1_____ the
  upper-airway structures
  during BVM
- to prevent the tongue from
  2_____ the airway
- to protect a patient with
  possible spinal injury
- to prevent vomiting during
  attempts at intubation ◄

3_____ _____
is used to prevent patients from
4_____ during intubation.

> a. visualize; b. vomiting; c. Sellic's
> manoeuvre; d. blocking

Case study 20

Traumatic aortic rupture usually occurs as a result of 1_____ of the aorta at the:

- pulmonary artery
- ligamentum teres
- 2_____ nuchae
- ligamentum arteriosum ◀

Ligamentum arteriosum is the most common area for an 3_____ _____ secondary to trauma.

> a. aortic rupture; b. transection;
> c. ligamentum

Vocabulary 7

adjust /əˈdʒʌst/
alkalize /ˈælkəˌlaɪz/
arteriosum /ɑːˌtiə.riˈɒs.əm/
ligamentum /ˌlɪg.əˈmen.təm/
atelectasis /ˌætəˈlek.tə.sɪs/
carina /kəˈraɪn.ə/
condensation /ˌkɒn.denˈseɪ.ʃən/
continue /kənˈtɪn.juː/
contractile /kənˈtræk.taɪl/
CPR, Cardiopulmonary /ˌkɑː.di.əʊˈpʊl.mə.nə.ri/
Resuscitation /rɪˌsʌs.ɪˈteɪ.ʃən/
end-tidal /ˈtaɪ.dəl/
farther /ˈfɑː.ðər/
hear /hɪər/ (**heard, heard**)
heartbeat /ˈhɑːt.biːt/
improperly /ɪmˈprɒp.ər.li/
initiate /ɪˈnɪʃ.i.eɪt/
innervate /ˈɪn.ə.veɪt/
laryngectomy /ˌlær.ɪnˈdʒek.təm.i/
leak /liːk/
ligament /ˈlɪg.ə.mənt/
main /meɪn/
mainstem /meɪn.stəm/
bronchus /ˈbrɒŋ.kəs/

MI, Myocardial /maɪ.əˌkɑː. di.əl/ **Infarction** /ɪnˈfɑːk.ʃən/
multifocal /mʌl.tiˈfəʊ.kəl/
nonperfusing /ˌnɒn.pər.fjuːz.ɪŋ/
nucha /njuːkə/
oesophageal /iːˌsɒfəˈdʒiːəl/
orally /ˈɔː.rə.li/
original /əˈrɪdʒ.ɪ.nəl/
pass /pɑːs/
position /pəˈzɪʃ.ən/
proven /ˈpruː.vən/
PVCs, Premature /ˈpremə.tjʊə/
Ventricular /venˈtrɪk.jə.lər/
Contractions /kənˈtrækʃəns/
reach /riːtʃ/
recording /rɪˈkɔː.dɪŋ/
resolve /rɪˈzɒlv/
slump /slʌmp/
stroke /strəʊk/ **volume** /ˈvɒl.juːm/
teres /tiːˈriːz/ pl **teretes**
through /θruː/
tip /tɪp/
visualize /ˈvɪʒ.u.əl.aɪz/
watch /wɒtʃ/

Unit 8

Case study 1

What is the clinical significance of a first-degree AV block?

- It signals the onset of rapid cardiovascular 1_____.
- It indicates that the 2_____ _____ may drop if action is not taken.
- It can lead to syncope and angina if not corrected quickly.

- It may foreshadow development of a 3____ _____ dysrhythmia. ◄

First-degree AV block in itself calls for 4_____ only; however, it may indicate the development of a more advanced heart block.

a. heart rate; b. observation;
c. decompensation; d. more advanced

Case study 2

In the 1_____ of baseline neurological status these should be included: 2_____ to sensory stimulation, 3_____ reaction, 4_____ function. ◄

a. response; b. pupillary; c. documentation;
d. motor

Case study 3

These are signs/symptoms of an 1_____ cerebral vascular accident: 2_____ of the speech, facial 3_____, drooling, weak 4_____ _____ on the affected side. ◄

a. slurring; b. motor response; c. droop;
d. acute

Case study 4

Which term best describes the following definition? Disease of arterial vessels marked by 1_____, 2_____, and loss of elasticity in the arterial walls – Arteriosclerosis ◄
3_____ is the most common form of

arteriosclerosis, usually involving medium-sized and large arteries.

Arterionecrosis is destruction (4_____) of the arteriole.

Angina is chest 5_____ associated with a deficiency of oxygen supply to the heart muscle.

a. thickening; b. hardening; c. necrosis;
d. discomfort; e. Atherosclerosis

Case study 5

The point of maximal impulse (PMI) can usually be felt on the:

1. left 1_____ chest ◄
2. in the 2_____ line
3. at the fifth intercostals space

This is an excellent place to auscultate heart sounds and 3_____ _____.

a. apical pulse; b. anterior; c. midclavicular

Case study 6

Central neurogenic hyperventilation is commonly associated with: CNS trauma ◄
1_____ _____ hyperventilation is characterized by rapid, deep, noisy breathing and is associated with lesions of the central 2_____ _____. Cheyne-Stokes is the pattern commonly seen with 3_____ _____.

a. Central neurogenic; b. diabetic
emergencies; c. nervous system

Case study 7

The 1_____
of Type II diabetes mellitus
includes polydipsia, polyuria
and: polyphagia. ◄

Polydipsia (excessive 2_____),
polyuria (excessive 3_____)
and polyphagia (excessive 4_____)
are just a few symptoms of
5_____ diabetes mellitus.

a. hunger; b. urination; c. untreated; d. thirst;
e. pathophysiology

Case study 8

Diabetic patients may 1_____
hypoglycaemia if they take too much
2_____ or if they: exercise too
much with limited food intake. ◄

Hypoglycaemia develops
in patients with diabetes when
they take too much insulin or get
too much 3_____ for the
4_____ __ _____ they eat

a. amount of food; b. exercise; c. insulin,
d. develop

Case study 9

You are called to treat a patient
who is unconscious and responsive
to painful stimuli only. Which of
the following treatment modalities
is appropriate for this patient?

- 1_____ _____ test,
- dextrose (if indicated),
- thiamine,
- monitor, 2_____, IV,
- rapid transport

This choice gives the most
appropriate treatment protocol

for this patient. Because he is
3_____, he may be treated
under 4_____ _____.
Treatment in this case is 5_____
__ ruling out the most treatable
cause for coma-diabetes.

a. aimed at; b. unconscious; c. oxygen;
d. implied consent; e. blood glucose ◄

Case study 10

A risk factor for the
formation of atherosclerosis
is: diabetes mellitus. ◄

1____ _____ for
atherosclerosis include
diabetes, 2_____ ____,
obesity, 3____ __ _____,
hypertension, and smoking.

a. lack of exercise; b. Risk factors;
c. advanced age

Case study 11

A patient with hypoglycaemia
may present with the following
signs or symptoms?

- bizarre behaviour *
- blurred vision
- gradual onset
- bradycardia

Changes in behaviour are
the 1____ _____ signs of
hypoglycaemia. Other signs and
symptoms include 2_____,
tachycardia, and 3_____.

a. diaphoresis; b. headache; c. most common

Case study 12

You have 1_____ the airway and 2_____ the cervical spine for your patient with an altered mental status.

- What is your next priority of care? – 3____ _____ for glucose assessment and 4_____ __ __. *

The first priority for patients with 5_____ _____ _____ of unknown cause is a blood glucose determination to 6____ ___ hypoglycaemia as a potential cause.

a. rule out; b. Draw blood; c. altered mental status; d. secured; e. immobilized; f. establish an IV

Case study 13

General management for a patient with altered mental status should include the following procedure: 1_____ blood glucose levels. ◄

Patients who 2_____ ____ altered mental status should 3__ _____ high-flow oxygen, IV access, and blood glucose levels 4_____. D50 should be administered when hypoglycaemia 5__ _____.

a. present with; b. be provided; c. is suspected; d. determine; e. measured

Case study 14

What are the 1_____ _____ for the development of hyperosmolar hyperglycaemic nonketotic coma (HHNK)?

- old age, type II diabetes, coexisting cardiac or renal disease, and increased insulin requirements. ◄
- 2_____ age, type I diabetes, coexisting cardiac or respiratory disease, and decreased insulin requirements
- 3_____, type II diabetes, viral infections, chronic alcoholism, and poor carbohydrate metabolism
- coexisting kidney disease, type I diabetes, narcotics use, and 4_____ with insulin regimen

The most significant predisposing factors are old age, type II diabetes, coexisting cardiac or renal disease, and increased insulin requirements

a. young; b. predisposing factors; c. noncompliance; d. obesity

Case study 15

This statement about hypoglycaemia is correct: Hypoglycaemia may occur in 1_____ patients, especially in chronic alcoholics. ◄

Hypoglycaemia may occur in nondiabetic patients, especially in 2_____ _____ who have poor diet and the inability to properly 3_____ carbohydrates. Except in cases of alcoholism and prolonged lack of 4____ _____, nondiabetics seldom have problems with hypoglycaemia. Signs and symptoms of hypoglycaemia

have a 5_____ _____. In early
stages of hypoglycaemia, the
patient may complain of extreme
6_____ ___ _____.

a. rapid onset; b. hunger and thirst;
c. metabolize; d. food intake; e. nondiabetic;
f. chronic alcoholics

Case study 16

For which of the following
conditions would you be likely
to receive an order to administer
intravenous thiamine?

- in status 1_____
- in 2_____ shock
- hyperventilation
- profound intoxication ◄

Intravenous thiamine is
used to reverse the effects of
acute thiamine deficiency,
which may lead to seizures and
encephalopathy in 3_____.

a. alcoholics; b. metabolic; c. epilepticus

Case study 17

A patient in a very 1_____
_____ of hypoglycaemia may
complain of: hunger. ◄
The earliest 2_____
of hypoglycaemia are hunger,
anxiety, and 3_____.

a. restlessness; b. manifestations; c. early
stage

Case study 18

In a patient with 1_____
_____, assessment of he
abdomen should be performed

in the following order: inspect,
auscultate, palpate, percuss. ◄
2_____ is the obvious
first step since you are going
to look before you do anything.
3_____ may not provide
much useful information but if
you are going to auscultate, it must
be performed before palpation.
4_____ is the third step.
You can gain a lot of information
through palpation. 5_____ (if
performed) is the last assessment step.

a. Auscultation; b. Percussion; c. Palpation;
d. Inspection; e. abdominal pain

Case study 19

You respond to a 20-year-old
female complaining of dizziness
and weakness. She is slow to
1_____ to your questions but
admits to taking several diet pills a
day in an effort to quickly 2____
_____. Vitals are blood pressure
98/54, pulse 184, respirations 32,
the skin 3_____ ___ _____.

- Immediate treatment
  should include: IV,
  oxygen, Adenocard 6
  mg rapid IV push. ◄

a. loose weight; b. pale and moist; c. respond

Case study 20

Focused examination of
the abdomen of a patient who is
complaining of abdominal pain
should consist of: gentle palpation
of the entire abdomen. ◄
Use only gentle palpation 1__
___ _____. Properly performed

auscultation for _____ 2_____
takes several minutes and is of little
value to your overall treatment
3_____. Correctly performed
4_____ requires a relatively
quiet environment and an experienced
hand to be of any diagnostic value.
Continued assessment for rebound
tenderness will aggravate the patient's
5_____ and is unnecessary
once you have determined the
patient has abdominal distress.

---
a. discomfort; b. in the field; c. regimen;
d. percussion; e. bowel sounds

Vocabulary 8

Adenocard, adenosine /ə.den'ə.sin/
advanced /əd'vɑːnst/
aggravate /'æg.rə.veɪt/
aim /eɪm/ **at** /ət/
apical /'eɪ.pɪ.kəl/
arrhythmia /ə'rɪð.mi.ə/
carbohydrate /ˌkɑː.bəʊ'haɪ.dreɪt/
coexist /ˌkoʊ·ɪg'zɪst/
consent /kən'sent/
decompensation /diːˌkɒm.pen'seɪ.ʃən/
depressant /dɪ'pres.ənt/
determination /dɪˌtɜːˌmɪ'neɪ.ʃən/
dextrose /'dek.strəʊs/
encephalopathy /enˌsef.ə'lɒp.ə.θi/
female /'fiː.meɪl/
foreshadow /fɔː'ʃæd.əʊ/
formation /fɔː'meɪ.ʃən/
gentle /'dʒen.tl/
HHNK, Hyperosmolar
Hyperglycaemic Nonketotic Coma
hyperglycaemic /ˌhaɪ.pə.glaɪ.'siː.mɪk/
hyperosmolar /ˌhaɪ.pə.ɒz.
mɒ.lər/ **coma** /'kəʊmə/
hypertension /ˌhaɪ.pə'ten.ʃən/
hypoglycaemia /ˌhaɪ.pəʊ.glaɪ'siː.mi.ə/
implied /ɪm'plaɪd/

insulin /'ɪn.sjʊ.lɪn/
intercostals /ˌɪn.tə'kɒs.təlz/
interior /ɪn'tɪə.ri.ər/
intoxication /ɪnˌtɒk.sɪ'keɪ.ʃən/
loose /luːs/ **weight** /weɪt/
maximal /'mæk.sɪ.məl/
medium /miː.di.əm/
metabolize /mɪ'tæbəˌlaɪz/
modality /məʊ'dæl.ə.ti/
noncompliance /ˌnɒn.kəm'plaɪəns/
nonketotic /ˌnɒn.ke.tɒt.ɪk/
obesity /əʊ'biː.sɪ.ti/
observation /ˌɒb.zə'veɪ.ʃən/
pathophysiology /ˌpæθ.əˌfɪz.i'ɒl.ə.dʒi/
polydipsia /ˌpɒl.ɪ'dɪp.sɪ.ə/
polyphagia /ˌpɒl.ɪ'feɪ.dʒə/
present /'prez.ənt/
rebound /riː'baʊnd/
tenderness /'ten.dər.nəs/
regimen /'redʒ.ɪ.mən/
requirement /rɪ'kwaɪə.mənt/
significance /sɪg'nɪf.ɪ.kəns/
thiamine /'θaɪ.ə.miːn/
untreated /ʌn'triː.tɪd/
vasodilator /ˌveɪ.zə.daɪ'leɪ.tər/

Unit 9
Case study 1

Which is the best way to examine
a patient with abdominal pain? –
Begin palpation of all four quadrants
ending with the painful area ◄
1_____all quadrants of the
abdomen, ending where the patient
says it 2_____. Because of the
need for a quiet environment and
several minutes to 3_____ this
successfully, you should not perform
abdominal 4_____
or 5_____ in the field.

a. Palpate; b. perform; c. auscultation;
d. hurts; e. percussion

Case study 2

Which organs are contained
in the right upper quadrant of the
abdomen? – Liver, gall bladder, head
of 1_____, part of 2_____,
and part of the 3_____. ◄

a. duodenum; b. colon; c. pancreas

Case study 3

A patient who complains of
pain in the left upper abdominal
quadrant may be suffering from
which of the following?

- pancreatitis ◄
- appendicitis
- hepatitis
- diverticulitis

Pain in the left upper
quadrant is most often due to
1_____, 2_____ or
diseases of the 3_____ _____.
Appendicitis often results
in right-lower-quadrant pain, but
the actual location of the area of
the appendix that is 4_____
may result in left-lower-quadrant
or even flank pain. 5_____
results in dull right-upper-quadrant
pain that is independent of the
presence of food in the GI tract.
Diverticulitis presents much like
appendicitis, but it is generally
localized to the left lower abdomen.

a. inflamed; b. pancreatitis; c. gastritis; d. left
kidney; f. Hepatitis

Case study 4

What do orthostatic vital
sign changes suggest for a patient
with acute abdominal pain?

- the patient has
  1_____
- the patient is
  hypovolaemic ◄
- the patient has
  2_____
- the patient is a diabetic

A positive tilt test in a patient
with acute abdominal pain suggests
that the patient is 3_____
and may have impending shock.

a. hypovolaemic; b. appendicitis; c. peritonitis

Case study 5

A patient with left shoulder pain
may have a: ruptured spleen.◄
Bleeding within the abdominal
cavity can 1_____ the abdominal
surface of the 2_____, causing
3_____ _____ to the shoulder.

a. irritate; b. referred pain; c. diaphragm

Case study 6

A patient with an acute
abdomen who shows no signs of
1_____ and has stable
vital signs should be positioned:
in whatever position is 2_____
_____ for the patient. ◄
Medical patients who
are 3_____ should be in
a position of comfort.

a. stable; b. haemorrhage; c. most comfortable

Case study 7

An unrestrained driver of a small car struck a tree at high speed. He has a distended abdomen that is tender when palpated. Vital signs are pulse, 120 beats per minute; respirations, 20 per minute; and blood pressure 116/90 mmHg.

- What would be most likely cause of the 1_____ _____? – Organ damage.◄

2_____ _____ from the mechanism of injury may 3_____ __ inflammation and bleeding, resulting in the 4_____ vital signs.

a. Organ damage; b. result in; c. abdominal tenderness; d. compensatory

Case study 8

If your patient has an open abdominal wound with a loop of bowel obtruding, you should treat this with: a wet sterile dressing and an occlusive dressing. ◄

The most appropriate dressing for an evisceration is the application of a 1___ _____ _____ (which keeps the organs moist) and an 2_____ dressing (which provides a barrier against further contamination and 3___ _____).

a. wet sterile dressing; b. occlusive; c. heat loss

Case study 9

A patient has been stabbed in the back. Which of the following signs would most likely make you suspect that the patient has a 1_____ _____?

- abdominal tenderness
- haematuria ◄
- thirst
- ecchymosis to the flank

Frank blood in the 2_____ is a strong sign of injury to the kidney. 3_____ _____ is unlikely, since the kidneys are located in the retroperitoneal space. 4_____ may provide indirect information about organ involvement but is not as specific as haematuria.

a. kidney injury; b. Bruising; c. urine; d. Abdominal tenderness

Case study 10

The signs of uraemia resulting from chronic renal failure include which of the following?

- pale skin, diaphoresis, and oedematous extremities
- pasty, yellow skin and wasting of the extremities ◄
- anxiety, delirium, nausea, and hallucinations
- anorexia, watery diarrhoea, nausea, and vomiting

Signs of 1_____ _____ are pasty, yellow skin and thin extremities, urea frost is a late sign. These signs result from jaundice, poor nutrition, and 2_____ _____ in the tissues. In 3_____ _____, the potassium level can be 4_____ _____.

Pericardial tamponade and uremic encephalopathy may also be present. Coupled with 5_____ _____, non-cardiac pulmonary oedema, severe dyspnoea, ascites, neck vein distension, rales in the bases may also be seen.

a. uraemia; b. extreme cases; c. kidney failure; d. dangerously elevated; e. protein loss

Case study 11

Patients with 1_____ inflammatory disease often complain of which of the following?

- diffuse lower-abdominal pain ◄
- severe vaginal 2_____
- tearing pain in the 3_____
- 4_____ upon urination

The most common presentation of PID is 5_____, moderate to severe lower-abdominal pain, which makes 6_____ difficult.

a. pelvic; b. uterus; c. itching; d. ambulation; e. bleeding; f. diffuse

Case study 12

You respond for a 44-year-old male diabetic who is complaining of a general feeling of weakness. During your questioning, you learn that he has been "constantly 1_____ ___ _____." His breath has a 2_____ _____, and his level of consciousness appears to be diminishing.

- What 3_____ _____ is this patient

most likely suffering from? – Diabetic ketoacidosis. ◄

- What vital signs would you expect from this patient? – Warm, dry skin; tachycardia; 4_____ ◄ _____.

This patient's symptoms are most likely due to: low levels of 5_____.

- This statement is the most accurate: He has not taken his 6_____ ____ of insulin or is ill. ◄

During transport, this patient slips into unconsciousness, and his breathing becomes very deep and rapid.

- What is this pattern called? – Kussmaul's respirations. ◄

Kussmaul's respirations are very 7____ ___ _____ and represent the body's attempt to 8_____ ___ the metabolic acidosis produced by the ketones and organic acids in the blood.

- What does appropriate treatment for this patient include? – A 9_____ _____ test, IV normal saline, and a fluid bolus. ◄

a. deep and rapid; b. compensate for; c. blood glucose; d. diabetic emergency; e. insulin; ◄ f. thirsty and hungry; g. correct dose; h. fruity odour; i. increased respirations

Case study 13

What is the primary treatment of metabolic acidosis? – Ventilating the patient adequately with oxygen.◄

Treatment of 1_____ _____ consists mainly of adequate 2_____. Identification of the cause of acidosis is not as critical as identifying that it is present and beginning 3_____ _____ to prevent its worsening.

a. ventilation; b. corrective measures; c. metabolic acidosis

Case study 14

Signs of 1_____ include:

- 2_____, rapid pulse, ◄
- cold, clammy skin, ◄
- headache, ◄
- 3_____,
- Coma ◄

a. hypoglycaemia; b. irritability;◄ c. weak ◄

Case study 15

Which rhythm is likely to foreshadow the development of other, more serious 1_____? – Accelerated junctional rhythm.◄

Because the 2_____ _____ is usually ischaemia, 3_____ junctional rhythm can 4_____ into more serious dysrhythmias.

a. deteriorate; b. accelerated; c. underlying cause; d. dysrhythmias

Case study 16

What is a possible cause of pulseless electrical activity? – Hypovolemia. ◄

1_____ _____ _____ may occur secondary to a variety of 2_____ and carries a grave prognosis.

3_____ _____ include pulmonary, tension embolus pneumothorax, acidosis, cardiac tamponade, hypovolemia, hypoxia, hypothermia, hyperkalemia, AMI, and drug overdose.

Hypokalemia may cause dysrhythmias but does not usually cause PEA. Tachycardia is not considered a cause of PEA simply because the definition of PEA is a pulseless patient with a rhythm that you would normally expect to find a pulse with. In other words, tachycardia 4_____ a pulse is PEA.

a. conditions; b. without; c. Common causes; d. Pulseless electrical activity

Case study 17

Paroxysmal 1_____ _____ (PND) is commonly a sign of: left-side heart failure.◄

Left-side heart failure with pulmonary oedema is often 2_____ _____ PND. PND manifests as difficulty 3_____ when the patient 4_____ _____. As the condition worsens, many patients will report the need to sleep 5_____ ___ in a recliner.

a. lies flat; b. sitting up; c. associated with;
d. nocturnal dyspnoea; e. breathing

Case study 18

Which set of 1_____ _____ is
suggestive of left ventricular heart
failure with pulmonary oedema?

- BP elevated, pulse fast and
  2_____, respirations
  rapid and 3_____.◄

a. vital signs; b. laboured; c. irregular

Case study 19

What feature distinguishes
dissecting aortic aneurysm from
acute myocardial infarction?

- The pain of dissecting
  aortic aneurysm is severe
  from the outset ◄
- The pain of dissecting
  aortic aneurysm usually
  migrates to the right arm
- Patients with dissecting
  aortic aneurysm have
  equal peripheral pulses
- Patients with dissecting
  aortic aneurysm show signs
  of periacdial tamponade

Patients with 1_____
_____ _____ describe their
pain as 2_____ severe from
the outset, whereas the pain of
AMI tends to build 3_____.

a. extremely; b. dissecting aortic aneurysm;
c. slowly

Case study 20

These statements about
the pain that accompanies a
myocardial infarction are correct:

- Patients often describe the
  pain as "crushing" ◄
- The pain is present only
  during exertion or stress. ◄
- Pain due to AMI radiates
  like anginal pain. ◄

The pain of MI is not generally
relieved by sublingual nitroglycerin,
and intravenous morphine or
nitroglycerin, is usually necessary.
It may have all of the 1_____
_____ of angina,
making a diagnosis by 2___
_____ relatively difficult.
The pain caused by myocardial
infarction is usually relieved only
by the use of: 3_____

a. morphine; b. same characteristic; c. EMS
providers

Vocabulary 9

accelerate /əˈksel.ə.reɪt/
acute /əˈkjuːt/
ambulation /ˈæm.bjʊ.lən.ʃən/
AMI, Acute /əˈkjuːt/
Myocardial /ˌmaɪ.əˈkɑː.di.əl/
Infarction /ɪnˈfɑːk.ʃən/
barrier /ˈbær.i.ər/
breathing /ˈbriː.ðɪŋ/
build /bɪld/ (**built, built**)
colon /ˈkoʊ.lən/
constantly /ˈkɒn.stənt.li/
contamination /kənˌtæm.ɪˈneɪ.ʃən/
corrective /kəˈrek.tɪv/
crushing /ˈkrʌʃ.ɪŋ/
dangerously /ˈdeɪn.dʒər.əs.li/

delirium tremens /dɪˌlɪr.i.əmˈtrem.ənz/
dissecting /daɪˈsekt.ɪŋ/ **aortic** /eɪˈɔː.tɪk/ **aneurysm** /ˈæn.jʊə.rɪ.zəm/
duodenum /ˌdjuː.əˈdiː.nəm/
dyspnoea /dɪs.pniː.ə/
ecchymosis /ˌeki'məʊ.sɪs/
evisceration /ɪˌvɪs.əˈreɪ.ʃən/
fruity /ˈfruː.tɪ/
gastritis /gæsˈtraɪ.tɪs/
grave /greɪv/
haematuria /ˌhiː.mə.t'jʊə.ri.ə/
hallucination /həˌluː.sɪˈneɪ.ʃən/
hurt /hɜːt/ **(hurt, hurt)**
identification /aɪˌden.tɪ.fɪˈkeɪ.ʃən/
infarction /ɪnˈfɑːk.ʃən/
involvement /ɪnˈvɒlv.mənt/
irritate /ˈɪr.ɪ.teɪt/
itching /ˈɪtʃ.ɪŋ/
jaundice /ˈdʒɔːn.dɪs/
late /leɪt/
loop /luːp/
migrate /maɪˈgreɪt/
morphine /ˈmɔː.fiːn/
nitroglycerin /ˌnaɪ.trəʊˈglɪs.ər.iːn/
nocturnal /nɒkˈtɜː.nəl/
normal /ˈnɔː.məl/
obtrude /əbˈtruːd/
odour /ˈəʊdə/
orthostatic /ˌɔː.θəˈstæt.ɪk/
outset /ˈaʊt.set/
pasty /ˈpæs.ti/
PEA, Pulseless /pʌls.ləs/ **Electrical** /ɪˈlek.trɪ.kəl/ **Activity** /ækˈtɪv.ɪ.ti/
PID, Pelvic /ˈpel.vɪk/ **Inflammatory** /ɪnˈflæm.ə.tər.i/ **Disease** /dɪˈziːz/
PND, Paroxysmal /ˌpær.ɒk.ˈsɪz.məl/ **Nocturnal** /nɒkˈtɜː.nəl/ **Dyspnea** /dɪs.pniː.ə/
protein /ˈprəʊ.tiːn/
provider /prəˈvaɪ.dər/
pulseless /pʌls.ləs/
recliner /rɪˈklaɪ.nər/
retroperitoneal /ˌret.rəʊˌper.ɪ.təʊ.ˈniː.əl/

slip /slɪp/
stable /ˈsteɪ.bl̩/
suggestive /səˈdʒes.tɪv/
unrestrained /ˌʌn.rɪˈstreɪnd/
uraemia /jʊəˈriː.mi.ə/
urea /jʊəˈriː.ə/ **frost** /frɒst/
uremic /jʊəˈriː.mɪk/
ventilate /ˈven.tɪ.leɪt/

Unit 10

Case study 1

Which of the following conditions would result in an increase in a patient's PaCO$_2$?

- airway obstruction ◄
- hypoventilation ◄
- physical exertion ◄

PaCO$_2$ measures carbon dioxide levels in the 1_____, which are influenced by alterations in CO$_2$ production or 2_____.
Such levels would be increased by physical 3_____ of muscles, by hypoventilation, or by an airway 4_____.

a. elimination; b. obstruction; c. blood; d. exertion

Case study 2

The pharyngo-tracheal lumen airway should be removed if the patient: regains consciousness ◄

If the patient is unconscious and vomits, the PTL will help prevent 1_____. Instead, if a gag reflex returns, the PTL will have to 2_____ _____ before the patient 3_____.

a. vomits; b. aspiration; c. be removed

Case study 3

Which of the following patient presentations would best be managed by a nasal intubation?

- The patient is unconscious and apnoeic with a pulse
- The patient is unconscious, apnoeic, and pulseless
- The patient is unconscious, is breathing slowly, and has a gag reflex ◄
- The patient is semiconscious, is breathing slowly, and has a pulse

There must be some 1_____ respiratory effort for the 2_____ _____ to have a good chance of successful 3_____. The presentation in the last choice can probably be managed by basic airway manoeuvres.

a. placement; b. spontaneous; c. blind insertion

Case study 4

The digital intubation method used for patients who: have suspected spinal injury.◄

Because the 1_____ _____ does not require hyperextending the patient's 2_____, it is used for patients with suspected 3_____ ___ _____ injury.

a. spinal or cervical; b. digital method; c. neck

Case study 5

You are called to the home of a 26-year-old male who is having difficulty breathing. Your assessment reveals a pulse rate of 100 with a strong and regular radial pulse, a blood pressure of 132/78, and a respiratory rate of 36, laboured with audible wheezes.

The patient's skin is pale, moist, and at a normal temperature. He is having difficulty exhaling and says that he has experienced this before. He rates this event as a 9 on a 1-10 severity scale. He states that this event was unprovoked and that he has been having dyspnoea for 20-30 minutes.

- This patient is most likely suffering from which condition? – Asthma. ◄

This patient shows the clinical symptoms of 1_____. Due to the repeat nature of this episode, it is 2_____ that this is pulmonary oedema, upper-airway obstruction, or simple pneumothorax. If he were suffering from 3_____ _____, you would also expect haemoptysis.

A spontaneous (or 4_____) pneumothorax would also present with a sudden 5_____, but would most likely not also have wheezing or a history of 6_____.

- Treating this patient with nebulized steroids would: provide no immediate relief of the bronchospasm. ◄

7_____ _____ would provide no immediate relief of this

patient's bronchospasm, as they will not prevent or lessen attacks in progress. Steroid therapy is useful as a long-term 8_____ treatment.

- This patient's respiratory distress is due to: constriction of the smaller airways. ◄

9_____ of the smaller airways is causing air to be trapped in the alveoli.

- This patient's disease is regarded as: a chronic inflammatory disease. ◄

Asthma is regarded as chronic 10_____ _____. Chronic obstructive pulmonary diseases commonly include emphysema and chronic bronchitis.

This patient's respiratory distress may have been caused by one of several triggers. These 11_____ include allergens, irritants, and which of the following?

- viral infections
- hot weather
- exercise ◄
- bee stings

12_____, exercise, and irritants are common triggers of asthma attacks. Cold weather, 13_____, and anxiety are lesser triggers.

a. pulmonary oedema; b. triggers; c. simple; d. Constriction; e. inflammatory disease; f. stress; g. asthma; h. onset; i. Nebulized steroids; j. recurrence; k. suppressive; l. unlikely; m. Allergens

Case study 6

Your patient is a 51-year-old male with a history of COPD. He states that he has called EMS because he "can hardly breathe." On 1_____ assessment you 2_____ that the patient is in obvious respiratory 3_____ but not too hypoxic.

- You should: 4_____ low-flow oxygen at a rate of 2-6 L/min via 5_____ cannula. ◄

a. determine; b. administer; c. distress; d. nasal; e. initial

Case study 7

You patient is a 29-year-old female complaining of the sudden onset of severe shortness of breath and chest pain. She indicates that she 1__ _____ from surgery to her left femur after an automobile crash.

- What is this patient most likely suffering from? – Pulmonary embolism. ◄
- You would expect to find: bradycardia ◄
- You would expect to see this patient in tachycardia rather than in bradycardia due to the increasing dyspnoea and hypoxia resulting from the 2_____ _____.
- This patient s physiological problems are most likely due to what cardiac problem? – The right side of the heart pumping against increased resistance. ◄

The pulmonary embolism has caused the right side of the heart to have to pump harder against a 3_____ caused by the 4_____ _____.
This result is the severe shortness of breath and hypoxia.

- Proper management for this patient includes: – Transport in shock position. ◀
- This patient should be transported in the position in which it is easiest for her to breathe (i.e. the 5_____ _____).
- What condition is a common cause of this patient's problem? – Placement of a central line. ◀

> a. pulmonary embolism; b. is recovering; c. partial blockage; d. shock position; e. resistance

Case study 8

You are called by the police department to a neighbourhood where you encounter a male patient approximately 20-30 years old. The police officer states that neighbours called because the patient was "freaking out." 1_____ say they saw him smoking something just before he started acting in a 2_____ _____.

During your assessment, you notice that the patient is 3_____ and anxious. His pupils are 4_____, and he is hypertensive and tachycardic.

Dilated pupils, hyperactivity, tachycardia, and hypertension are classic signs of 5_____ ___. (Narcotic use would result in lethargy, stupor, and respiratory depression).

The appropriate treatment for this patient consists of oxygen, IV, ECG, monitoring and: transport. ◀
Transport is the only other treatment required for this patient. Be prepared to provide 6_____ _____ if needed.

Naloxone is used with narcotic ingestion to restore respirations and is not indicated in this patient. Activated charcoal and ipecac are indicated for 7_____ __ _____ via the oral route. This patient was reported to have inhaled (smoked) something that appears to be a 8_____.

When treating this patient, you should be prepared for which of the following complications?

- Tachycardia and 9_____ _____
- 10____ _____ any hypoglycaemia
- Dysrhythmias and seizures ◀
- Bradycardia and tachypnoea

Dysrhythmias and seizures are both serious possible 11_____ of stimulation effects from cocaine use.

a. Witnesses; b. hyperactive; c. CNS depression; d. complications; e. stimulant; f. septic shock; g. dilated; h. respiratory support; i. cocaine use; j. bizarre manner; k. poisoning or overdose

Case study 9

Which of the following requires intermediate-level 1_____ through the use of a solution of bleach and water?

- routine 2_____ measures in your station and bunkroom
- any items that have come into contact with 3_____ _____
- any 4_____ that were used in any invasive procedures
- all items that have come into contact with intact skin ◄

Intermediate-level disinfection is used for all instruments and supplies that have come into contact with 5_____ ____.

a. mucous membranes; b. intact skin; c. house cleaning; d. disinfection; e. instruments

Case study 10

Why must your assessment be especially diligent in an intoxicated patient?

- Alcohol can decrease pain tolerance in the patient.
- Alcohol can mask signs and symptoms of injury. ◄
- Alcohol can increase the patient's willingness to 1_____.

- Alcohol can 2_____ an injury's effect on the patient's level of consciousness

As a mild anaesthetic, ethanol can reduce the patient's 3_____ of pain. It will be important to carefully and completely 4_____ the patient for any 5_____ _____.

a. unnoticed injuries; b. examine; c. perception; d. cooperate; e. decrease

Case study 11

Early symptoms of overdose of tricyclic 1_____ include which of the following?

- tachycardia and a wide QRS complex ◄
- 2_____, vomiting, and severe diarrhoea
- psychosis and bizarre behavioural changes
- altered mental status and 3_____ _____
- 4_____ with wide QRS complex is an important early sign of 5_____. High doses of sodium bicarbonate IV drip will help control dysrhythmias.

a. toxicity; b. antidepressants; c. tachycardia; d. slurred speech; e. nausea

Case study 12

What do the symptoms of acetaminophen 1_____ include?

- 2_____, vomiting, malaise, diaphoresis, and right-upper-quadrant pain ◄
- nausea, 3_____, confusion, lethargy, seizures, and dysrhythmias
- altered 4_____ _____, hypotension, slurred speech, and bradycardia
- nausea, dilated 5_____, rambling speech, lethargy, headache, and dizziness

a. mental status; b. overdose; c. vomiting;
d. nausea; e. pupils

Case study 13

1_____ administration of sodium bicarbonate may be ordered for a patient who has overdosed on which of the following drugs?

- acetaminophen
- benzodiazepines
- narcotics
- antidepressants ◄

2_____ _____ is sometimes ordered in the field for ingestions of tricyclic 3_____ with cardiac symptoms (wide-complex tachycardias).

a. Prehospital; b. Sodium bicarbonate;
c. antidepressants

Case study 14

An adult patient has overdosed on an unknown medication in a 1_____ _____. She is 2_____, oriented, and refusing treatment and transport.

- What is your most appropriate next action? – Consult with 3_____ _____ to transport the patient. ◄

This patient may not have the right to 4_____ _____ and transport due to the actions she has taken. Consulting with medical direction on how to 5_____ _____ this patient may be helpful.

a. best approach; b. medical direction;
c. suicide attempt; d. refuse treatment; e. alert

Case study 15

What are the classic symptoms of 1_____ overdose? – Respiratory depression and constricted pupils. ◄
2_____ _____ and 3_____ ("pin-point") pupils are classic symptoms of narcotic overdose.

a. constricted; b. Respiratory depression;
c. narcotic

Case study 16

Chest pain associated with stable angina may be caused by: a built up of lactic acid and CO_2 ◄
1_____ _____ is caused by a temporary low flow state in the 2_____ _____ that does not lead to 3_____ _____ __ _____ (infarction). During hypoperfusion, lactic acid and excessive carbon dioxide are not 4_____ _____, causing irritation and pain.

a. Stable angina; b. coronary arteries;
c. carried away; d. cell injury or death

Case study 17

The pain of 1_____
_____ is brought on by:

- exercise or stress ◄
- imminent AMI
- difficulty breathing
- 2_____ of nitroglycerin

3_____ of stable angina are brought on by exercise or by stress and are usually easily managed.

a. Attacks; b. overuse; c. stable angina

Case study 18

A patient's signs and symptoms include orthopnoea, spasmodic coughing, agitation, cyanosis, rales, jugular vein distention, and elevated blood pressure, pulse, and respirations. What 1_____ should you suspect?

- left heart failure ◄
- right heart failure
- 2_____ infarction
- 3_____ shock

Listed are 4_____ signs and symptoms of left heart failure with 5_____ oedema.

a. cardiogenic; b. classic; c. pulmonary;
d. condition; e. myocardial

Case study 19

A primary reason for administering oxygen to a patient with AMI is to:

- help limit the infarct size ◄
- 1_____ pulmonary oedema

- reduce 2_____ and fear
- treat ventricular dysrhythmias

3_____ can help limit the size of the infarct by 4_____ oxygen delivery to the heart muscle.

a. Oxygen; b. increasing; c. prevent;
d. anxiety

Case study 20

You have just started an IV lifeline, but the fluid is not flowing properly.

- What is the first thing you should do troubleshoot this situation? – Make sure the constricting band has been removed.◄

Proper flow cannot be achieved if the constriction band (1_____) is not removed.
Care of the patient with 2_____ _____ is similar to care for the patient with:
3_____ _____
Patients with cardiac contusion can present with the symptoms of myocardial infarction, including 4____-_____ dysrhythmias. Care is similar to care of any cardiac patient.

a. myocardial infarction; b. tourniquet; c. life-
threatening; d. cardiac contusion

Vocabulary 10

acetaminophen /əˌsiː.təˈmɪn.ə.fen/
anaesthetic /ˌæn.əsˈθet.ɪk/
antidepressant /ˌæn.ti.dɪˈpres.ənt/

213

asthma /ˈæs.mə/
attack /əˈtæk/
band /bænd/
bee /biː/
benzodiazepines /benˈzɒ.dɪ.azˈe.pɪːnz/
bleach /bliːtʃ/
bunkroom /bʌŋk.rʊm/
carry /ˈkær.i/
charcoal /ˈtʃɑːr.koʊl/
cocaine /kəʊˈkeɪn/
cooperate /kəʊˈɒp.ər.eɪt/
diligent /ˈdɪl.ɪ.dʒənt/
disinfection /ˌdɪs.ɪnˈfek.ˈʃən/
drip /drɪp/
ethanol /ˈeθ.ə.nɒl/
freak /friːk/
haemoptysis /hiːˈmɒ.ptɪ.sɪs/
instead /ɪnˈsted/
instrument /ˈɪn.strə.mənt/
intermediate /ˌɪn.təˈmiː.di.ət/
invasive /ɪnˈveɪ.sɪv/
ipecac /ˈɪp.ɪ.kæk/
irritant /ˈɪr.ɪ.tənt/
item /ˈaɪ.təm/
life-threatening /ˈlaɪfˌθret.ən.ɪŋ/
lumen /ˈlu.mən/ pl -mina
malaise /mælˈeɪz/
manner /ˈmæn.ər/
Naloxone /nəˈlɒksəʊn/
narcotic /nɑːˈkɒt.ɪk/
ordered /ˈɔː.dəd/
overuse /ˌəʊ.vəˈjuːz/
perception /pəˈsep.ʃən/
progress /ˈprəʊ.gres/
rambling /ˈræm.blɪŋ/
rate /reɪt/
recover /rɪˈkʌv.ər/
recurrence /rɪˈkʌr.əns/
refuse /rɪˈfjuːz/
relief /rɪˈliːf/
restore /rɪˈstɔːr/
scale /skeɪl/
septic /ˈsep.tɪk/
spasmodic /spæzˈmɒd.ɪk/
station /ˈsteɪ.ʃən/

stimulant /ˈstɪm.jʊ.lənt/
stupor /ˈstjuː.pər/
suppressive /səˈpres.ɪv/
surgery /ˈsɜː.dʒər.i/
tourniquet /ˈtʊə.nɪ.keɪ/
troubleshoot /ˈtrʌb.ḷ.ʃuːt/
unnoticed /ʌnˈnəʊ.tɪst/
unprovoked /ˌʌn.prəˈvəʊkt/
willingness /ˈwɪl.ɪŋ.nəs/

Unit 11
Case study 1
What factor would 1_____ a patient from receiving thrombolytic therapy after an AMI? – He or she has had recent ulcer or gastrointestinal bleeding. ◀

Any condition that would present a significant 2_____ _____ excludes a patient from receiving 3_____ therapy.

> a. thrombolytic; b. bleeding hazard; c. exclude

Case study 2
In which of the following situation should a paramedic perform an 1_____ _____ first? –

- During cardiac arrest at a swimming pool. ◀
- When the patient is in a toxic environment.
- When the scene is not yet secured by law enforcement.
- During a rescue from a fully involved structure fire.

Before assessing 2_____,

_____, ___ _____,

it is necessary to remove the

patient (and yourself) to a
place of relative 3_____.

a. safety; b. airway, breathing, and
circulation; c. initial assessment

Case study 3

What are the signs of
1_____ _____ in a
patient who is receiving IV fluids?
– Dyspnoea, rales, and rhonchi.◀
2_____, rales, and rhonchi
are classic signs of fluid overload,
which is usually first 3_____
__ pulmonary oedema.

a. manifested as; b. Dyspnoea; c. circulatory
overload

Case study 4

When caring for a patient
with a pulmonary contusion, it
is essential not to: overload the
patient with IV fluids ◀
1_____ _____
involves bruising of the lung tissue.
It is essential not to 2_____ a
patient suffering from pulmonary
contusion with fluids, as this can
quickly lead to pulmonary 3_____.
The patient should be given high-flow
oxygen and intubated if necessary.
Immobilization on a 4_____
may be necessary depending on the
mechanism of injury. If so, the head
of the board may be elevated slightly
to improve 5_____ _____.

a. Pulmonary contusion; b. respiratory effect;
c. overload; d. backboard; e. oedema

Case study 5

A single-lead ECG
tracing is useful for obtaining
information about the heart.

- What can be determined
  from a single-lead ECG
  tracing? – Timing of
  electrical impulse travel. ◀

A single-lead ECG, used
for1_____ _____, can
be used to determine the 2_____
_____, 3_____ and the length
of time it takes for the 4_____
to travel through the heart.

a. heart rate; b. impulse; c. routine
monitoring; d. regularity

Case study 6

What does the treatment for a
patient whose ECG shows premature
1_____ _____ include?
– Observation only as long as the
patient remains asymptomatic ◀
If the patient is
2_____, this arrhythmia
requires 3_____ only.

a. observation; b. asymptomatic; c. atrial
contractions

Case study 7

Why are 1_____ _____
and 2_____ _____ considered
major goals for prehospital care
of MI patients? – Both anxiety
and pain increase heart rate and
myocardial oxygen demand.◀
Anxiety and pain can increase
the heart rate and, therefore, the3
_____ _____ of the myocardium.

a. oxygen demand; b. relieving pain; c. easing anxiety

Case study 8

Some treatments for suspected 1__ _____ mask the elevated cardiac enzyme levels that are used to diagnose MI in the hospital setting.

- To prevent this, you should NOT administer: any drugs via the IM route ◄

2_____ injections can injure muscle tissues, causing the release of 3_____ that may mask the cardiac enzymes that are locked for to confirm a 4_____ of MI.

a. Intramuscular; b. diagnosis; c. enzymes; d. MI patients

Case study 9

Patients who 1____ _____ and have altered mental status are best transported: left-lateral recumbent. ◄

There is significant opportunity for the loss of 2_____ _____ for this patient. A lateral recumbent position will allow 3_____ _____ of the airway in the case of vomiting, as well as 4____ _____ for suctioning.

a. easy access; b. airway control; c. passive draining; d. have overdosed

Case study 10

Blood flows from the pulmonary veins into which structure?

- left atrium of the heart. ◄
- right atrium of the heart
- capillaries of the lungs

- right ventricle of the heart

Oxygenated blood flows from the lungs, 1___ the pulmonary veins, into the 2_____ _____. From there, it passes through the mitral (3_____) valve into the left 4_____. It passes through the aortic 5_____ then enters into the 6_____.

a. via; b. ventricle; c. left atrium; d. valve; e. bicuspid, f. aorta

Case study 11

Blood enters the right atrium of the heart through which of the following structures?

- tricuspid valve
- right ventricle
- left pulmonary arteries
- superior and inferior vena cava ◄

Blood enters the right atrium through the superior and inferior 1____ ____ and is pumped through the 2_____ _____ into the right ventricle. From there, it passes through the pulmonic valve into the 3_____ _____ and into the lungs.

Simultaneous palpation of the apical impulse and the 4_____ _____ allows you to assess the relationship between the: ventricular contractions and pulse.

Determining the relationship between the 5_____ _____ and the carotid pulse may give you

the first indication of a 6_____
_____, such as a
dysrhythmia. To assess central and
7_____ circulation, you
should assess 8_____ (central)
and 9_____ (peripheral) pulses.

Remember that the cardiovascular
system requires three factors to work
effectively: intact and functioning
pump, an adequate circulating blood
volume, and a container (vascular
vessels) of the appropriate size to
10_____ the blood effectively.

An apical pulse indicates
the pump is functioning, and
a carotid pulse shows you that
the circulating blood volume
is reaching target tissues.

a. peripheral; b. apical impulse; c. circulate; d. tricuspid valve; e. carotid; f. cardiac irregularity; g. carotid pulse; h. pulmonary arteries; i. vena cava; j. radial

Case study 12

What do the signs and symptoms
of hypertensive crisis include?

- 1_____ oedema,
  tachycardia, tachypnoea,
  and venous 2_____
- paralysis, seizures,
  headache, and 3_____
  level of consciousness
- severe 4_____
  distress, apprehension,
  cyanosis, and diaphoresis
- restlessness, confusion,
  blurred vision, nausea,
  and vomiting ◄

a. congestion; b. respiratory; c. pitting; d. altered

Case study 13

These statements are true
regarding 1_____:

- It may cause a reflex
  hypothermia. ◄
- 2_____ may result
  which can lead to a rise
  in core temperature. ◄
- 101.84° F (38.8° C) should be
  used as a target temperature
  to prevent overcooling. ◄

Using of ice or cold water may
cause a 3_____ _____
and cause the patient to shiver which
will raise the body temperature
again. Hypothermia can result
from: an increase in 4____ _____, a
decrease in 5____ _____, or
a combination of these two factors.

a. heat loss; b. reflex hypothermia; c. heat production; d. overcooling; e. Shivering

Case study 14

In case of 1_____:
Do not 2____ if there is any
possibility of refreezing. ◄
A golden rule for the
treatment of 3_____ _____ is
to never thaw it if there is any
possibility of 4_____.

a. refreezing; b. frostbite; c. frozen flesh; d. thaw

Case study 15

A 17 year-old male complains
of a steadily worsening headache

several days after being struck in the head during football practice.

- What injury best describes this patient's presentation? – Subdural haematoma. ◄

A subdural bleed occurs when a 1_____ ____ bleeds into the area below the 2____ _____. It may take some time before 3_____ from the bleeding is high enough 4__ _____ clinical signs and symptoms.

> a. dura mater; b. pressure; c. to cause; d. small vein

Case study 16

1_____ _____ allows you to continuously record: pulse rate and oxygen saturation. ◄

Once it is attached to the patient's 2_____, the pulse oximeter will continuously record the 3_____ ____ and oxygen saturation level.

> a. pulse rate; b. finger; c. Pulse oximetry

Case study 17

What would a pulse oximetry reading of 88% indicate for your patient with acute respiratory distress?

- normal oxygenation
- mild hypoxia
- moderate 1_____
- severe hypoxia ◄

A pulse oximetry 2_____ around 90% for a patient in a normal 3_____ indicates that severe hypoxia is present. 4_____ pulse oximetry readings

are from 93% to 100%, with 93-95 considered the lower end of normal.

> a. atmosphere; b. reading; c. Normal; d. hypoxia

Case study 18

Pulsus paradoxus means: an abnormal decrease in the systolic pressure during inspiration compared with expiration.◄

Pulsus paradoxus is an 1_____ _____ in systolic blood pressure that drops more than 10 to 15 mmHg during inspiration 2_____ ____ expiration. Normally, the systolic pressure decreases 5 to 10 mmHg during inspiration, however, in patients with asthma, COPD, pericardial tamponade, pulmonary embolism or tension pneumothorax, the 3_____ _____ may decrease 10 to 20 mmHg or more during 4_____.

> a. systolic pressure; b. inspiration; c. compared with; d. abnormal decrease

Case study 19

Bradycardia refers to a heart rate that is less than how many beats per minute? – 60.

- What 1_____ is considered normal in an athletic adult? – Bradycardia.◄

Sinus 2_____, or a heartbeat slower than 60 BPM, is often 3_____ _____, particularly in an 4_____ adult.

a. athletic; b. considered normal;
c. dysrhythmia; d. bradycardia

Case study 20

The wheezing associated with left-sided 1_____ _____ results from: fluid in the lungs.◄

The wheezing, due to 2_____ of smooth muscle in the lung, is a reaction to 3_____ in the lung spaces.

Which of the following are signs and symptoms of right-side heart failure? Tachycardia, 4_____ _____, and 5_____ ____ distention.

a. fluid; b. heart failure; c. jugular vein;
d. bronchoconstriction; e. peripheral oedema

Vocabulary 11

aorta /eɪˈɔː.tə/
asymptomatic /əˌsɪmp.təˈmæt.ɪk/
atmosphere /ˈæt.mə.sfɪər/
atrial /ˈeɪ.tri.əl/
bicuspid valve /baɪˈkʌs.pɪdˌvælv/
board /bɔːd/
circulate /ˈsɜː.kjʊ.leɪt/
continuously /kənˈtɪn.ju.əs.li/
core /kɔːr/
drain /dreɪn/
dura mater /ˌdjuə.rəˈmeɪ.tə/
easing /ˈiː.z.ɪŋ/
frostbite /ˈfrɒst.baɪt/
golden /ˈɡəʊl.dən/ **rule** /ruːl/
hypertensive /ˌhaɪ.pəˈten.sɪv/
impulse /ˈɪm.pʌls/
irregularity /ɪˌreg.jəˈlær.ə.ti/
law /lɔː/ **enforcement** /ɪnˈfɔːs.mənt/
lead /liːd/
mitral valve /ˈmaɪ.trəlˌvælv/
overcooling /ˌəʊ.vəˈkuː.lɪŋ/
paralysis /pəˈræl.ə.sɪs/

production /prəˈdʌk.ʃən/
pulse /pʌls/
pump /pʌmp/
regularity /ˌreg.jʊˈlær.ə.ti/
relationship /rɪˈleɪ.ʃən.ʃɪp/
routine /ruːˈtiːn/
saturation /ˌsæt.jʊˈreɪ.ʃən/
severe /sɪˈvɪə/
simultaneous /ˌsɪm.əlˈteɪ.ni.əs/
smooth /smuːð/
steadily /ˈsted.ɪ.li/
structure /ˈstrʌk.tʃər/
superior /suːˈpɪə.ri.ər/
target /ˈtɑː.gɪt/
thrombolytic /ˌθrɒm.bɒˈlit.ɪk/ **therapy** /ˈθer.ə.pi/
timing /ˈtaɪ.mɪŋ/
tracing /ˈtreɪ.sɪŋ/
travel /ˈtræv.əl/
tricuspid valve /traɪˈkʌs.pɪdˌvælv/
ulcer /ˈʌl.sər/
vena cava /ˌviː.nəˈkeɪ.və/

Unit 12

Case study 1

Why is 1_____ sulphate used in the management of AMI patients? – To relieve pain and reduce myocardial 2_____ _____. ◄

Morphine relieves pain, decreases venous return, and reduces the oxygen demand of the 3_____.

a. oxygen demand; b. morphine;
c. myocardium

Case study 2

If it is not treated, left ventricular failure results in:

- ischemic heart disease
- pulmonary oedema.◄

219

- chronic hypertension
- cor pulmonale

Because the left ventricle fails to function as an effective forward 1_____, left ventricular failure results in pulmonary oedema as blood 2_____ __ _____ the pulmonary circulation. Left-side failure is common 3_____ an 4_____ myocardial infarction and can also lead to cardiogenic 5_____.

a. acute; b. shock; c. following; d. pump, e. back up into

Case study 3

What is the most common cause of cardiogenic shock? – Left ventricular failure.◄

Cardiogenic shock 1_____ most often from 2____ _____ _____ following acute MI.

- Management of left-side heart failure 3_____ high-flow oxygen, IV of crystalloid solution, ECG monitoring, and the administration of: morphine sulphate and nitroglycerin. ◄

a. includes; b. left ventricular failure; c. results

Case study 4

Which of the following indicates that of 1____ _____ is developing cardiogenic shock?

- increasing pain

- narrowing pulse pressure
- falling blood pressure ◄
- sinus bradycardia

2_____ _____ _____, especially a systolic pressure lower than 80 mmHg together with decreasing level of consciousness, is a sign of 3_____ _____ in an AMI patient. Reflex 4_____ may develop as the patient's body attempts to compensate for the shock.

a. AMI patient; b. Falling blood pressure; c. cardiogenic shock; d. tachycardia

Case study 5

A patient is complaining of chest pressure and shortness of breath. He has jugular venous distension and pedal oedema. His lung sounds are clear and equal.

- What condition most likely causes these findings? – 1_____-____ heart failure ◄

Reduced 2_____ _____ of the right ventricle causes 3_____ _____ to "back up" into the 4_____ vascular system, causing 5_____ as evidenced by the pedal oedema and JVD. Lung fields that are past the cardiac 6_____ remain free from fluid.

a. systemic; b. congestion; c. pumping capacity; d. Right-side; e. insufficiency; f. blood flow

Case study 6

What is the most common complication of an acute 1_____ _____? – The onset of a dysrhythmia. ◄

The most common complication of MI is 2_____, and some dysrhythmias are or become 3_____ _____. Cardiogenic shock may develop 4_____ an AMI, especially when the site of infarction is the 5_____ _____. 6_____ is a complication of arterosclerosis and coronary artery vasoconstriction or vasospasm.

> a. left ventricle; b. life threatening;
> c. myocardial infarction; d. following;
> e. dysrhythmia; f. Angina

Case study 7

What is the 1_____ _____ of management for a patient with left ventricle failure and pulmonary oedema? – Decrease venous return. ◄

The primary goal for patients with left ventricular failure and pulmonary oedema is to reduce 2_____ _____ to the heart, or preload, and thus reduce pressure on the 3_____ _____.

- What set of vital signs is suggestive of left ventricular 4_____ _____ with pulmonary oedema? – BP elevated, pulse 5_____ _____ _____, respirations 6_____ ____ _____. ◄

> a. fast and irregular; b. pulmonary
> circulation; c. heart failure; d. rapid and
> laboured; e. venous return; f. primary goal

Case study 8

You arrive to a golf course to find a 45-year-old male unconscious and 1_____ ____ _____ but only with movement. The patient was 2_____ in the head by a golf ball travelling at 3_____ _____. His eyes are closed; 4_____ _____ reveals his left pupil is 2 mm, and the right is 8 mm and not reactive to light.

This patient moves upper extremities to localized pain and moves lower extremities spontaneously. He is breathing full deep respirations at a rate of 24 per minute.

- You would expect the vital signs of this patient generally to follow the following grouping: RR increased, HR decreased, BP increased. ◄

This set of vitals, known as Cushing's 5_____ (respiratory rate increased, heart rate decreased, blood pressure increased) is common in close head injuries.

- Treatment of this patient would include: placing the patient in the sniffing position to facilitate airflow. ◄

Placing the victim in the 6_____ _____ manipulates the head and neck, facilitating airflow.

- A patient with a closed head injury should be closely 7_____ ____ all of the following: hypovolemic shock, respiratory alkalosis, hypoxic seizures. ◄

a. monitored for; b. triad; c. pupil examination; d. responsive to pain; e. sniffing position; f. high velocity; g. struck

Case study 9

Which group of vital signs changes is associated with Cushing's reflex?

- Increased 1_____ pressure, decreased 2_____ _____, decreased 3_____ ____, increased temperature. ◄

a. blood; b. pulse rate; c. respiratory rate

Case study 10

For which of the following procedures is a gown most necessary?

- Emergency childbirth ◄
- Drawing blood
- Suctioning the airway
- Cleaning instruments

Wearing a 1____ is considered part of your BSI precautions with 2_____ _____. It may be recommended in some circumstances when 3_____ instruments or 4_____ _____, but is not generally needed.

a. drawing blood; b. cleaning; c. emergency childbirth; d. gown

Case study 11

All of the following statements about use of disposable gloves and infection control are true:

- Gloves should be worn for 1_____ _____ contact. ◄
- Gloves should be 2_____ for each new patient contact. ◄
- Gloves cannot protect healthcare workers from 3_____ _____. ◄

Gloves cannot protect you from food-or-airborne-infectious agents. 4_____ should not eat or drink inside the ambulance.

a. changed; b. needle sticks; c. Personnel; d. every patient

Case study 12

How should you maintain respiratory isolation when transporting a patient 1_____ __ having tuberculosis? - Have both patient and personnel wear the appropriate masks. ◄

Both the patient and all 2_____ who come in contact with him or her should wear the appropriate masks in order to maintain 3_____ _____. For you own legal protection and for the optimal patient care you should never transport a patient unattended in your Unit.

a. suspected of; b. personnel; c. respiratory isolation

Case study 13

For which procedure is it necessary to wear gloves, gown, mask, and protective eyewear? – 1_____ with an emergency childbirth. ◄

Childbirth can be extremely messy and involve blood, 2_____ _____, urine, and 3_____, so maximum 4_____ should be taken to include gloves, gowns, mask, and 5___ _____.
For routine IV starts and IM drug administration gloves alone should be appropriate BSI.

a. amniotic fluid; b. faeces; c. eye protection; d. precautions; e. Assisting

Case study 14

The use of alcohol-based wash is encouraged in the 1_____ _____ when hot water and soap are not readily available.

- To be most effective, you should also: 2_____ gross matter from your hands, since alcohol cannot penetrate protein. ◄

Alcohol can never take the place of thorough hand washing, but when 3____ _____ is not possible, it can offer some protection. To be 4____ _____, you should first remove debris, as alcohol cannot penetrate large protein molecules. Saturate your hands and use 5_____ to remove particulate matter. Let your hands 6___ ___ immediately, but do not wipe them dry, as this 7_____ the effectiveness of the alcohol.

a. friction; b. diminishes; c. hand washing; d. field setting; e. most effective; f. air dry; g. remove

Case study 15

For what procedure is it necessary to wear a mask and protective eyewear? – Endotracheal intubation. ◄

Commonly accepted infection-control guidelines, call for all personnel to wear 1_____ and 2_____ _____ for any procedure that carries the risk of 3_____ ___ blood, 4_____, or other fluids.

a. vomitus; b. splashing of; c. masks; d. protective eyewear

Case study 16

When you are 1_____ ___ more than one 2_____ _____ at a time, you should change your gloves: for each new patient. ◄

Changing gloves for 3____ new patient contact prevents 4_____-_____.

a. each; b. caring for; c. cross-contamination; d. trauma patient

Case study 17

Which form of hepatitis poses the lowest risk to paramedics? – Hepatitis A.◄

Hepatitis A is 1_____ (or food-borne) and poses the least risk for 2_____ _____.

Hepatitis B virus (HBV) is the 3_____ occupational blood-borne pathogen risk for paramedics.

Hepatitis C occurs most frequently in 4__ ____ _____ and paramedics are at risk of contracting this disease from accidental needle sticks.

Hepatitis D occurs only in individuals who currently have or had HBV infection, and who, therefore also pose a 5____ ____ to EMS providers.

a. IV drug abusers; b. enteric; c. high risk; d. healthcare providers; e. major

Case study 18

Which type of hepatitis is spread via the faecal or oral route? – Hepatitis A.◄

Hepatitis A is spread by the 1_____-____ _____ and is most commonly acquired from eating 2_____ ____. Hepatitis B, C, and D are all 3_____-_____ diseases.

a. blood-borne; b. contaminated food; c. faecal-oral route

Case study 19

Which infection is transmitted through contact with blood or body secretions? – Hepatitis B.◄

1_____ _ is a blood-borne disease that is transmitted through contact with blood or 2____ _____.

• What is the most common job-related source of HIV infections among healthcare workers? – An accidental needle stick. ◄

3_____ _____ _____ are the most common source of work-related 4____ and hepatitis B infections in healthcare workers.

a. Accidental needle sticks; b. Hepatitis B; c. HIV; d. body secretions

Case study 20

What does the initial symptom of infection with HIV primarily consist of? – Mild fatigue and 1_____.◄

Although symptoms of full-blown AIDS include Kaposi's sarcoma and opportunistic infections, 2_____ _____ of infection with the AIDS virus often consist only of 3____ _____ and fever.

a. initial symptoms; b. mild fatigue; c. fever

Vocabulary 12

accidental /ˌæk.sɪˈden.təl/
acquire /əˈkwaɪər/
ambulance /ˈæm.bjʊ.ləns/
blood-borne /bɔːn/
blow /bləʊ/ **(blew, blown)**
BSI, British /ˈbrɪt.ɪʃ/ **Standards** /ˈstæn.dədz/ **Institution** /ˌɪnstɪˈtjuːʃən/
capacity /kəˈpæs.ə.ti/
childbirth /ˈtʃaɪld.bɜːθ/
common /ˈkɒmən/
consist /kənˈsɪst/
contract /kənˈtrækt/
cor /kɔːr/ **pulmonale** /ˈpʊl.mə.nə.l/
effectiveness /ɪˈfek.tɪv.nəs/
eyewear /ˈaɪweər/
faeces /ˈfiː.siːz/
food /fuːd/ **-borne** /bɔːn/
full-blown /ˌfʊlˈbləʊn/
gross /grəʊs/
ischemic /ɪsˈkiː.mɪk/

Kaposi's /kæˈpəʊ.sɪz/
sarcoma /sɑːˈkəʊ.mə/
matter /ˈmæt.ər/
messy /ˈmes.i/
needle /ˈniː.dl̩/ **stick** /stɪk/
occupational /ˌɒk.jʊˈpeɪʃən.əl/
opportunistic /ˌɒp.ə.tjuːˈnɪs.tɪk/
particulate /pəˈtɪ.kjuː.lət/
primarily /praɪˈmer.ɪ.li/
sarcoma /sɑːˈkəʊ.mə/
saturate /ˈsæt.jʊ.reɪt/
splash /splæʃ/
sulphate /ˈsʌl.feɪt/
triad /ˈtraɪ.æd/
wear /weər/
wipe /waɪp/
wiper /ˈwaɪp.ər/
worker /ˈwɜː.kər/

Unit 13

Case study 1

When performing
1_____-_____ rescues, use of
personal 2_____ _____
is required when: the rescuer
works in any and all water. ◄
No matter the 3_____
_____ of the rescuer, personal
safety is absolute.

```
a. competency level; b. flotation device;
c. water-related
```

Case study 2

1_____ may be best defined
as: a general feeling of uneasiness. ◄
Anxiety is a general feeling of
uneasiness or 2_____ that
results from 3_____ _____.

```
a. apprehension; b. Anxiety; c. continued
stress
```

Case study 3

Hyperventilation syndrome most
often occurs in a patient who is:

- anxious and upset ◄
- asthmatic
- in shock from 1_____
- a heavy smoker

2_____
syndrome which is characterized
by rapid breathing, is most
often caused by 3_____,
though it is also associated
with many organic diseases.

```
a. anxiety; b. Hyperventilation; c. trauma
```

Case study 4

When interviewing patients who
are distraught or potentially violent,
you should do all of the following:

- Remove the patient from
  the crisis situation as
  quickly as possible. ◄
- 1_____ the patient
  to explain the situation in
  his or her own words. ◄
- Avoid 2_____ ____
  or shouting at the person
  who is distraught. ◄

The purpose of the interview is to
3_____ the patient and to 4_____ as
much information as possible, not to
tell the patient what you think. There
is a time to reorient patients to reality,
but first you must work to calm them
down and 5____ _____ _____.

```
a. gain their trust; b. calm; c. obtain;
d. arguing with; e. Encourage
```

Case study 5

Your partner and you are evaluating a patient experiencing a behavioural emergency. Your patient is visibly 1_____ and is pacing back and forth. He is verbally confrontational, and his hands are in fists. At times, he displays 2_____ _____, both physical, and verbal.

- What action is most appropriate for this situation? – Observe the scene for danger. ◀

Given the circumstances, not enough personnel are available 3__ _____ this patient if he becomes violent. 4_____ a hands-on assessment may not be possible given the state of the patient's 5_____. Constantly being aware of your surroundings will provide the greatest 6_____ __ _____.

a. level of safety; b. aggressive actions; c. upset; d. behaviour; e. to restrain; f. Conducting

Case study 6

This is an example of 1_____ and labelling the patient's feelings: "You seem angry. Do you want to tell me about it?" ◀
This is one way to acknowledge what a patient is feeling, and to 2_____ him or her to 3_____ those feelings without passing 4_____ or getting too personal.

a. encourage; b. judgement; c. express; d. acknowledging

Case study 7

Your patient is a 46-year-old male with a 1____ _____ of mental illness. He appears depressed and 2_____. Suddenly, he begins to sob uncontrollably.

- What should you do?
  – Maintain _ 3____, _____, and non-judgemental attitude.◀

a. a quiet listening; b. long history; c. withdrawn

Case study 8

Your friend experiences severe 1_____ when crossing bridges. She 2_____ to cross any bridges and alters her travel routes accordingly. This is an example of which of the following conditions?

- psychosis
- neurosis
- delirium
- phobia ◀

An intense fear of something is called a phobia. A 3_____ can be disabling and its 4_____ is often unknown.

a. cause; b. phobia; c. anxiety; d. refuses

Case study 9

Depression is an example of a(n):

- psychiatric 1_____
- psychosis
- mood disorder ◀
- 2_____ disease

Depression is a 3_____ _____; depressed patients feel 4_____ and helpless and manifest many physical symptoms as well.

a. hopeless; b. illness; c. mood disorder; d. organic

Case study 10

What term best describes a patient who talks nonstop and is restless and 1_____?

- manic ◄
- depressed
- demented
- schizophrenic

A patient who is displaying manic symptoms is 2_____ or extremely active and 3_____ constantly. The patient may be extremely 4_____ or violent. If the patient has bipolar disorder, he or she may swing between periods of 5_____ and depression.

a. talks; b. overactive; c. suspicious; d. restless; e. mania

Case study 11

A patient with bipolar disorder usually suffers from which of the following?

- frequent 1_____
- delusional behaviour
- wide mood swings ◄
- 2_____ thoughts

A patient with 3_____ _____ (manic-depressive disorder) suffers from wide

mood swings from 4_____ to debilitating depression.

a. euphoria; b. bipolar disorder; c. hallucinations; d. psychotic

Case study 12

You are interviewing a 43-year-old woman with a long history of schizophrenia. She appears to try to cooperate, but there are long periods of 1_____ in your conversation while she listens to her "voices". How should you respond during her silence?

- 2_____ your last question.
- Restate her last 3_____
- Remain quietly attentive. ◄
- Tell her an interesting 4_____.

During silences, remain relaxed and attentive and wait to hear what the patient has to say. This will 5_____ the patient to talk.

a. story; b. Repeat; c. response; d. encourage; e. silence

Case study 13

What is the difference between bulimia and anorexia nervosa?

- They are basically the same disorder.
- Bulimia is an intense fear of 1_____, whereas anorexia is the insatiable 2_____ for food.
- Anorexia is less severe and rarely life-threatening.

- Bulimia is more
  often associated with
  binge eating ◄

Bulimia and anorexia nervosa
are both common 3_____
_____. They both have similar
features such as misperceptions
of 4____ _____. Bulimia is
characterized by 5_____ _____
followed by self-induced vomiting.

> a. eating disorders; b. binge eating; c. body
> image; d. obesity; e. craving

Case study 14
Which statement about
suicide is correct?

- People who talk about
  suicide rarely attempt
  it by deadly means.
- Suicidal patients are
  1_____ ____ and require
  institutionalization.
- The 2_____ _____ is
  lowest during holiday
  seasons or birthdays.
- There is a high correlation
  between suicide attempts and
  alcohol consumption. ◄

3_____ is a CNS depressant.
People who do not frequently
drink often do so before killing
themselves; furthermore, alcoholics
are 4_____ __ commit suicide.
Suicidal patient may or may not
openly discuss suicide, but you
should 5____ _____ any
discussion of it by your patient.
Most 6_____ _____ are
depressed, not mentally ill. Holidays

and important personal times such
as anniversaries, birthdays, or death-
days are high times for suicide.

> a. suicide rate; b. take seriously; c. prone to;
> d. suicidal patients; e. mentally ill; f. Alcohol

Case study 15
There are many factors to
consider when assessing a patient
for suicide risk. Which of the
following accurately accounts
for one 1_____ ____ factor?

- Young women 2_____
  _____ more often
  than young men do.
- Generally men 3_____
  attempt suicide more
  often than women do.
- Caucasian males, over
  85 years of age have the
  highest suicide rate. ◄

Women attempt suicide
more often, but men are 4_____
_____ at it. Also, men
choose more 5_____ _____.
About 60% of the people who
successfully commit suicide have
a history of 6_____ attempts

> a. more successful; b. deadly means;
> c. commit suicide; d. suicide risk; e. attempt;
> f. previous

Case study 16
Hyperextension of the neck,
followed by hyperflexion, is
common in: rear-end impacts.◄
A strong force 1_____ the
car from behind causes the head
to 2____ _____. If the head

restraint is not properly placed, it can actually act as a fulcrum, causing the neck to 3_____. Then the head snaps forward, with the chin pointing toward the chest. This 4_____ a severe 5_____ of the neck.

a. Hyperextend; b. results in; c. hyperflexion; d. move backward; e. striking

Case study 17

On reaching the scene of a single-motor vehicle accident, you note that the driver is pinned behind the 1_____ _____. You also note the presence of two sets of spiderweb patterns on the 2_____.

- What does this alert you to? - Look for a second 3_____ in this accident. ◄

The spiderweb pattern is made when a victim's head 4_____ the windshield. Two spiderweb patterns 5_____ that there is a second victim somewhere on the scene

a. victim; b. windshield; c. hits; d. indicate; e. steering wheel

Case study 18

Your Unit is dispatched to a single automobile crash. The patient's car hit a large tree 1_____-__. The patient, a young adult woman, is found conscious and alert but 2_____ in the car. The 3___ ___ deployed and she denies any head or neck pain, although she does 4_____ of hip and leg pain.

After a difficult, 20-minute 5_____, the patient is finally released from the car. Suddenly, your patient's vital signs begin to 6_____.

- This patient is most likely transitioning from: compensated shock to decompensated shock ◄

This patient's body is showing signs that it can no longer 7_____ for the damage done by the traumatic event. In addition, 8_____ metabolic products may have been trapped in the injured tissues and now be circulating back toward the heart. These toxins may result in cardiac dysrhythmias or cardiac arrest.

a. extrication; b. head-on; c. air bag; d. collapse; e. trapped; f. complain; g. toxic; i. compensate

Case study 19

Your patient is a middle-aged female who has been in a car accident. Because the initial assessment showed no immediate 1_____ _____, you are now treating her most serious injuries, which include a 2_____ broken femur and kneecap.

- After 3_____ the injured leg and rechecking the pulse, motor responses, and sensation, you should: repeat the initial assessment. ◄

Quickly repeat the initial assessment after every 4_____ _____.
You and your partner have had your attention on her lower extremity for a few minutes, and now you should refocus and repeat an 5___ _____.

Cervical immobilization with a collar should be completed 6_____ ____ treatment of the leg. Proximal pulse check is part of the reassessment that occurs immediately after stabilizing and 7_____ the leg.

> a. life threats, b. prior to, c. stabilizing, d. significant intervention, e. suspected, f. splinting, g. ABC assessment

Case study 20
Cardiogenic shock can result in all of the following:
1_____, respiratory failure, an elevated heart rate. ◄
2_____ _____ is the most severe form of pump 3_____ that often results in dysrrhythmias, hypotension, respiratory failure, and possibly organ failure. The heart rate is initially elevated as the body attempts to 4_____ for the shock.

> a. compensate; b. Cardiogenic shock; c. failure; d. dysrhythmias

Vocabulary 13

acknowledge /ək'nɒl.ɪdʒ/
angry /'æŋ.gri/
anniversary /ˌæn.ɪ'vɜː.sər.i/
anorexia nervosa / æn.əˌrek.si.ə.nə'vəʊ.sə/

argue /'ɑːg.juː/
attentive /ə'ten.tɪv/
attitude /'æt.ɪ.tjuːd/
aware /ə'weər/
back /bæk/ **and forth** /fɔːθ/
backward /'bæk.wəd/
binge eating /bɪndʒ i:.tɪŋ/
bipolar disorder /baɪ'pəʊ.lə.dɪˌsɔː.dər/
bulimia /buˌlɪm.i.ə/
calm (sb) /kɑːm/ **down** /daʊn/
Caucasian /kɔː'keɪ.ʒən/
collar /'kɑl.ər/
commit /kə'mɪt/
competency /'kɒmpɪtənsi/
confrontational /ˌkɒn.frʌn'teɪ.ʃən.əl/
consumption /kən'sʌmp.ʃən/
correlation /ˌkɒr.ə'leɪ.ʃən/
craving /'kreɪ.vɪŋ/
crossing /'krɒs.ɪŋ/
deadly /'ded.li/
debilitating /dɪ'bɪl.ɪ.teɪt.ɪŋ/
decompensated /diː'kɒmpenˌseɪt.əd/
delusional /dɪ'luː.ʒən.əl/
demented /dɪ'men.tɪd/
deploy /dɪ'plɔɪ/
disable /dɪ'seɪbl/
distraught /dɪ'strɔːt/
euphoria /juː'fɔː.ri.ə/
feeling /'fiː.lɪŋ/
fist /fɪst/
fulcrum /'fʊl.krəm/
furthermore /ˌfɜː.ðə'mɔːr/
hands-on /ˌhænd.'zɒn/
helpless /'helplɪs/
hit /hɪt/
hopeless /'həʊp.ləs/
image /'ɪm.ɪdʒ/
insatiable /ɪn'seɪ.ʃə.bḷ/
institutionalization /ˌɪnt. stɪˌtjuː.ʃən.əl.aɪ'zeɪ.ʃən/
kneecap /'niː.kæp/
label /ˌleɪ.bəl/
manic /'mæn.ɪk/
means /miːnz/
mentally /'men.təl.i/

misperception /ˌmɪs.pəˈsep.ʃən/
mood /muːd/
mood /muːd/ **swing** /swɪŋ/
neurosis /njʊəˈrəʊ.sɪs/
no matter /ˈmætə/
overactive /ˈəʊ.vərˈæk.tɪv/
pace /peɪs/
phobia /ˈfəʊ.bi.ə/
psychiatric /ˌsaɪ.kiˈæt.rɪk/
psychosis /saɪˈkəʊ.sɪs/
psychotic /saɪˈkɒt.ɪk/
rate /reɪt/
rear-end /ˈrɪə.rend/
recheck /riː.tʃek/
relaxed /rɪˈlækst/
reorient /riː.ˈɔː.ri.ənt/
restate /ˌriːˈsteɪt/
restrain /rɪˈstreɪn/
schizophrenic /ˌskɪt.səˈfren.ɪk/
self-induced /ˌself.ɪnˈdjuːst/
seriously /ˈsɪə.ri.əs.li/
silence /ˈsaɪ.ləns/
snap /snæp/
sob /sɒb/
spiderweb /ˈspaɪ.dəz.web/
striking /ˈstraɪ.kɪŋ/
suicidal /ˌsuː.ɪˈsaɪdəl/
surroundings /səˈraʊn.dɪŋz/
swing /swɪŋ/
thought /θɔːt/
toward /təˈwɔːd/
toxin /ˈtɒk.sɪn/
trust /trʌst/
uncontrollably /ˌʌn.kənˈtrəʊ.lə.bli/
uneasiness /ʌnˈiː.zi.nəs/
upset /ʌpˈset/
visibly /ˈvɪz.ɪ.bli/
windshield /ˈwɪnd.ʃiːld/
withdrawn /wɪðˈdrɔːn/

Unit 14

Case study 1

Why are patients who present with pulmonary oedema usually assumed to have had a 1_____ _____? – An AMI is frequently a 2_____ _____ of left ventricle failure. ◄

Myocardial infarction is a common cause of left ventricular failure, which is closely associated with 3_____ _____.

a. pulmonary oedema; b. common cause; c. myocardial infarction

Case study 2

A patient suspected of showing early signs of shock should usually be placed 1_____ with his or her feet 2_____.

- When is this position 3_____?
  – When a head injury is suspected. ◄

The shock position is used only if 4_____ _____ is not suspected.

a. Contraindicated; b. elevated; c. head injury; d. supine

Case study 3

What is a differential sign or symptom of 1_____ _____ associated with trauma? – Warm, dry skin distal to the 2_____ _____. ◄

This condition reflects a specific sign that points directly to the 3_____ _____ of hypoperfusion.

a. Underlying cause; b. spinal shock; c. injury site

Case study 4

You are called to a rooftop for a 17-year-old female who was sunbathing. She is alert and oriented and states she was using lotion without any SPF protection to "speed up her tan". She was in the sun from 9 A.M. to 2 P.M. She is in 1_____ _____ and requests that you help her off the rooftop. She has blisters 2_____ the entire front of her body. You should 3_____ this patient to have:

- first-degree burns
- minor burns
- critical burns ◄

This should be classified as a 4_____ _____ with over 50% body surface area containing 5_____-_____ _____.

a. critical burn; b. consider; c. second-degree burns; d. significant pain; e. covering

Case study 5

This statement is true regarding 1_____ burns: Both 2_____ _____ _____ cause burns by 3_____ cell membranes and damaging tissues on contact. ◄

a. chemical; b. disrupting; c. acids and alkalis

Case study 6

The first step in managing a burn patient is to: stop the burning process. ◄

The first step 1__ _____ a burn is to stop the 2_____ _____ or the burn will continue to 3_____ more tissue. Then attention should be turned toward ensuring and maintaining an 4_____ _____.

a. destroy; b. in managing; c. adequate airway; d. burning process

Case study 7

A burn wound that blisters is an example of a: Second-degree burn. ◄
1_____ _____ is characteristic of 2_____-_____ burns.

a. Second-degree; b. Blister formation

Case study 8

An adult who has burns over both sides of one arm and both sides of one leg would be 1_____ to have total burns over what percentage of body surface area? - 27%. ◄
Using the 2_____ __ _____, this patient has burns over 27% of her body 3_____ _____ (both sides of one arm = 9%, 4_____ _____ of one leg = 18%).

a. both sides; b. surface area; c. rule of nines; d. estimated

Case study 9

Your patient has a chemical burn to her face and eyes. How should you treat this? – Brush the chemical away and then flush the area with 1_____ _____ of clean cold water. ◄

The correct treatment for most chemical burns is to 2_____ the area with 3____ _____ immediately and to continue this treatment even during the transport.

a. cool water; b. copious amounts; c. flush

Case study 10

A child has 1_____-_____ burns over the front of her trunk and the entire front of her right leg.

- According to the rule of nines, what 2_____ of her body surface area is affected? – 25%. ◄

According to the rule of nines as applied to 3_____ _____, the front or back of the trunk each represents 18% of the body surface and the front of one leg represents 7% with the entire leg 4_____ ___ 14%.

a. counting for; b. paediatric injuries; c. percentage; d. third-degree

Case study 11

How should you treat a patient who has sustained dry lime burns to the hand and arm? – Brush the lime away and then flood the skin with cool water. ◄

Brush away as much of the 1_____ as possible, then flood the 2_____ ____ with water. 3_____ chemicals are generally not recommended because the use of one chemical to neutralize another usually 4_____

__ the release of heat and the 5_____ of a third chemical.

a. formation; b. Neutralizing; c. burned area; d. results in; e. lime

Case study 12

An adult patient has burns 1_____ her 2_____ and upper back.

- Using the rule of nines, this patient's burns cover: 18% of her body surface area. ◄

The head and 3_____ _____ are each equal to 9% of body surface area.

a. covering; b. upper back; c. head

Case study 13

How would you 1_____ a burn that is pearly white and almost 2_____? - Third-degree burn. ◄

This is often appearance of a 3_____-_____ burn, which is painless because of 4_____ of nerve cells.

a. third-degree; b. classify; c. destruction; d. painless

Case study 14

In a patient with a 1_____ ____ to the airway, it is 2_____ to watch for signs and symptoms of the development of:

- laryngeal oedema ◄
- shock
- respiratory arrest
- bronchiolitis

A burn to the highly vascularized tissue of the airway can lead to 3_____ _____ and a 4_____ airway.

| a. blocked; b. laryngeal oedema; c. critical; d. thermal burn |

Case study 15

An adult with burns over the front of both arms and the chest is burned over what percentage of her body area (BSA)? - 18% ◄

Using the rule of nines, the 1_____ of each arm 2_____ 4.5% BSA, and the 3_____ _____ equals 9%; the 4_____ ____ covers 18% of the BSA.

| a. total burn; b. anterior chest; d. equals; e. front |

Case study 16

How will the skin over a second-degree burn appear?

- bright red
- mottled red ◄
- pearly white
- charred black.

The skin over a second-degree burn will most frequently appear 1_____ ____ and contain 2_____. A first-degree burn will appear 3_____ ____ and a third-degree burn will be 4_____ __ _____.

| a. charred or white; b. bright red; c. blisters; d. mottled red |

Case study 17

Which patient is most likely to need burn centre care versus 1_____ _____ care:

- female, age 34, second-degree burn over 10% of BSA (body surface area)
- male, age 46, third-degree burn over a small area of the back
- female, age 52, second-degree burns to face and right hand. ◄
- male, age 27, second-degree burn over entire left arm excluding hand

Severe partial 2_____ or full thickness burns to the face, hands, feet, and perineum often 3_____ burn centre care, even if they are 4___ _____.

| a. not extensive; b. warrant; c. thickness; d. trauma centre |

Case study 18

Prehospital care for a patient who has moderate to severe burns includes: dry sterile dressings, two IV lines with large-bore catheters held at a TKO rate. ◄

Cover the burns with dry 1_____ _____ and be ready to institute aggressive 2_____ _____ as ordered. 3___ _____ offer comfort but 4_____ the body temperature in a severely burned patient. 5___-____ dressings are being used with some success, but the standard of care is still dry sterile dressing.

a. Gel-type; b. lower; c. fluid therapy;
d. sterile dressings; e. Wet dressings ◄

Case study 19

What 1_____ _____ involves
a fracture of both the 2_____
and 3_____ bone? – LeFort II. ◄

a. maxillary; b. facial injury; c. nasal

Case study 20

The next two questions are
based on the following scenario:

You are called to the scene of a
22-year old man who was playing in a
softball tournament. He was hit in the
eye with a hard-hit line-drive softball.
According to his teammates he was
knocked to the ground and had a brief
1_____ __ _____ that
lasted approximately seven seconds.

While assessing the injured eye
you notice a collection of blood in
front of the patient's pupil and iris.

- What is your differential
  diagnosis? – Hyphema.◄

2_____ is a collection of
blood in the 3_____ _____
of the eye due to trauma. This type
of injury is a potential threat to the
patient's 4_____ and requires
5_____ by an ophthalmologist.

- How would you transport
  this patient to the hospital?
  – Immobilized on a
  6_____ with the head
  of backboard elevated. *

A c- spine injury should
be suspected with any injury

to the head. Treatment of this
patient would include 7____
_____ _____. The
preferred position of transport of a
hyphema is with the head elevated,
therefore, you should 8_____
the head of the backboard.

a. backboard; b. anterior chamber;
c. full body immobilization; d. elevate;
e. Hyphema; f. evaluation; g. vision; h. loss of
consciousness

Vocabulary 14

bright /braɪt/
brush /brʌʃ/
BSA, Body /ˈbɒd.i/ **Surface** /
ˈsɜː.fɪs/ **Area** /ˈeərɪə/
charred /tʃɑːd/
classify /ˈklæs.ɪ.faɪ/
count /kaʊnt/ **for**
covering /ˈkʌv.ər.ɪŋ/
degree /dɪˈgriː/
drive /draɪv/
ensure /ɪnˈʃɔːr/
excluding /ɪkˈskluː.dɪŋ/
extensive /ɪkˈsten.sɪv/
flood /flʌd/
gel /dʒel/
hard /hɑːd/
held /held/
institute /ˈɪn.stɪ.tjuːt/
iris /ˈaɪrɪs/
large-bore /lɑːdʒ/, /bɔː/
last /lɑːst/
LeFort II fracture / ˈfræk.tʃə/
lime /laɪm/
line /laɪn/
lotion /ˈləʊ.ʃən/
maxillary /mækˈsɪl.ər.i/
ophthalmologist /ˌɒf.θælˈmɒl.ə.dʒɪst/
painless /ˈpeɪn.ləs/
pearly /ˈpɜː.li/
percentage /pəˈsen.tɪdʒ/

rooftop /'ruːf.tɒp/
rule/ ruːl/ of nines /naɪnz/
speed up /'spiːd.ʌp/
tan /tæn/
therapy /'θer.ə.pi/
TKO, To Keep venous /'viː.nəs/
infusion / ɪn'fjuː.ʒən/ line /laɪn/ open
trunk /trʌŋk/

Unit 15
Case study 1

You are called to a scene of a motor vehicle collision (MVC). During your initial assessment, you find an 1_____32-year-old male with multiple 2_____ to his face and head. He has 3_____ respirations and a weak, 4_____ peripheral pulse.

• Your first action would be: to open the airway with a jaw thrust and immobilize the 5_____ _____. ◄

Always remember ABCs.

a. thready; b. cervical spine; c. contusions; d. snoring; e. unresponsive

Case study 2

Intracranial haemorrhage can cause vital sign changes characterized by an 1_____ systolic blood pressure and 2_____ pulse pressure, bradycardia, and 3_____ respiratory rate.

• These changes are collectively 4_____: Cushing's reflex. ◄

Change in vital signs that are associated with increased 5_____ _____ is termed Cushing's reflex.

a. widening; b. intracranial pressure; c. termed; d. increasing; e. irregular

Case study 3

A patient suspected of showing early signs of shock should usually be placed 1_____ with his or her feet 2_____.

• When is this position 3_____? – When a head injury is suspected.◄

The shock position is used only if 4_____ _____ is not suspected.

a. Contraindicated; b. elevated; c. head injury; d. supine

Case study 4

Your patient is a victim of an assault, is experiencing malocclusion and numbness to the chin. There is also a suspected nasal fracture, and significant facial bleeding and bruising.

• What treatment is appropriate for this patient? – 1_____ the cervical spine, control the airway but avoid the use of a nasopharyngeal airway, control bleeding, and transport ◄

Patients with 2_____ _____ also have suspected

3_____ _____ and should be immobilized appropriately.

Avoid the use of any 4_____ _____ manipulations in a patient with facial fractures, as the device could be introduced directly into the brain __ 5_____ through the area of the fracture.

Cardiac (6___) monitoring, pulse oximetry, and other 7_____ _____ are always appropriate when you have a 8_____ injured patient.

> a. Monitoring devices; b. nasopharyngeal airway; c. by perforating; d. spinal trauma; e. Secure; f. ECG; g. facial fractures; h. seriously

Case study 5

The presence of marked purplish-red racoon eyes on a patient in prehospital environment should lead you to suspect: significant previous head injury. ◄

Periorbital ecchymosis or 1_____ ____, presents as bruises, 2_____ _____ the eyes. It often indicates basal or other 3_____ _____, but when seen in the prehospital environment, it suggests significant 4_____ _____ because this condition takes time to develop after injury.

The earliest finding you would note with a newly developing skull injury is 5_____ _____ of the soft tissues around each eye that may make it difficult even to open the eyes to check 6_____.

> a. Extreme swelling; b. skull fracture; c. previous injury; d. racoon eyes; e. circling around; f. pupils

Case study 6

The collective change in vital signs associated with the 1____ _____ of increasing 2_____ pressure consists of: slowing pulse rate, deep or erratic respirations, 3_____ blood pressure. ◄

> a. intracranial; b. increasing; c. late stages

Case study 7

Your patient is a car-crash victim who was unconscious prior to your arrival but is now awake. As you examine the patient, you notice that he is becoming 1_____.

- What should you suspect? – Epidural haematoma formation.◄

The symptoms are indicative of a mass-forming 2_____ in the head, such as an epidural or subdural 3_____. When a patient has a simple concussion, his or her mental status will continue to 4_____ with time.

> a. improve; b. lesion; c. haematoma; d. disoriented

Case study 8

The 1_____ _____ of a patient experiencing the later stages of increased intracranial pressure will be characterized by: increased blood pressure, 2_____ pulse and 3_____ ____. ◄

a. respiratory rate; b. decreased; c. vital signs

Case study 9

Your patient suffers a head trauma that results in a 1_____ loss of consciousness followed by a complete 2_____ __ _____.

- What is the term for this condition? – Cerebral concussion. ◄

A concussion is a 3_____ loss of consciousness in response to 4____ _____.

a. head trauma, b. brief, c. transient, d. return of function

Case study 10

An injury to the brain 1_____ the site of a blunt force impact is called: Contrecoup ◄
During significant force to the head, the brain can 2_____ ___ _____ the opposite side of the skull away from the 3_____ _____. This mechanism can cause a contrecoup injury.

a. opposite; b. original force; c. shift and strike

Case study 11

A 1_____ _____ is a brain injury that: is on the opposite side of the head from the impact site.◄
A contrecoup injury is an injury to the brain opposite the 2_____ _____; it results from the brain's 3_____ movement against the skull wall following the initial

impact. The 4____ _____ is noted at the site of the actual impact.

a. coup injury; b. impact site; c. countrecoup contusion; d. rebounding

Case study 12

What is the management for a patient with a head injury and an unusual respiratory pattern? – Rapid transport because of possible brain stem injury. ◄
1_____ respiratory patterns indicate the possibility of 2_____ _____ injury and call for rapid transport of the patient. Hyperventilation should be used only when you strongly suspect herniation is 3_____. It is not indicated for the 4_____ _____ of increasing ICP. You should ventilate the patient at a normal rate with 100% oxygen.

a. brain stem; b. Unusual; c. routine treatment; d. occurring

Case study 13

Battle's sign and periorbital ecchymosis are classic signs of: a basilar skull fracture. ◄
Battle's sign is the 1_____-___-_____ discoloration just behind the ears. 2_____ _____ is black-and-blue discoloration around the eyes, also known as raccoon eyes. Both are classic signs of a 3_____ _____ _____.

a. basilar skull fracture; b. Periorbital ecchymosis; c. black-and-blue

Case study 14

What is a positive Battle's sign an indication of? – Basilar skull fracture.◄

1_____ _____ is noted as discoloration of the 2_____ _____ behind the ear. It is an indication that blood has collected there following a 3_____ _____ _____. Periorbital ecchymosis (racoon's eyes) is noted with 4_____ ____ _____ trauma and fractures. 5_____ _____ may have no external manifestations or signs.

a. Subarachnoid bleeding; b. basal skull fracture; c. facial and orbital; d. mastoid area; e. Battle's sign

Case study 15

The signs and symptoms of 1_____ _____ include which of the following:

- disorientation and confusion, decreased pulse and blood pressure, and cyanosis
- transient loss of consciousness, headache, 2_____, nausea, and 3_____. ◄
- 4_____ of cerebrospinal fluid, headache, and bleeding from the nose or ears
- headache, Battle's sign, confusion, lethargy, and rapid loss of 5_____

a. consciousness; b. vomiting; c. drowsiness; d. cerebral haemorrhage; e. leakage

Case study 16

What is the greatest concern when a person experiences blunt force trauma to the head?

- It can interrupt the integrity of the blood brain barrier.
- It can cause a significant increase in intracranial pressure. ◄
- It can cause significant ringin in the ears.
- It can lacerate the scalp, causing bleeding.

Increased ICP after a 1_____ _____ trauma to the head is potentially 2_____ and will need close monitoring and management both 3_____ and within the 4_____ department.

a. emergency; b. lethal; c. prehospital; d. blunt force

Case study 17

A patient who complains of a 1_____ ___ _____ complete loss of vision in one eye is most likely suffering from: retinal detachment. ◄

The 2_____ captures the image that is projected by the 3____ of the eye. It can spontaneously 4_____ from the inner surface of the eye, causing sudden and painless loss of vision.

a. lens; b. separate; c. retina; d. sudden and painless

Case study 18

Your patient, a car accident victim, 1_____ __ seeing

"a dark " in front of one eye.
What should you suspect? –
Retinal detachment ◄

A patient with a detached
2_____ will often complain of
3_____ a dark curtain in front
of part of the field of vision.

a. seeing; b. retina; c. complains of

Case study 19

An unconscious patient who has
one 1_____ _____ that is reactive
to light is showing early signs to:
increased intracranial pressure. ◄

A unilaterally dilated pupil may
be an 2_____ _____ of increased
intracranial pressure. As 3_____
increases in the brain, it puts
pressure on the 4_____ _____ that
is located near the area of swelling.

a. swelling; b. early sign; c. optic nerve;
d. dilated pupil

Case study 20

Lifting improperly may
most likely result in an injury
to: lumbar part of the back ◄
The 1_____ _____ will
be most impacted from an
2_____ _____
_____; the 3_____ _____ is
also at risk for injury, although
such injuries are less likely.

a. cervical spine; b. unevenly distributed
load; c. lumbar spine

Vocabulary 15

basal /ˈbeɪsəl/
Battle's /ˈbætəl/ **sign** /saɪn/

brief /briːf/
capture /ˈkæp.tʃər/
cerebrospinal /ˌser.ɪ.brəˈspaɪ.nəl/
circle /ˈsɜː.kl̩/
collectively /kəˈlek.tɪv.li/
curtain /ˈkɜː.tən/
department /dɪˈpɑːt.mənt/
detached /dɪˈtætʃt/
discoloration /dɪˌskʌl.əˈreɪ.ʃən/
distribute /dɪˈstrɪb.juːt/
environment /ɪnˈvaɪ.rən.mənt/
examine /ɪgˈzæm.ɪn/
external /ɪkˈstɜː.nəl/
ICP, Intracranial /ɪn.trəˈkreɪ.ni.əl/ **Pressure** /ˈpreʃ.ər/
integrity /ɪnˈteg.rə.ti/
interrupt /ˌɪn.təˈrʌpt/
introduce /ˌɪn.trəˈdjuːs/
jaw /dʒɔː/ **thrust** /θrʌst/
lacerate /ˈlæs.ər.eɪt/
leakage /ˈliː.kɪdʒ/
lens /lenz/
lumbar /ˈlʌm.bər/
malocclusion /ˌmæl.əˈkluː.ʒən/
manipulation /məˌnɪp.jʊˈleɪ.ʃən/
mastoid /ˈmæs.tɔɪd/
MVC, Motor /ˈməʊtə/ **Vehicle** /ˈviː.ɪ.kl̩/ **Collision** /kəˈlɪʒ.ən/
numbness /ˈnʌm.nəs/
opposite /ˈɒp.ə.zɪt/
perforate /ˈpɜː.fər.eɪt/
periorbital /ˌper.ɪˈɔːbɪtəl/
projected /prəˈdʒek.tɪd/
purplish /ˈpɜː.pl̩.ɪʃ/
reactive /riˈæk.tɪv/
respiratory /rɪˈspɪr.ə.tər.i/
pattern /ˈpæt.ən/
ringing /ˈrɪŋ.ɪŋ/
showing /ˈʃəʊ.ɪŋ/ v
subarachnoid /ˌsʌb.əˈræk.nɔɪd/
term /tɜːm/
transient /ˈtræn.zi.ənt/
unevenly /ʌnˈiː.vən.li/
unilaterally /ˌjuː.nɪˈlæt.ər.əl.i/
widen /ˈwaɪ.dən/

Unit 16

Case study 1

A patient has fallen off a 20-foot (6.1 m) ladder, striking his back on a railing. He is experiencing pain at the injury site and a loss of bladder control.

- Which part of the 1_____ ____ is most like affected by this mechanism? – Sacral.◄

Nerves that assist in 2_____ _____ exit from the 3_____ _____, located above the 4_____.

a. sacral spine; b. bladder control; c. spinal cord; d. coccyx

Case study 2

Your patient is a 65-year-old male who is complaining of pain in his abdomen, back, and flanks. His blood pressure is 90/60. On examination, you note that the 1_____ _____ are markedly the weaker than radial pulses.

- What should you do next? – Treat for hypovolemia and transport rapidly. ◄

The patient is showing signs and symptoms of abdominal 2_____ _____. Do not palpate the abdomen 3_____; treat decreased tissue perfusion and transport.

a. unnecessarily; b. aortic aneurism; c. femoral pulses

Case study 3

Moving the outstretched forearm so that the anterior surface is facing downward is called: pronation. ◄

Pronation is rotating the forearm so that the 1_____ _____ is facing down.

Supination is the 2_____ movement.

Rotation is the type of movement required to 3_____ the extremity.

4_____ occurred when the arm was moved out from the midline of the body.

a. Extension; b. reposition; c. anterior surface; d. opposite

Case study 4

The posterior tibial pulse can 1__ _____ near the: medial ankle bone. ◄

The posterior tibial pulse is assessed just 2_____ ___ _____ to where the 3_____ bone protrudes medially. The pulse located on the top of the foot is the 4_____ _____. The popliteal pulse is located 5_____ the knee.

a. dorsalis pedis; b. behind; c. below and posterior; d. be palpated; e. ankle

Case study 5

Where would you expect to see a wound that is described as 1_____ to the knee? – Calf ◄

Distal refers to a location that is 2_____ from the trunk of the body than the 3_____ _____.

a. reference point; b. further; c. distal

Case study 6

Which type of wound would most likely require a tourniquet?

- 1_____ of the hand at the forearm
- bilateral open 2_____ of the femurs
- below-the-knee amputation by a machine
- tearing injury ot the upper arm ◄

Because a tearing wound can tear multiple large 3_____ _____, bleeding may be particularly difficult to control, and a 4_____ may be necessary. Clean amputations often do not require a tourniquet.

a. tourniquet; b. blood vessels; c. amputation; d. fractures

Case study 7

Your patient has a suspected hand injury.

- How can you best immobilize the hand in the position of function? – Place a roll of 1_____ _____ into the palm and 2_____ the hand to a splint. ◄

The 3_____ _____, or position of function, for the hand 4__ _____ by using a gauze roller bandage (or similar material) placed inside the 5_____ with the 6_____ curled around it. The hand, 7_____, ___ _____ should then be splinted with a board, wire ladder, or 8_____-_____ splint.

a. palm; b. neutral position; c. vacuum-type; d. gauze bandage; e. wrist and forearm; f. secure; g. fingers; h. is achieved

Case study 8

A greenstick fracture is one that is: partial ◄
A 1_____ _____ is a partial fracture that is on only one side of the 2____ ____.
These fractures are noted most frequently 3__ _____ but may also be seen in adults.

a. long bone; b. in children; c. greenstick fracture

Case study 9

An injury to the 1_____ surrounding a joint that is marked by pain, swelling, and bruising is called: a sprain ◄
A sprain is a partial tearing of a ligament caused by a sudden twisting or 2_____ of a joint beyond its normal range of motion. It results in 3_____ and discoloration caused by bleeding into the 4_____.
A strain is an injury to the muscle or 5_____ and usually does not result in discoloration.
A dislocation occurs when the normal 6_____ of two bones is disrupted.
Arthritis is 7_____ of joints characterized by pain and swelling but does not result in discoloration.

a. articulation; b. inflammation; c. stretching; d. ligaments; e. tissue; f. swelling; g. tendon

Case study 10

When 1_____ a limb with a suspected fracture, one caregiver applies the splint while another: holds the limb and monitors distal pulse, motor, and sensation ◄

2_____ of a suspected fracture is best accomplished with two 3_____. After positioning the limb properly, one EMS provider 4_____ the splint, while the other holds the 5_____ in position and 6_____ the distal pulse, motor, and 7_____ _____.

a. limb; b. rescuers; c. splinting;
d. Immobilization; e. sensory responses;
f. applies; g. monitors

Case study 11

What is the proper 1_____ for aligning a fractured long bone? –Stabilize the proximal portion, and then bring the distal portion into alignment.◄

Use gentle 2_____ to bring the distal part of the limb 3_____ _____ with the proximal part.

a. into alignment; b. procedure; c. traction

Case study 12

When would you 1_____ ___ _____ limb injuries on scene? – Only if the patient does not need rapid transport ◄

If the patient's condition is such that 2_____ _____ is necessary, you would care for limb injuries while 3__ _____, rather than completing a detailed physical exam and bandaging and splinting on scene.

a. en route; b. rapid transport; c. bandage and splint

Case study 13

What should you always do if your 1_____ of a limb suggests that it is fractured? – Treat it as if a fracture exists and immobilize it to prevent further injury. ◄

You cannot 2____ a patient by immobilizing a limb properly, but you may possibly 3_____ further injury 4__ _____ __ immobilize a fracture. Always assess the 5_____ _____ before and after 6_____.

a. by failing to; b. harm; c. distal pulse;
d. cause; e. splinting; f. examination

Case study 14

A wrestler feels his shoulders "pop" when his opponent 1_____ his arm during a hold. There is immediate pain and loss of 2_____ __ _____ in the shoulder. What is the patient's likely injury?

- Subluxation ◄
- Muscle 3_____
- 4_____ ligament
- Torn rotator cuff

A 5_____ of the shoulder is a partial dislocation of the 6_____, due to injuries sustained by the 7_____ _____ during a severe twisting force to the joint.

a. subluxation; b. strain; c. rotator cuff;
d. twists; e. range of motion; f. Torn; g. joint

Case study 15

A driver who follows a "down and under" pathway of injury

after a collision is most likely to have what type of injury?

- fractured ribs
- ruptured diaphragm
- fractured femur ◀
- lacerated liver or spleen

The "1_____ ___ _____"
pathway results in injury to the
2_____ ___ _____ rather than to the
abdominal and thoracic organs. These
injuries are caused as the patient's
knees strike the lower part of the
3_____ and energy forces travel
along the 4_____ to the pelvis and
maybe even into the 5_____ _____.

a. femur; b. dashboard; c. pelvis and legs;
d. down and under; e. lower spine

Case study 16

Which of the following
patients is most critical in terms of
age and mechanism of injury?

- An 86 year-old-female with a fractured clavicle
- A 28-year-old male with a fractured femur
- A 43-year-old female with a fractured rib
- A 56-year-old male with a pelvic fracture ◀

Each fracture has a potential
1_____ _____ of one or more
Units per fracture site. Because
of its ring shape, the 2_____
frequently has two or more fractures
present. In addition, nerve and
blood vessel 3_____ and injury

to 4_____ organ can
complicate the severity of this injury.
Patients with pelvic
fractures are always considered
5_____-_____ patients and
should be rapidly 6_____
and transported. If a patient has
bilateral 7_____ _____, he or
she is also a high-priority patient.

a. high-priority; b. genitourinary; c. femur
fractures; d. blood loss; e. damage;
f. stabilized; g. pelvis

Case study 17

Which patient is most likely to
require 1_____ transport?

- 25-year old male, 2_____ wrist
- 45-year-old male, fractured pelvis ◀
- 38-year-old female, fractured 3_____
- 52-year-old female, fractured 4_____

Because of the possibility of
severe 5_____ _____, patients with
fractures of the pelvis are most
likely to need immediate transport.

a. fractured; b. blood loss; c. immediate;
d. tibia; e. humerus

Case study 18

The patient has a closed fracture
of the left ankle and the pelvis is
stable. There is no penetrating trauma
noted in the chest or abdomen,
and the patient denies pregnancy.
Which of the following chambers
of the PASG should be inflated?

- Both legs and the abdominal compartment
- The right leg and the abdominal compartments
- The left leg and the abdominal compartments
- None. PASG is not indicated in this patient ◄

PASG is no longer indicated for 1_____ _____ of shock patients. If this patient has an unstable 2_____ _____ in addition to the presence of shock. PASG could be used as an 3___ _____ to assist in stabilizing the fractured pelvis.

Because the pelvis is intact, it would be better to rapidly transport her (after full-body and 4_____ _____ immobilization) to a well-padded long 5_____ _____.

Shock can be managed with oxygen, positioning (elevate lower end of long board), rapid transport, and careful 6_____ _____.

Some services use pulmonary oedema and penetrating 7_____ _____ as the only contraindications to the use of PASG. If that is the case in your service area, then PASG could be used for this patient, but in that case, all compartments should be 8_____.

You would never inflate only the leg and then the abdominal section. Most likely, the 9_____ would not help stabilize the ankle fracture and additional 10_____ would be required.

a. pelvic fracture; b. splinting; c. air splint; d. cervical spine; e. garment; f. inflated; g. spine board; h. fluid administration; i. routine management; j. chest trauma

Case study 19

Knee, femur, and hip dislocation and fracture caused by the 1_____ hitting the firewall and absorbing initial impact are common in 2_____ _____ with a: "down and under" pathway ◄

"3__ __ ____" refers to injuries sustained in the head, neck, and chest region. In the "down and under" pathway, the body 4_____ forward and downward. This can be limited by the correct use of 5___ _____.

a. slides; b. frontal collisions; c. seat belts; d. Up and over; e. Knees

Case study 20

- What should you do to care for a patient with a suspected pelvic fracture? – Apply the PASG/MAST, titrate two IVs to effect, and monitor for 1_____ __ _____. ◄

This is the current field treatment regimen for 2_____ _____. The PASG/MAST is used as an 3___-_____ to contain the fractured pelvis and 4_____ further injury.

a. Prevent; b. air-splint; c. pelvic fractures; d. signs of shock

Vocabulary 16

align /əˈlaɪn/
alignment /əˈlaɪn.mənt/

245

amputation /ˌæm.pjʊˈteɪ.ʃən/
arteria /aːˈtiə.riə/ dorsalis /
dɔr.sə.lɪs/ pedis /ped.ɪs/
arthritis /ɑːˈθraɪ.tɪs/
articulation /ɑːˌtɪk.jʊˈleɪ.ʃən/
bandage /ˈbæn.dɪdʒ/
caregiver /ˈkeəˌɡɪv.ər/
coccyx /ˈkɒk.sɪks/
curl /kɜːl/
dislocation /ˌdɪs.ləˈkeɪ.ʃən/
face /feɪs/ down /daʊn/
firewall /ˈfaɪə.wɔːl/
forearm /ˈfɔː.rɑːm/
genitourinary /ˌdʒen.ɪ.təʊˈjʊə.rɪ.nər,i/
greenstick /griːn.stɪk/
fracture / ˈfræktʃə/
ligament /ˈlɪɡ.ə.mənt/
limb /lɪm/
markedly /ˈmɑː.kɪd.li/
medial /ˈmiː.di.əl/
opponent /əˈpəʊ.nənt/
outstretched /ˌaʊtˈstretʃt/
palm /pɑːm/
pathway /ˈpɑː.θ.weɪ/
pelvis /ˈpel.vɪs/
pop /pɒp/
popliteal /ˌpɒp.lɪˈtiː.əl/
pronation /prəʊˈneɪ.ʃən/
railing /ˈreɪ.lɪŋ/
roller /ˈrəʊ.lər/ bandage /ˈbæn.dɪdʒ/
rotate /rəʊˈteɪt/
rotator /rəʊˈteɪt.ər/ cuff /kʌf/
rotator /rəʊˈteɪt.ər/
sacral /ˈseɪ.krəl/
strain /streɪn/
subluxation /ˌsʌb.lʌkˈseɪ.ʃən/
supination /ˈsuː.pɪn.əɪ.ʃən/
tendon pl. tendines /ˈten.dən/
titrate /ˈtaɪ.treɪt/
twist/twɪst/
wire /waɪər/ ladder /ˈlæd.ər/
wrestler /ˈres.lər/

Unit 17
Case study 1
Knee injuries and 1____ _____ that occur during a motor vehicle crash are often the result of what pathway of 2_____ _____? – "Down and under" ◄

During a frontal crash, the "down and under" pathway causes the 3_____ __ _____ the lower dashboard violently, causing the described 4_____ _____.

a. knees to strike; b. injury pattern; c. energy transfer; d. hip dislocations

Case study 2
You suspect that a trauma patient has a pelvic injury. She is cool and diaphoretic, with a heart rate of 134 and blood pressure of 100/72.

• What 1_____ is most appropriate in the management of her condition? – Application of PASG. ◄

The use of the MAST/PASG as a splint in the stabilization of suspected pelvic fractures is 2_____ for this patient.
Since the systolic blood pressure is greater than 90-100 mmHg, any IV fluid should 3__ _____ __ a slow, of "keep open," rate. This may 4_____ any additional bleeding from the dilution of 5_____ _____.

a. Clotting factors; b. reduce; c. indicated; d. be restricted to; e. procedure

Case study 3

A conscious adult who falls 1_ _____ of 20 feet (6.1 m) is most likely to 2____ __ his or her:

- head
- hands
- back
- feet ◄

Conscious adults who fall more that three times their height tend to land on their feet; this tends to cause bilateral 3_____ fractures, hip 4_____, and 5_____ _____ of the spinal column.

---
a. Compression fractures; b. dislocations; c. a distance; d. land on; e. calcaneous
---

Case study 4

A 25-year-old female complains of 1_____ lower-abdominal pain, vaginal 2_____, and low-grade fever.

- What condition best describes the patient's presentation? – Pelvic 3_____ disease. ◄

PID causes lower-abdominal 4_____ that is difficult to localize and often has an associated fever. Pain associated with an ectopic pregnancy is more 5_____, as is the pain associated with solid organ involvement.

---
a. inflammatory; b. localized; c. discharge; d. discomfort; e. diffuse
---

Case study 5

A 28-year-old woman is complaining of a sudden onset of 1_____ abdominal pain that 2_____ to her shoulder. Her BP = 88/60, P = 110, and R =20. Her skin is cool, pale, and 3_____. She states that her last normal menstrual period was 6 – 8 weeks ago.

- What condition best describes the patient presentation? – Ectopic pregnancy ◄

A sudden rupture of an ectopic pregnancy would result in a loss of blood that would place the patient in 4_____ shock.

---
a. compensatory; b. radiates; c. severe; d. clammy

Case study 6

Your patient is a 28-year-old female who reports that she is nine weeks pregnant. She is complaining of severe abdominal pain, shoulder pain, and vaginal 1_____. Vital signs are within normal limits, and a physical exam reveals 2_____ in the lower-left quadrant.

- What should you suspect is occurring? - Ectopic pregnancy ◄

Most ectopic pregnancies implant within the 3_____ _____ and have attained a large enough size around nine weeks to 4_____ the tube, resulting in intense pain and bleeding.

The bleeding may or may not be present from the vagina. Most cases of spontaneous 5_____ are undetected by the mother, who doesn't even know she is pregnant, and present as an "abnormal menstrual cycle."

a. abortion; b. bleeding; c. rupture; d. fallopian tube; e. tenderness

Case study 7

Your patient is a 32-year-old woman who reports that she is nine weeks pregnant. She is complaining of 1_____ abdominal pain, slight vaginal bleeding, and 2_____ pain. Abdominal examination reveals 3_____ tenderness in the lower right quadrant. The patient is somewhat 4_____ and tachycardic.

- You should suspect developing 5_____ from what condition? – Ectopic pregnancy. ◄

Signs and symptoms of ectopic pregnancy include lower-abdominal pain that is often referred to the shoulder, abdominal tenderness, and rapidly developing shock.

a. significant; b. shock; c. agitated; d. shoulder; e. severe

Case study 8

Your patient is a 33-year-old woman who is nine months pregnant. She 1_____ of severe abdominal pain and 2_____

tenderness. She 3_____ there is no vaginal bleeding at this time.

- What should you suspect? – Abruptio placentae (premature 4_____ of the placenta). ◄

a. reports; b. separation; c. abdominal; d. complains

Case study 9

Answer the next three questions on the basis of the following information.

You respond to a 25-year-old female who is complaining of vaginal bleeding and abdominal pain.

The patient states that she is 33 weeks pregnant and that this is her first pregnancy. She says that when the pain started, it felt like "something was tearing." She 1_____ vaginal bleeding during the pregnancy prior to this event. Upon 2_____, you notice what appears to be approximately 500 cc of dark, almost black, blood.

- What 3_____ is this patient most likely suffering from? – Abruptio placentae ◄

The tearing feeling and the 4_____-_____ blood are classic signs and symptoms of abruptio placentae.

Placenta praevia often has bleeding that is contained within the uterus due to the placenta blocking the os (opening or mouth) of the 5_____.

- This condition is 6_____ to both the mother and the baby. ◄

Both lives are at stake. Oxygen is passed from the mother to the baby via the placenta. A separation greatly decreases the blood 7_____ to the infant and the uncontrolled bleeding is dangerous to the mother.

- In addition to high-flow oxygen and continuous 8_____ of the mother's vital signs and the baby's foetal heart tones, you should treat this patient with: one or two large-bore IVs of normal saline or Ringer's lactate ◄

Administering one or two large-bore IVs of normal saline or Ringer's lactate is 9_____ when combined with rapid transport.

You should titrate the BP to 100-110 so as not to 10_____ the circulation, causing pulmonary oedema and further compromising the oxygen supply to the infant.

a. condition; b. denies; c. overload;
d. dangerous; e. assessment; f. uterus;
g. dark-coloured; h. supply; i. monitoring;
j. appropriate

Case study 10

- What is the usual clinical 1_____ of placenta praevia? –2_____ bright red bleeding ◄

Placenta praevia usually presents as painless bright red bleeding that occurs in the 3_____ trimester of pregnancy. The blood may be 4_____ within the uterus.

a. Painless; b. contained; c. third;
d. presentation

Case study 11

Your patient is a 32-year-old woman who reports that she is 14 weeks pregnant. She complains of abdominal 1_____ and vaginal bleeding.

- How should you proceed? – Treat for signs and symptoms of 2_____, provide 3_____ support, and transport. ◄

The patient is most likely suffering a 4_____. Treat her for signs and symptoms of shock due to 5_____ _____, provide emotional support, retain any clumps of tissue she passes, and transport.

a. miscarriage; b. emotional; c. cramping;
d. blood loss; e. hypovolemia

Case study 12

- Which are the only two 1_____ in which a prehospital provider should place a gloved hand into the vagina? – 2_____ cord and 3_____ presentation ◄

In both of these cases, relieving pressure off the trapped umbilical cord (prolapsed) or the face and airway passages (trapped breech) may be the 4_____ _____ measure provided by the paramedic.

a. Prolapsed; b. breech; c. life-saving; d. situations

Case study 13

Signs and symptoms of a pregnant patient with preeclampsia include: elevated BP, visual disturbance, headache, and oedema. ◄

Common signs and symptoms of 1_____ include headache, 2_____, confusion, 3_____ _____, nausea, vomiting, proteinuria, hypertension, and 4_____.

a. dizziness; b. blurred vision; c. oedema; d. preeclampsia

Case study 14

- The normal 1_____ period is: 40 weeks. ◄

2___ _____ delivery usually occurs within the 40th week of pregnancy. These are normal 3_____ changes that occur in vital signs during pregnancy: a woman's blood pressure usually 4_____ during the first two trimesters and her pulse rate 5_____.

a. gestation; b. Full-term; c. physiological; d. rises; e. falls

Case study 15

You are recording vital signs for a 34-year-old woman who is eight months pregnant. Her blood pressure is 100/70, pulse rate is 80, and respirations are 17 per minute and normal. Upon 1_____ of her chest, you hear a mild systolic flow 2_____.

- How should you treat this patient? – The murmur is not a 3_____ of concern; document these findings on the patient-care report. ◄

A mild systolic murmur in a pregnant patient whose vital signs are normal is not a cause of 4_____.

a. murmur; b. finding; c. concern; d. auscultation

Case study 16

Answer the next four questions on the basis of the following information.

You respond to a 19-year-old female who is 25 weeks pregnant and is complaining of a severe headache and 1_____ vision. Upon initial assessment, you notice that she has substantial 2_____, especially in her feet and hands. She states that she has not been under the regular care of a physician during this pregnancy.

- What 3_____ would you expect to see in this patient's vital signs? – Hypertension. ◄

This is toxaemia, a 4_____ disorder of pregnancy.

- This patient is most likely suffering from the condition known as: preeclampsia. ◄

Treatment for this patient includes rapid transport without light and sirens, an IV of normal saline or Ringer's lactate, and oxygen.

- It may also call for the administration of: magnesium sulphate. ◄

Magnesium sulphate is the appropriate medication for the suppression of seizures in a 5_____ patient. Valium may help control seizures, but magnesium suppresses them.

- If left untreated, this patient's condition may worsen and she may begin to experience: grand mal seizures. ◄

Seizures indicate that the patient's condition has worsened. The condition is then called 6_____.

a. oedema; b. blurred; c. hypertensive;
d. eclampsia; e. abnormality; f. preeclampsia

Case study 17
Your patient is a 35-year-old woman who is eight months pregnant. You note that her blood pressure is 140/90 and oedema is present all over her body. The patient is 1_____ and complains of seeing spots and having a 2_____.

- From this information, what condition should you suspect is present? – Preeclampsia ◄

The patient shows symptoms and signs of preeclampsia (or 3_____ of pregnancy) and should be transported to the hospital. The distinction between eclampsia and preeclampsia is the presence of 4_____ and/or 5_____.

a. coma; b. anxious; c. seizures; d. toxaemia;
e. headache

Case study 18

- Which of the following signs and symptoms would be present in a pregnant patient with preeclampsia? – High blood pressure, headaches, oedema, and visual disturbances. ◄

Patient with preeclampsia (or toxaemia of pregnancy) 1_____ all the signs and symptoms of the hypertensive disorders of pregnancy except 2_____. Once the patient begins to 3_____ seizures, the condition has changed from preeclampsia to eclampsia.

a. manifest; b. seizures; c. experience

Case study 19
Causes of third-trimester bleeding include: 1_____ placentae, placenta 2_____, 3_____ rupture.

a. praevia;◄ b. abruptio;◄ c. uterine ◄

251

Case study 20

Your patient is a 29-year-old woman who is nine months pregnant with her third child. She reports the onset of painless 1_____ ____ vaginal bleeding in the last half hour.

- How should you treat this patient? – Treat her for signs and symptoms of shock and transport immediately.◄

Bright red bleeding in late pregnancy is assumed to be 2_____ praevia, which is a true 3_____ _____ that is life threatening to both mother and baby. Treat the mother for shock and transport 4_____.

---

a. immediately; b. medical emergency;
c. placenta; d. bright red

Vocabulary 17

at /ət/ **stake** /steɪk/
attain /əˈteɪn/
block /blɒk/
breech /briːtʃ/
clot /klɒt/
clump /klʌmp/
dangerous /ˈdeɪn.dʒər.əs/
dilution /daɪˈluːʃən/
distinction /dɪˈstɪŋk.ʃən/
grade /greɪd/
heart /hɑːt/ **rate** /reɪt/
implant /ɪmˈplɑːnt/
in addition /əˈdɪʃ.ən/
intense /ɪnˈtens/
land /lænd/
life-saving /ˈlaɪfˌseɪ.vɪŋ/
miscarriage /ˈmɪsˌkær.ɪdʒ/
murmur /ˈmɜː.mər/
os /ɒs/ pl. **ossa** kost

physician /fɪˈzɪʃ.ən/
PID, Pelvic /ˈpel.vɪk/ **Inflammatory** /ɪnˈflæm.ə.tər.i/ **Disease** /dɪˈziːz/
proceed /prəˈsiːd/
restricted /rɪˈstrɪk.tɪd/
retain /rɪˈteɪn/
somewhat /ˈsʌm.wɒt/
substantial /səbˈstæn.ʃəl/
support /səˈpɔːt/
suppression /səˈpreʃ.ən/
tear /tɪər/
tend /tend/ **to the needs of sb**
tone /təʊn/
toxaemia /tɒkˈsiː.mi.ə/
trimester /trɪˈmes.tər/
undetected /ˌʌn.dɪˈtekt.əd/
Valium /ˈvæl.i.əm/
violently /ˈvaɪə.lənt.li/
vital /ˈvaɪ.təl/ **signs** /saɪnz/

Unit 18

Case study 1

A pregnant patient complains of painful, irregular 1_____ _____. The patient states that she is 37 weeks pregnant and her 2_____ membranes ruptured two days ago.

- Based on this information, you would: 3_____ immediate transport. ◄

Immediate transport is 4_____ for this patient's condition. Without the intact protective amniotic sac, the foetus is at risk of being 5_____.

---

a. indicated; b. amniotic; c. infected; d. labour contraction; e. initiate

---

Case study 2

The use of PASG/MAST is indicated: to 1_____ lower-extremity 2_____ in a hypotensive patient. ◄

Third trimester pregnancy, impaled objects, and dyspnoea are all 3_____ for use of the PASG/MAST. In addition, the PASG/MAST is contraindicated with any 4_____ bleeding occurring above the site of the garment.

> a. contraindications; b. uncontrolled;
> c. stabilize; d. fractures

Case study 3

What is the cause of the supine-hypotensive syndrome in the pregnant patient? –1_____ of the uterus on the inferior vena cava ◄

Supine-hypotensive syndrome, a normal 2_____ during late pregnancy, is caused by the pressure of the pregnant uterus on the inferior vena cava when the patient is 3_____.

> a. supine; b. occurrence; c. Pressure

Case study 4

You arrive at the scene of an 1_____ delivery in the field. The first 2_____, who called for 3_____, reports that the patient is a 32-year-old female who is "G4 P3."

- What does this mean? – The patient has been pregnant four times and 4_____ three live children. ◄

- What does it mean if a woman is described as 5_____? – She has delivered more than one live baby ◄

> a. responder; b. assistance; c. delivered;
> d. imminent; e. multipara

Case study 5

Which of the following signs most likely indicates 1_____ birth?

- painful uterine contraction
- urge to have a bowel movement ◄
- ruptured membranes
- dilation of the cervix

When the foetus is close to the 2_____ of the birth canal, the head presses down on the internal 3_____ _____, resulting in the urge to have a 4_____ _____. Painful uterine contractions can start well in advance of 5_____ delivery.

> a. imminent; b. bowel movement; c. anal
> sphincter; d. physical; e. entrance

Case study 6

When should you examine a woman who is about to give birth for crowning? – During 1_____. ◄

Look for 2_____, or the appearance of the baby's head at the 3_____ of the vagina, only during a contraction

> a. crowning; b. opening; c. contraction

Case study 7

During delivery a loop of umbilical cord presents from the 1_____ _____.

- You should: 2_____ the cord with a moist and sterile dressing,◄

Covering the exposed cord will 3_____ drying of the cord. Additionally, you should try to 4_____ two fingers into the birth canal and try to keep pressure from the baby's 5_____ away from the cord.

> a. birth canal; b. minimize; c. insert; d. head; e. cover

Case study 8

- During a normal delivery, you would tell the mother to stop 1_____ when what occurs? – The head is 2_____. ◄

To avoid a 3_____ delivery, tell the mother to 4_____ pushing after the head is delivered.

> a. pushing; b. stop; c. precipitous; d. delivered

Case study 9

Answer the next four questions on the basis of the following information.

You are called to the home of a 21-year-old female in 1_____ labour. She is two weeks from her 2_____ ____ date and is having contractions of 1.5 minutes 3_____, which are three minutes apart. This is her second pregnancy. Her first child was delivered vaginally at 4_____ _____.

- What is your first course of action for this patient? – Place her on the 5_____ in high Fowler's or comfortable position and examine her for crowning. ◄

In this situation, the first step would be to 6_____ the patient for 7_____ to determine if you need to assist with delivery on the scene or if you can attempt to transport her.

Your patient suddenly tells you she feels something slippery between her legs. Upon visual examination, you notice a two-inch (5 cm) segment of the umbilical cord 8_____ from the vagina.

- What is this condition called? – Prolapsed cord. ◄
- What are appropriate treatment options for this patient? – Provide high-flow oxygen and rapidly transport the mother in 9_____-_____ position, take pressure off the cord by placing your fingers into the vagina and gently 10_____ the infant, 11_____ the cord in a moist sterile dressing, provide supplemental oxygen, and transport quickly. ◄

If you opt to position the patient for transport, you should place her in the left-lateral 12_____ position to 13_____ uterine blood flow and return.

You are ready to transport this patient.

- If the umbilical cord is still exposed, how can you use it to evaluate the infant's perfusion? – Gently feel the cord for 14_____ to determine the infant's 15_____ ____. ◄

The umbilical vein, found within the umbilical cord, provides 16_____ blood to the infant. The vein is large enough for you to feel the pulsations as blood flows from the placenta to the 17_____.

> a. duration; b. full term; c. examine;
> d. oxygenated; e. active; f. crowning;
> g. expected due; h. stretcher; i. knee-chest;
> j. heart rate; k. protruding; l. lifting; m. wrap;
> n. recumbent; o. improve; p. pulsations;
> r. foetus

Case study 10

A patient who is 37 weeks pregnant is having contractions and states that her 1_____ _____ about 20 minutes ago. The vaginal exam 2_____ that the baby's foot is present in the birth canal.

- Your next action would be to: 3_____ the patient to the cot and initiate rapid transport.◄

A single-limb presentation is considered 4_____ vaginally and requires rapid caesarean

section to successfully deliver the infant. Rapid transport is indicated.

> a. reveals; b. move; c. water broke;
> d. nondeliverable

Case study 11

What are the blood vessels in the 1_____ ____? – Two arteries and one vein.◄

The umbilical cord contains two 2_____ and one vein; only the umbilical 3_____ is used for 4_____ _____.

> a. arteries; b. vascular access; c. vein;
> d. umbilical cord

Case study 12

What does the term effacement refer to? – 1_____ of the cervix during the first stage of 2_____ ◄

Effacement refers to the stretching and thinning of the 3_____, which occurs during the 4_____ stage of normal labour.

> a. labour; b. cervix; c. Thinning; d. first

Case study 13

What does the presence of meconium on the 1_____ or in the 2_____ _____ indicate? – The infant may have been distressed. ◄

The presence of meconium indicates that the foetus may have been 3_____ before birth.

> a. amniotic fluid; b. distressed; c. neonate

255

Case study 14

When does the 1_____ stage of labour begin? – Immediately 2____ the birth of the baby. ◄

The third stage of labour 3_____ with the birth of the foetus and 4____ with the delivery of the placenta.

```
a. begins; b. third; c. ends; d. upon
```

Case study 15

What is the appropriate treatment for a prolapsed cord? – Place two fingers to 1_____ the presenting part of the 2_____ off the cord, place the mother in 3____-_____ position, 4_____ oxygen, and transport. ◄

A 5_____ cord should be treated by placing two fingers of a gloved hand into the vagina to raise the presenting part of the foetus off the 6____, then place the mother in Trendelenburg or knee-chest position, administer high-flow oxygen, and 7_____ immediately.

```
a. knee-chest; b. foetus; c. administer;
d. transporting; e. prolapsed; f. cord; g. raise
```

Case study 16

Regarding a single limb presentation during an emergency delivery, this statement is true: this is a nondeliverable presentation and requires immediate transport to an appropriate receiving facility. ◄

A 1____ presentation during delivery requires a 2_____ _____ to 3_____ the delivery.

Provide high-flow oxygen and 4____ to the mother during transport.

```
a. limb; b. care; c. complete; d. caesarean
section
```

Case study 17

What is the order of care for a newborn born with evidence of meconium staining? – Suction with the 1____ _____ first, then remove remaining meconium under direct 2_____. ◄

Do not resuscitate or stimulate further until the meconium is 3_____ ____ the respiratory tree by direct visualization of the cords.

```
a. bulb syringe; b. cleared from;
c. visualization
```

Case study 18

What is the correct 1_____ for cutting the umbilical cord after the birth of the baby? – Clamp the cord in two places 5 cm 2_____ and cut it between the clamps. ◄

Generally, you want to 3_____ the first clamp several 5 – 7 inches, (13 -18 cm) away from the 4_____.

```
a. apart; b. place; c. procedure; d. infant
```

Case study 19

Immediately after delivery, how should you 1_____ a neonate? – At the 2_____ of the mother's vagina, with its head slightly 3_____ than the body. ◄

Position the neonate at the level of the mother's vagina, with his or her head slightly lower

than the body to 4_____
drainage of 5_____.

---

a. secretions; b. level; c. lower; d. position;
e. facilitate

Case study 20

You would perform chest
compressions on any newborn:
whose heart is less than 60
beats per minute. ◄

1_____ _____ are
required when a newborn's heart
rate is 2_____ than 60, or between 60
and 80 after 30 seconds of positive-
pressure 3_____.

Remember to perform each
4_____ for approximately
30 seconds, then 5_____ for the
need to continue resuscitation.

- The appropriate range for
  the heart rate of a healthy
  neonate immediately
  after birth is 150 – 180
  beats per minute. ◄

---

a. intervention; b. ventilation; c. less;
d. reassess; e. chest compressions

Vocabulary 18

apart /əˈpɑːt/
bulb /bʌlb/
cervix /ˈsɜː.vɪks/ pl **cervices** /-vɪs.iːz/
distressed /dɪˈstrest/
duration /djʊəˈreɪ.ʃən/
effacement /ɪˈfeɪs.mənt/
Fowler's /foʊ'ler/ **position** /pəˈzɪʃ.ən/
in advance /ədˈvɑːns/
inch /ɪntʃ/
internal /ɪnˈtɜː.nəl/
lift /lɪft/
multipara /mʌl.tiˈpær.ə/

nondeliverable /ˌnɒn.dɪˈlɪv.ər.ə.bl̩/
precipitous /prɪˈsɪp.ɪ.təs/
pulsation /pʌlˈseɪ.ʃən/
responder /rɪˈspɒnd.ər/
slippery /ˈslɪp.ər.i/
Trendelenburg position /pəˈzɪʃ.ən/

Unit 19
Case study 1

- What is the 1_____
  for administering positive
  pressure ventilations to
  a Central newborn? –
  Cyanosis 2_____
  while oxygen is given. ◄

Apnoea and tachycardia
may 3_____ be present in
the newborn, but once they are
corrected, you do not need to
4_____ to progress further
inverted into the pyramid.

---

a. persists; b. initially; c. criterion; c. continue

Case study 2

1_____ and drugs are
most often delivered to a newborn
through the use of which circulatory
2_____? – Umbilical vein ◄
The 3_____ ____,
located in the umbilical cord, is
used for this purpose. If the cord is
left untreated at the hospital, it may
be cannulated for a week or even
longer. It enters immediately into
the 4_____ _____.

---

a. hepatic circulation; b. umbilical vein;
c. vessel; d. Medications

Case study 3

You are assessing a neonate who has a pink body and blue 1_____, a pulse rate of 90, positive grimace response, active 2_____, and 3_____ respiratory efforts.

- What is the Apgar score for this infant? – 6.◄

The score would consist of one point each for appearance, pulse rate, grimace, and respiratory 4_____, and two points for activity.

a. motion; b. extremities; c. effort; d. irregular

Case study 4

During an 1_____ delivery, the newborn's head presents in the canal.

- After suctioning, how can you 2_____ with the delivery of the anterior shoulder? – Gently guide the infant's head downward ◄

The head will 3_____ ____ drop down as the shoulders begin to pass through the birth canal. The paramedic can gently 4_____ the head to help with the process.

a. assist; b. tend to; c. guide; d. emergency

Case study 5

During a normal delivery, you would 1_____ the infant's mouth and nose just 2_____:

- the head is out of the vagina ◄
- the entire infant is delivered
- the head and chest are delivered
- you clamp the cord

Suction the infant's mouth and nose immediately after the head is delivered and you can 3_____ the mouth and nose. Suctioning of the infant's mouth and nose should be performed after the head has been 4_____.

Remember to suction the mouth first, 5_____ the nose.

a. after; b. access; c. then; d. suction; e. delivered

Case study 6

You are assisting in a delivery 1__ ___ _____. As the baby's head is born, you realize that the umbilical cord is 2_____ around the baby's neck.

- What is your first step in the 3_____ of this problem? – Attempt to 4_____ the cord _____ the baby's head.◄

First, attempt to slip the cord over the baby's head. If this is impossible you should 5_____ the cord in two places, and carefully to 6___ it between the clamps, then 7_____ with the delivery.

a. slip over; b. cut; c. management; d. wrapped; e. continue; f. clamp; g. in the field

Case study 7

What is the appropriate 1_____ for the heart rate of a healthy neonate 2_____ after birth? – 150 – 180 beats 3____ _____. ◄

Heart rate at birth is normally 150 – 180 beats per minute, 4_____ to 130 – 140 within a few minutes.

> a. slowing; b. immediately; c. range; d. per minute

Case study 8

The first step in the 1_____ of a distressed neonate is to: ventilate with 100% oxygen for 15-30 seconds. ◄

2_____ with 100% oxygen, and then 3_____ the heart rate and initiate 4_____ compressions is necessary.

> a. Ventilate; b. chest; c. evaluate; d. resuscitation

Case study 9

You have just delivered a baby girl. 1_____ reveals that the infant 2_____ loudly and has a heart rate of 140, her 3_____ is pink, but the extremities are blue, and she is actively moving all extremities.

- Her APGAR score is: 9 ◄

With the exception of the blue extremities, the infant scores a "2" on 4_____, _____, _____, and 5_____. Her "Appearance" scores as a 1.

> a. Evaluation; b. body; c. cries; d. activity, pulse, grimace; e. respirations

Case study 10

All of the following statements about supplying supplemental oxygen to a neonate are correct:

- Do not withhold oxygen from a neonate in the 1_____ setting. ◄
- Administer 2_____ oxygen by blowing it across the neonate's face. ◄
- Oxygen should be 3_____ if possible prior to administration. ◄

Oxygen 4_____ occurs only if oxygen is administered for several days.

> a. toxicity; b. supplemental; c. warmed; d. prehospital

Case study 11

Children of what age are in the greatest danger from airway 1_____ caused by aspirated 2_____ objects? – 1-3 years. ◄

Children between 1 and 3, who tend to 3____ things into their mouths, are in greatest danger of 4_____ of foreign objects.

> a. aspiration; b. foreign; c. obstruction; d. put

Case study 12

You should 1_____ to remove foreign material from a patient's airway with forceps only in what situation? – You are able to visualize the obstruction directly. ◄

To prevent tissue 2_____, you should attempt to physically

3_____ foreign material only if you can actually see the obstruction with a 4_____.

a. laryngoscope; b. remove; c. damage; d. attempt

Case study 13

Until ruled out by a physician, documented fever in an infant younger than three months old is always considered to 1_____ _____: meningitis. ◄

Fever in a child younger than 2_____ months old is considered to be 3_____ unless proven otherwise; transport all infants with fever 4_____.

a. meningitis; b. three; c. promptly; d. result from

Case study 14

What volume of fluid bolus should be given initially to severely dehydrated child? – 20 ml/kg ◄

Give a 1_____ dehydrated child an 2_____ bolus of 20 cc/kg of normal 3_____ or Ringer's solution. Reassess for 4_____ and repeat with 10 or 20 cc/kg boluses as long as the child continues to 5_____ and you do not detect any signs of fluid 6_____.

a. initial; b. severely; c. response; d. overload; e. improve; f. saline

Case study 15

The best place to assess for cyanosis in an infant or child is the: oral mucosa ◄

The best place to assess for 1_____ in an infant or child is the 2____ _____, lips, or tongue. Nail beds of an infant may not be an 3_____ indicator of central circulation 4_____even when they appear cyanotic.

a. accurate; b. oral mucosa; c. status; d. cyanosis

Case study 16

This statement 1_____ febrile seizures is true: febrile seizures occur because of a rapid rise in skin temperature ◄

2_____ _____ occur in children because of a 3_____ rise in temperature and not necessarily the 4_____of the fever itself.

- All paediatric patients who have had seizures should be: transported to a hospital for evaluation. ◄

The cause of seizure activity can be determined only in the hospital.

a. rapid; b. severity; c. Febrile seizures; d. regarding

Case study 17

Unilateral wheezing in a 14-month-old child is suggestive of: aspiration of a foreign body. ◄

Wheezing localized into one lung only minimizes the 1_____ of asthma or other 2_____ disease. If a foreign body is small enough to pass through the glottic 3_____ and carina, it will eventually carina somewhere in either the 4_____ _____ or the bronchioles.

If the obstruction is not complete air moving past the restricted lung passage will 5_____ a wheeze.

---

a. main bronchi; b. pulmonary; c. opening; d. produce; e. likelihood

---

Case study 18

A 2-year-old female presents with lethargy and poor feeding. The parent states that the patient has had a 1_____ fever for the past seven days, with 2_____, nausea, and vomiting for the past four days.

She presents with pale, cool skin, a pulse rate of 180, and a respiratory rate of 40. She cries weakly when a painful stimulus 3__ _____. The ECG shows a rapid narrow complex dysrhythmia.

Based upon this information, what is the patient's 4_____ problem?

- respiratory distress
- respiratory failure
- hypoperfusion ◀
- dysrhythmia

The history of diarrhoea, nausea, and vomiting indicates a strong 5_____ situation resulting in the tachycardia and dyspnoea.

---

a. moderate; b. is applied; c. dehydration; d. primary; e. diarrhoea

---

Case study 19

A 3-year-old female is unresponsive and not breathing. Parents state that she was eating grapes when she suddenly made a high-pitched whistling noise and turned blue.

- Your immediate action would be: start 1_____ resuscitation. ◀

The high-pitched whistling 2_____ and cyanosis 3_____ the patient is suffering from an airway obstruction.

Back blows and chest thrusts are performed only on infants. Since the patient is 4_____, your immediate step should be to start CPR.

Abdominal thrusts are performed only on conscious 5_____ victims. For unresponsive victims suspected of having an airway obstruction, you should begin CPR but look in the mouth to see if you visualise the object 6_____ __ each ventilation attempt.

---

a. unresponsive; b. cardiopulmonary; c. indicates; d. prior to; e. choking; f. noise

---

Case study 20

Answer the next three questions on the basis of the following information.

You respond to a 4-year-old female who has taken an 1_____ quantity of children's aspirin.

Upon arrival, you find the patient conscious, crying, and lethargic. Her mother states that she found the child playing in the bathroom.

A flavoured children's aspirin bottle was found nearby with only a few tablets in it.

- In this situation, you should make the 2_____ that: the aspirin bottle was full and treat accordingly. ◄

Unless you know otherwise, always assume a medication bottle was full. There is nothing in this situation to indicate child abuse.

Although today the quantity of pills packaged has been reduced, in order to lessen the likelihood of 3_____ by accidental ingestion, this child's 4_____ LOC (level of consciousness) suggests there is a serious overdose situation here.

- Children's aspirin is in which class of medications? – Salicylates. ◄
- Correct treatment for this patient may include: IV, oxygen, ECG, and activated 5_____. ◄

The appropriate treatment is IV, oxygen, ECG, and activated charcoal. Be prepared to treat dysrhythmias and to provide a fluid challenge if ordered. Sodium bicarbonate may also be ordered by medical direction.

```
a. unknown; b. overdose; c. decreasing;
d. charcoal; e. assumption
```

Case study 21
Tertiary injuries from a blast include:

- Extremity 1_____
- 2_____ lacerations
- Impaled objects
- Lung injuries ◄

Tertiary blast injuries are caused by the victim being 3_____ ____ from the blast and into objects on the ground. Injuries from this are 4_____ __ those sustained from ejection from an automobile.

Primary blast injuries result from compression of hollow organs such as the lungs.

Secondary blast injuries are caused by flying debris propelled by the force of the 5_____.

```
a. similar to; b. blast; c. fractures; d. Organ;
e. propelled away
```

Vocabulary 19

accordingly /əˈkɔː.dɪŋ.li/
Apgar /ˈæpɡɑː/ **score** /skɔːr/
assumption /əˈsʌmp.ʃən/
blowing /ˌbləʊ.ɪŋ/
cardiopulmonary /ˌkɑː.di.əʊˈpʊl.mə.nə.ri/
criterion /kraɪˈtɪə.ri.ən/
dehydration /ˌdiː.haɪˈdreɪ.ʃən/
downward /ˈdaʊn.wəd/
ejection /ɪˈdʒekt.ʃən/
flavoured /fleɪ.vəd/
grape /ɡreɪp/
grimace /ˈɡrɪ.məs/
inverted /ɪnˈvɜː.tɪd/
laryngoscope /ˌlærɪŋˈɡɒ.skəʊp/
lip /lɪp/
loudly /ˈlaʊd.li/
mucosa /mjuːˈkəʊ.sə/
nail /neɪl/ **bed** /bed/
nausea /ˈnɔː.zi.ə/
passage /ˈpæsɪdʒ/

Salicylates /sə'lɪs.ɪˌleɪts/
warmed /ˌwɔːmd/
weakly /wiːk.li/

Unit 20

Case study 1

Your patient is a 4-year-old girl who 1_____ in the middle of the night with a cough that her mother describes as sounding "like a seal barking." The patient feels more comfortable 2_____ __. Vital signs are: respiration, 26/min; pulse, 100; temperature 101° F (38.3° C). On 3_____ ____, you hear stridor on inspiration.

- From this scenario, you should suspect what condition? – Croup ◄

The signs, symptoms, and assessment 4_____ of croup are described. The seal-bark cough is a classic presentation with croup.

```
a. awoke; b. physical exam; c. findings;
d. sitting up
```

Case study 2

Your patient is a 6-year-old child who is conscious but not breathing because of an airway obstruction.

- What is the first thing you should do for this patient? – Perform subdiaphragmatic abdominal thrusts.◄

The first step in treating a 1_____ child of this age with a complete airway obstruction is to perform the Heimlich 2_____ (i.e. subdiaphragmatic abdominal thrusts). Continue until the obstruction is 3_____ or the child becomes unconscious.

```
a. manoeuvre; b. relieved; c. conscious
```

Case study 3

Your patient is a 10-year-old boy who 1___ _____ off his bicycle.

- What should you do when obtaining the history of the 2_____? – Obtain as much information as possible from the child.◄

With a child of this age, obtain as much information as possible from the patient him- or herself; this will allow the child to feel respected and 3_____. The adult 4_____ can fill in relevant details.

```
a. has fallen; b. caretaker; c. mature;
c. accident
```

Case study 4

Answer the next three questions on the basis of the following information.

You respond to a 12-year-old male who is wheezing and having difficulty breathing. The patient has a long history of asthma and states that he used his 1_____ but that it didn't help much. Upon examination, you 2_____ that the patient is tachycardic and tachypnoeic with a 3___-_____ cough.

- What is the primary 4_____
in treating this patient? –
Correct hypoxia, 5_____
bronchospasms, and
decrease inflammation. ◀

This patient's condition
might have been triggered by
any of the following: allergens,
exercise, medications.

- Cold air is also a common
6_____ for asthma. ◀
- Treatment for this patient
includes the following
medications: albuterol,
terbutaline, and steroids.◀

a. inhaler; b. goal; c. non-productive;
d. reverse; e. trigger; f. discover

Case study 5

A 12-year-old unconscious male
is being brought to the edge of the
pool by two lifeguards. He is apnoeic.

- How would you establish
his airway? – Manual
1_____ _____
precautions, modified
jaw thrust. ◀

Since no information is presented
about the exact nature of the patient's
condition, one assumes that there is a
2_____ _____ involved and
manual precautions must be taken.
A modified jaw thrust can open an
airway without disturbing the in-line
3_____ of the cervical spine.

a. trauma mechanism; b. alignment;
c. cervical spine

Case study 6

Myocardial infarction may go
unrecognized in elderly patients.
Why is this true? – They lack
1_____ symptoms such as
frequent chest pain or discomfort. ◀
More than half of all elderly
patients who suffer MI do not
complain of 2_____ _____;
therefore, their AMI often goes
3_____. In the presence
of 4_____ _____ such
as diabetes, neuropathy prevents
them from sensing pain as
unaffected individuals would.

a. chronic diseases; b. unrecognized; c. chest
pain; d. typical

Case study 7

Which of the following
statements regarding falls among
the elderly is most accurate?

- The elderly have the
highest incidence of falls
- Fall-related injuries
represent the 1_____
_____ of accidental death
among the elderly ◀
- Falls account for the
highest percentage of
2_____ department
visits among the elderly
- A majority of falls are
3_____ related to
infrapatellar bursitis

Falls kill more elderly people
annually than any other trauma. It is
important to carefully 4_____
and manage these patients.

a. leading cause; b. evaluate; c. primarily;
d. emergency

Case study 8

These are typically characteristics of an abused elderly person:

- Multiple physical and mental 1_____, such as dementia ◄
- Incontinent, 2_____ _____, and over the age of 65 ◄
- 3_____ handicapped, over the age of 75, and frail. ◄

The typical abused elder is generally poor and 4_____ on the abuser.

a. dependent; b. impairments; c. physically;
d. mentally handicapped

Case study 9

Drug dosages are lower in elderly patients than in young adults primarily because elderly patients: have a slower rate of elimination of drugs. ◄

The 1_____ of many common 2_____ is up to 50% lower in elderly adults primarily because of a decreased rate of 3_____ of the drug by the liver and kidneys.

a. elimination; b. medications; c. dosage

Case study 10

Which of the following statements regarding treatment for the care of a patient who is suffering from complications of dialysis is correct?

- If possible, obtain a blood pressure reading on the arm on which the shunt is located.
- Watch for narrow complex tachycardia to develop as the patient becomes hypoxic.
- Monitoring for dysrhythmias is frequently unnecessary in a haemodialysis patient.
- To prevent exacerbation of the problem, start an IV only if ordered by medical control ◄

Fluid administration in dialysis patients should be under the 1_____ _____ of medical control.
Dysrhythmias are 2_____ and if present, are generally caused by electrolyte 3_____. To prevent accidental damage to the shunt, a BP should never be assessed on the arm with the 4_____.

a. imbalances; b. direct authority; c. common;
d. shunt

Case study 11

What is the leading cause of death among the elderly?

- metastatic 1_____
- 2_____ disease
- 3_____ and falls
- cardiac disease ◄

Because cardiac disease is so common, you should administer medications commonly prescribed for other types of emergencies with extreme 4_____.

a. caution; b. respiratory; c. accidents;
d. cancer

Case study 12

An elderly man is complaining of a 1_____ _____ of severe pain in his right leg. The 2_____ extremity is cool to the touch and pale. The temperature and pulse in the patient's left leg is normal.

- You suspect: arterial occlusion. ◀

A sudden loss of 3_____ _____ to the leg within the arterial bed would account for the sudden 4_____ in skin colour and temperature.

a. blood flow; b. change; c. affected; d. sudden onset

Case study 13

What does ascites refer to?

- 1_____ alcoholism
- fluid in the abdomen ◀
- 2_____ abdominal pain
- a ruptured aortic aneurysm

3_____ refers to an 4_____ of fluid in the abdomen.

a. Ascites; b. accumulation; c. chronic; d. severe

Case study 14

Answer the next two questions on the basis of the following information.

You arrive on the scene and find an elderly male complaining of severe abdominal and back pain. Upon further questioning, he states that the pain is "all over the left side". 1__ _____, you feel a pulsating mass in the abdomen.

- This patient is most likely suffering from: abdominal aortic aneurysm. ◀

This patient is exhibiting the classic signs and symptoms of an 2_____ _____ _____. Further palpation may cause the aneurysm to rupture, so be very careful in assessing this patient.

This patient's vital signs have been 3_____ steadily throughout the time he has been under your care.

- Treatment for this patient should include: cardiac monitoring. ◀

4_____ _____ should always be performed when you suspect an aneurysm is present.

a. Cardiac monitoring; b. worsening; c. On palpation; d. abdominal aortic aneurysm

Case study 15

You are called to the home of an elderly female who is having difficulty breathing. She has 1_ _____ of chronic congestive heart failure. (CHF) Which 2_____ ____ pattern is most likely for this patient?

- shallow, rapid 3_____; decreased pulse rate; cool, clammy skin
- deep laboured respirations, decreased 4_____ _____; hot, dry skin

- shallow, rapid respirations; increased pulse rate; cool clammy skin ◄
- increased respiratory rate, decreased pulse rate, flushed, dry 5____
- What are 6_____
  _____ associated with patients chronic CHF? – Diuretics, potassium, and digoxin.◄

a. a history; b. respirations; c. pulse rate; d. vital sign; e. skin; f. common medications

Case study 16
Which of the following areas of physical examination of an elderly patient is often the most difficult to accurately perform?

- 1_____ of the abdomen
- 2_____ of the lungs
- Blood pressure 3_____
- Examination of mental status ◄

Assessing the 4_____ _____ of an elderly patient is often difficult. It is often necessary to enlist the help of family and caregivers to accurately 5_____ if a patient's mental status is different from the norm.

a. measurement; b. auscultation; c. mental status; d. examination; e. determine

Case study 17
Your patient is a 60-year-old woman who has fallen down her front steps and has possibly 1_____ her ankle.

- Which assessment finding may be considered 2_____ in this patient? – Altered mental status ◄

Altered mental status is an abnormal finding in 3_____ _____ patients. The pulse rate does decrease somewhat with age but should 4_____ within the normal range of 60-100. Blood pressure often 5_____ with age and respiration rates increase slightly as patients use less of their lung tissues.

a. fractured; b. abnormal; c. healthy elderly; d. increases; e. remain

Case study 18
Your patient is a 66-year-old man who is extremely thin but has a noticeably distorted barrel-shaped chest. He reports a history of dyspnoea that has recently got worse. You note that he purses his lips when breathing, but hypoxia is 1____ _____.

- In addition to monitoring vital signs, breath sounds, and the ECG, starting an IV, and transporting the patient, what other 2_____ should you give to this patient? – 3_____ low-flow oxygen and a bronchodilator ◄

The patient is showing signs and symptoms of 4_____.

Administer low-flow oxygen to
5_____ his hypoxic drive.

a. treatments; b. preserve; c. Administer;
d. not apparent; e. emphysema

Case study 19

Your patient is a 67-year-old
female who complains of increasing
leg pain and tenderness. The skin
over the affected area is 1____ ____
___, and Homan's sign is positive.
Vital signs are 2_____.

- How should you treat this
  patient? – Elevate the leg
  and transport the patient
  for further evaluation. ◄

The 3_____ _____
suggests deep venous thrombosis. The
correct action is 4__ _____ the leg
and transport the patient for further
evaluation. Do not massage the area
or allow the patient to walk, since
pulmonary emboli may be 5_____.

a. to elevate; b. unremarkable; c. clinical
picture; d. warm and red; e. provoked

Case study 20

Dopamine can be used to:

- decrease 1_____ demand
- increase cardiac output ◄
- reduce blood pressure
- 2_____ dysrhythmias

3_____ is a potent
sympathomimetic agent, and in cases
of 4_____ _____, it may
be used to increase cardiac output.

a. oxygen; b. Dopamine; c. cardiogenic shock;
d. prevent

Case study 21

A patient is covered with
1_____-_____ material
after an accidental spill.

- An adequate level of
  shielding would be: a
  cloth uniform.◄

Alpha particles carry very
little energy. _ 2_____ is
adequate protection against
such a 3_____.

a. contaminant; b. A uniform;
c. alpha-radioactive

Vocabulary 20

abuser /əˈbjuː.zər/
account /əˈkaʊnt/
accumulation /əˌkjuː.mjʊˈleɪ.ʃən/
alpha /ˈæl.fə/
awoke /əˈwəʊk/
bursitis /bɜːˈsaɪ.tɪs/
caretaker /ˈkeəˌteɪ.kər/
caution /ˈkɔː.ʃən/
CHF, Congestive /kənˈdʒes.tɪv/
Heart /hɑːt/ **Failure** /ˈfeɪ.ljər/
dementia /dɪˈmen.ʃə/
dependent /dɪˈpen.dənt/
dialysis /daɪˈæl.ə.sɪs/
digoxin /dɪdʒ.ɒ k.sɪn/
discover /dɪˈskʌv.ər/
distorted /dɪˈstɔː.tɪd/
disturb /dɪˈstɜːb/
dosage /ˈdəʊ.sɪdʒ/
edge /edʒ/
enlist /ɪnˈlɪst/
flushed /flʌʃt/
frail /freɪl/
haemodialysis /ˌhiːmə.daɪˈælɪsɪs/

handicapped /ˈhæn.dɪ.kæpt/
Homans' /ˈhəʊ.mænz/ **sign** /saɪn/
impairment /ɪmˈpeər.mənt/
infrapatellar /ˌɪn.frə.pəˈtel.ər/
majority /məˈdʒɒr.ə.ti/
mature /məˈtjʊər/
measurement /ˈmeʒ.ə.mənt/
modify /ˈmɒdɪˌfaɪ/
neuropathy /ˌnjʊəˈrɒp.ə.θi/
non-productive /ˌnɒn.prəˈdʌk.tɪv/
noticeably /ˈnəʊ.tɪ.sə.bli/
occlusion /əˈkluː.ʒən/
particle /ˈpɑː.tɪ.kl̩/
provoke /prəˈvəʊk/
pulsate /pʌlˈseɪt/
purse /pɜːs/
shaped /ʃeɪpt/
shield /ʃiːld/
subdiaphragmatic /ˌsʌbˌdaɪə.frægˈmæt.ɪk/
sympathomimetic /ˌsɪm.pə.θə.mɪˈmet.ɪk/ **syndrome** /ˈsɪn.drəʊm/
throughout /θruːˈaʊt/
unaffected /ˌʌn.əˈfek.tɪd/
unrecognized /ʌnˈrek.əg.naɪzd/

Unit 21

Case study 1

Your patient is a 67-year-old male who is complaining of chest pain. The chest pain 1_____ after two doses of nitroglycerin. He reports a history of 2_____ and says that all his 3_____ _____ have been relieved by nitroglycerin.

- How should you treat this patient? – Treat the patient as though he is having an AMI and transport rapidly. ◄

A patient with angina whose pain does not respond to nitroglycerin is most likely suffering from MI and should be transported 4_____ _____.

a. angina; b. without delay; c. continues; d. previous attacks

Case study 2

Your patient is a 68-year-old male with a history of two 1_____ AMIs. Your assessment findings include a pulse rate of 124, peripheral oedema, and jugular vein distention. The patient 2_____ any chest pain or breathing difficulty.

- What condition should you 3_____? – Right ventricular failure ◄

The patient's 4_____, _____ ___ _____ suggest right ventricular failure.

a. history; signs and symptoms; b. denies; c. suspect; d. prior

Case study 3

Your patient is a 70-year-old male. He complains of chest pain that 1_____ while he was raking leaves. You perform an 2_____ assessment and a focused history and 3_____ _____ and administer oxygen and nitroglycerin. The patient then states that he feels much better.

- What is he most likely 4_____ ____? – Stable angina. ◄

The pain of stable angina is brought on 5__ _____, and 6_____ by rest, oxygen and nitroglycerin.

a. by exertion; b. suffering from; c. relieved; d. began; e. initial; f. physical examination

Case study 4

A 72-year-old male is found unconscious in his front yard after working in the yard for five hours without a break. He is tachycardic, with hot, dry skin and shallow respirations.

- Management should include what procedure? – Administer high-flow oxygen. ◄

This patient is experiencing a 1____ _____ and possible 2_____. It is important for him to receive 3_____, high 4_____ of oxygen, and active 5_____ _____ to reduce his body temperature.

a. Concentration; b. heat stroke; c. fluid; d. cooling measures; e. dehydration

Case study 5

Your patient is an obese 77-year-old woman who has called 1___ complaining of a 2_____ _____ __ dyspnoea, coughing, haemoptysis, and diaphoresis. __ 3_____, you note tachypnoea and tachycardia, an crackles d localized wheezing, and distended neck veins and varicose veins.

- You should suspect: pulmonary embolism.◄

This patient displays many of the risk factors for pulmonary embolism; her signs and symptoms also fit. The rapid onset of the problem should lead you to hypothesize acute 4_____ _____.

a. pulmonary embolism; b. EMS; c. sudden onset of; d. On examination

Case study 6

You are caring for a 77-year-old female who is in moderate respiratory distress. She is sitting in a tripod position with 1___-____ _____. She has a recent cold with increasing dyspnoea and a 2_____ _____ with yellow sputum. She denies chest pain. She has been smoking cigarettes for the past 40 years.

Vital signs are BP 150/80, pulse 100, respirations 36 and laboured. Her skin is 3_____ and she has 4_____ _____ in the legs. You hear expiratory wheezing upon auscultation of the lungs.

- Her pedal oedema is most likely caused by: cor pulmonale. ◄

Patients with COPD maintain chronic high levels of CO_2, which may result in 5_____ _____ and lead to right-sided heart failure, or cor pulmonale.

a. productive cough; b. cyanotic; c. pitting oedema; d. pulmonary hypertension; e. two-word dyspnoea

Case study 7

Your patient is a 78-year-old woman who is complaining of diffuse abdominal pain, nausea, and vomiting. Physical examination reveals abdominal distention and absent bowel sounds.

- You should suspect she has: bowel obstruction. ◄

1_____ signs and symptoms of myocardial infarction that are 2_____ ____ in elderly patients include all of the following: 3_____ ___ _____, syncope, 4_____ pain.
There are many atypical signs and symptoms of MI in elderly patients. A tearing sensation in the chest generally 5_____ a dissecting aneurysm is occurring.

a. Atypical; b. confusion and fatigue; c. indicates; d. commonly seen; e. neck

Case study 8

Your patient is an 82-year-old female with a suspected MI. While 1__ _____ to the hospital, you note that her systolic blood pressure, which had been stable, has started 2__ _____, and that she is becoming 3_____. At the same time, her 4_____ _____ converts to sinus tachycardia.

- What should you suspect is happening?

– She is developing cardiogenic shock. ◄

Signs of cardiogenic shock include a sudden drop in 5_____ blood pressure and increasing confusion.

a. to drop; b. confused; c. systolic; d. en route; e. heart rhythm

Case study 9

Your patient is a 67-year-old male who reports a 45-pack-a-year smoking history, 1_____ respiratory infections, and a 2_____ cough. He is overweight and has peripheral 3_____.
Auscultation of the chest reveals rhonchi. There is also noticeable jugular vein distention.

- What disease process should you suspect? – Chronic bronchitis. ◄

The patient's history, signs, and symptoms are consistent with 4_____ _____. The "blue bloater" frequently has peripheral oedema, cyanosis, and JVD due to right-side 5_____ _____ in addition to the respiratory problems.
Emphysema patients present with barrel chest and signs of wasting of the extremities.

a. heart failure; b. chronic bronchitis; c. chronic; d. frequent; e. cyanosis

Case study 10

A 72-year-old man trips and falls while walking to his bathroom.

Physical findings include a lateral 1_____ of the left foot and knee. The patient has 2_____ and a protrusion in the left groin area.

- You suspect: anterior dislocation of the hip. ◄

The outward rotation of the left extremity along with the 3_____ in the groin area points to an 4_____

_____ _____.

a. anterior dislocation injury; b. deformity; c. tenderness; d. rotation

Case study 11
Answer the next two questions on the basis of the following information.

You arrive to find a 65-year-old male in acute respiratory distress. You hear wheezes from across the room, and you note 1_____ accessory muscle use.

The patient has assumed a tripod 2_____ and is breathing through pursed lips. Your physical exam reveals a barrel chest and stained 3_____.

Vital signs are blood pressure, 160/90; pulse, 100 strong and irregular with atrial fibrillation on the cardiac monitor; and respiratory rate, 40, with shallow and 4_____ breathing.

Auscultation of the chest reveals wheezes and 5_____ lung sounds throughout all fields.

- What is this patient most likely suffering from? – Emphysema. ◄

- Why is this patient breathing through pursed lips? – To provide positive pressure to inflate the alveoli. ◄

Breathing through 6_____ ____ is a common compensatory mechanism COPD patients use to provide positive end-expiratory pressure, which forces more alveoli to inflate.

a. position; b. fingernails; c. laboured; d. diminished; e. pursed lips; f. extreme

Case study 12
Under what 1_____ could the pulse oximetry reading show a elevated reading in a patient? – When the patient is exposed to carbon monoxide. ◄

Carbon monoxide 2_____ can cause _ 3_____ high pulse oximetry reading

a. a falsely; b. poisoning; c. circumstance

Case study 13
Your patient is a 67-year-old male who smokes cigarettes and has a history of previous MI. He complains of sudden-onset severe pain in his right leg. He also relates numbness and diminished 1_____ _____ in the right leg.

Other assessment findings are diminished pulse, pallor, and lowered skin temperature in the right leg.

You should suspect which of the following?

- femoral artery aneurysm

- occlusion of the femoral artery ◀
- 2_____ _____ _____
- hypertensive encephalopathy

The patient is displaying signs and symptoms of 3_____ occlusion of the femoral artery.

Aneurysms generally do not occur in the femoral artery. If an aneurysm were present, the signs and symptoms would be 4_____ _____ those presented.

Deep-vein thrombosis would 5_____ __ vascular pooling distal to the site of occlusion, and oedema would be present or developing in the extremity, but arterial circulation would be 6_____.

a. deep venous thrombosis; b. acute; c. result in; d. different from; e. motor function; f. unaffected

Case study 14

Answer the next two questions on the basis of the following information.

You are called to the home of a 68-year-old female who is complaining of severe dyspnoea. She states that it started about 45 minutes ago and has been 1_____ progressively _____. She has a 2_____ _____ but denies chest pain at this time. Her breathing is very congested. During your assessment you notice accessory muscle use and rales bilaterally.

Which of the following conditions is this patient most likely suffering from?

- pulmonary embolism
- acute pulmonary oedema ◀
- pneumonia
- lung cancer

Rapid onset, rales, 3_____ _____ use, and dyspnoea are classic symptoms for a patient with acute pulmonary oedema.

- In addition to oxygen, this patient should also be treated with which medication? – Morphine sulphate ◀

Morphine sulphate would be an appropriate treatment for acute pulmonary oedema. It increases peripheral venous capacitance and decreases venous return, 4_____ _____ and decreasing myocardial oxygen demand.

a. getting worse; b. improving ventilation; c. accessory muscle; d. cardiac history

Case study 15

You have arrived on scene to find a 75-year-old female in respiratory distress. Your assessment reveals: BP 138/90, pulse 136/minute, and RR 34.

Upon auscultation, you note diffuse 1_____ _____ in the apices and diminished 2_____ _____ in the bases. Pulse oximetry is 82% on room air, and the patient appears fatigued.

What treatment guidelines should you follow for this patient?

- 3_____ an IV at a KVO rate ◀

- If possible, 4_____ via BVM at a rate of 24/min to maximize oxygenation ◄
- 5_____ orotracheal or nasotracheal intubation ◄

Because the patient appears 6_____, respiratory failure is imminent. Inadequate tidal volume may not permit good gas exchange without manual support.

a. bilateral wheezes; b. breath sounds; c. Attempt; d. ventilate; e. fatigued; f. Establish

Case study 16

Your patient is a 75-year-old man. His wife called EMS because he "has a terrible headache and is very confused." Vital signs: respirations, 26; pulse, 78; and blood pressure, 200/120. The 1_____ _____ you must address is most likely which of the following?

- hypertensive emergency ◄
- senile dementia
- cardiac tamponade
- cerebrovascular accident

Although the chief complaint was 2_____ ___ _____, it is likely that the primary problem to address is 3_____ _____. Senile dementia of new onset could have a variety of causes, but in this case, it may be connected to the hypertensive crisis. There is not enough information to determine if elder abuse or cardiac tamponade is present, but it is unlikely in this scenario.

Another possibility for this patient is a stroke. If 4_____ is occurring, prompt management of the hypertensive crisis can reduce 5_____.

a. stroke; b. primary problem; c. morbidity; d. headache and confusion; e. hypertensive crisis

Case study 17

You respond to a "shortness of breath" call. Upon arrival you find the first responders placing a 70-year old male on a nonrebreather mask. Family members state that the patient came back from the store approximately 45 minutes ago, complaining of moderate respiratory distress.

He has a history of "some sort of lung disease" for which he uses an inhaler.

The family does not know what type of medication the patient is taking. There is no history of fever or recent illness.

You observe that the patient is cyanotic. The oxygen reservoir on the mask does not appear to collapse, even though the litre flow is set correctly. Although he is sitting on the edge of the bed, his eyes are closed and he does not respond to verbal commands. There is accessory muscle use evident, with intercostals muscle retractions. His breath sounds are diminished in all fields and absent in both bases. Faint expiratory wheezing is auscultated at only the apices.

His heart rate is 140, respiratory rate 42, and BP 106/72. The pulse oximeter registers an SpO$_2$ of 75%. The rest of his physical exam is unremarkable.

- Based on the information given, what might be a suspected assessment? – Emphysema ◄

The timing of the onset, medical history, and physical findings point to emphysema as the 1_____ _____.

- What would be your initial priority in managing this patient's condition? – Instruct first responders to assist the patient's ventilations with a BVM and 100% oxygen. ◄

This patient has begun to 2_____ in terms of his ability to ventilate adequately, as evidenced by the decreased mental status and very poor skin signs. This patient will require aggressive 3_____ _____ in order to be ventilated.

- What airway adjunct(s) might you consider first for this patient? – Bag-valve mask.◄

The most immediate piece of ventilation equipment to use would be a CPAP. CPAP eliminates the need for 4_____. If CPAP is not available, a BVM would be the next choice. The patient will need 5_____ before any attempt of intubation. In addition, as

implied by the patient's presenting position, he will likely have an intact gag reflex, making the 6_____ of an OPA difficult, if not impossible.

- What medication may be used in the management of this patient's condition? – Albuterol. ◄

A beta agonist like albuterol is indicated in this situation. Morphine sulphate may worsen the patient's condition by potentially depressing 7_____ _____. Adenosine is a cardiac medication used to control supraventricular tachycardia. Epinephrine has significant cardiac 8_____ _____, especially in older patients.

a. primary suspect; b. decompensate;
c. airway management; d. intubation;
e. preoxygenation; f. insertion; g. respiratory drive; h. side effects

Case study 18
You are called to the home of a 78-year-old male who is having difficulty breathing. The patient is sitting upright in a tripod position and you note 1_____ accessory muscle use. His skin is pale, cool, and clammy. 2_____ _____ are: blood pressure, 180/72; heart rate, 90; and respiratory rate, 40. Breathing is 3_____ ____ _____ with a coarse rattling sound during expiration. Auscultation reveals coarse rales to the 4_____ _____ with no air movement in the bases. The patient can speak only in one-or-two-word 5_____.

Family members inform you that the patient was sleeping when this episode began and that this has happened several times since his 6____ one year ago. He has mild pedal oedema and neck veins are nondistended. His family first noticed the patient having dyspnoea about 25-30 minutes ago.

- This patient is exhibiting the signs and symptoms of: Congestive heart failure ◄
- Which medication should be used for this patient? - Morphine sulfate ◄
- Prior to an acute onset a patient with the symptoms and history described may 7_____: paroxysmal nocturnal dyspnoea. ◄

Paroxysmal nocturnal dyspnoea (PND), dyspnoea upon exertion, and increased dyspnoea are all signs of worsening CHF.

- 8_____ for the management of this patient include all of the following: increasing venous return to the heart, decreasing myocardial oxygen demand, improving oxygenation and ventilation.◄
- This patient would mostly 9_____ ____: giving him intermittent positive pressure ventilation.◄

Increased ventilatory pressures 10_____: in driving off some of the pulmonary oedema.

- If this patient were experiencing right-side heart failure, you would expect to find all of the following: tachycardia, profound peripheral oedema, jugular venous 11_____. ◄

a. profound; b. benefit from; c. distension;
d. shallow and laboured; e. nipple line;
f. Vital signs; g. sentences; h. exhibit; i. AMI;
j. Priorities; k. assist

Case study 19

Answer the next six questions on the basis of the following information.

You are called to a nursing home and find a bedridden 78-year-old male with insulin-dependent diabetes who is in acute respiratory distress. The staff reports that the patient has been ill for the last few days and has had a persistent productive cough with thick yellow sputum.

His blood pressure is 168/72. His respiratory rate is 40 and laboured with coarse rhonchi upon auscultation of lung sounds. Lung sounds are absent in the lower third of his lung fields. The patient is also febrile with 1____, ____ ____ _____ ____.

- This patient is most likely suffering from what condition? – Pneumonia. ◄

This patient shows signs and symptoms of pneumonia. The fever is the symptom that provides the differential diagnosis between the various choices.

- Treatment of this patient should include: oxygen ◄

In addition to oxygen, this patient needs 2_____.

What common infectious disease does this patient's clinical presentation mimic?

- meningitis
- HIV/AIDS
- tuberculosis ◄
- hepatitis B

3_____ _____ presents with fever, flulike symptoms, and productive cough. Meningitis presents with high fever and 4_____ _____, but does not have respiratory involvement. HIV may not have any symptoms, although AIDS can present as a 5_____ __ diseases, depending upon which opportunistic disease has caused infection. 6_____ _ will present primarily with GI problems (nausea, vomiting, pain) and upper-right-quadrant abdominal pain.

- What is most likely the cause of his decreased lung sounds? – Atelectasis from inactivity. ◄

Diabetic patients heal more slowly from pneumonia when it occurs, but it is not a common disease for them. CHF and pulmonary hypertension would certainly contribute to worsening his signs and symptoms, but the most likely cause of absent or decreased 7____ _____ in the lower lobes of a sick elderly patient in incomplete expansion and shallow respiration 8___ __ _____.

- In this patient required tracheal suctioning, what step should be followed? – Sterile technique is required for suctioning this patient. ◄

Because 9_____ _____ will be performed on this patient, 10_____ _____ is required. Suction should be performed only upon withdrawal of the 11_____. For protection of the 12_____, gloves, eye protection, and face mask should be worn during the procedure. If the patient is being 13_____ you should hyperventilate before and after suctioning.

- How should this patient be positioned for transport? – High Fowler's position. ◄

Position of comfort is always the 14_____ transport position for nontraumatic patients when the patient is 15_____ ___ _____. To 16_____ _____ and maximize efforts, the best position for this patient would be high Fowler's position

a. hot, dry, flushed skin; b. rescuer;
c. antibiotics; d. due to inactivity; e. optimal;
f. facilitate breathing; g. tracheal suctioning;
h. lung sounds; i. sterile technique;
j. Hepatitis B; k. conscious and oriented;
l. flulike symptoms; m. Active tuberculosis;
n. variety of; o. catheter; p. ventilated

You will see the systolic pressure drop dramatically (often to less than 80 mmHg) when this occurs.

a. absent or reduced; b. MI; c. pulmonary vessels; d. cardiogenic shock; e. oedema

Case study 20

Your patient is an 84-year-old man with extreme difficulty breathing, apprehension, cyanosis, and diaphoresis. Assessment findings include elevated pulse and blood pressure. Rales and rhonchi are heard on auscultation. There is no chest pain.

• What condition should treat this patient for? – Left-side failure secondary to MI. ◄

The patient is displaying signs and symptoms of left ventricular failure, which most often occurs secondary to 1__.

Hypertension and tachycardia is due in part to increased left atrial pressure that is transmitted to the 2_____ _____.

Rales and rhonchi indicate that pulmonary 3_____ is present.

Right-side failure can lead to left-side failure, but such a patient generally has dry lungs and dependent oedema (usually pedal) as the presenting sign.

A dissecting aneurysm will present with pain, syncope, stroke, 4_____ __ _____ pulses, heart failure, pericardial tamponade, and/or signs of AMI.

If the ventricular failure worsens, 5_____ _____ may develop.

Case study 21

Signs and symptoms of radiation sickness include: 1____ ____.

Hair loss, nausea and vomiting are 2_____ signs and symptoms of 3_____ _____.

a. radiation sickness; b. common; c. hair loss ◄

Vocabulary 21

bedridden /ˈbed.rɪ.dən/
blue bloater /ˈbləʊ.tər/
call /kɔːl/
cerebrovascular /ˌser.ɪ.brəˈvæskjʊlə/
chief /tʃiːf/
coarse /kɔːs/
convert /kənˈvɜːt/
CPAP, Continuous /kənˈtɪn.ju.əs/ **Positive** /ˈpɒz.ə.tɪv/ **Airway** /ˈeə.weɪ/ **Pressure** /ˈpreʃ.ər/
expiratory /ɪkˈspɪr.ə.tər.i/
faint /feɪnt/
falsely /ˈfɒls.li/
fibrillation /ˌfaɪ.brɪˈleɪ.ʃən/
fingernail /ˈfɪŋ.gə.neɪl/
flulike /ˈfluː.laɪk/
groin /grɔɪn/
hypothesize /haɪˈpɒθ.ə.saɪz/
inactivity /ˌɪn.ækˈtɪv.ɪ.ti/
leaf /liːf/ pl **leaves**
nonrebreather /ˌnɒn.rəbrə.ðər/ **mask** /mɑːsk/
nursing /ˈnɜː.sɪŋ/
OPA, Oropharyngeal /ˈɔː.rə.fəˈrɪn.dʒɪ.əl/ **Airway** /ˈeə.weɪ/
overweight /ˌəʊ.vəˈweɪt/

278

productive /prəˈdʌk.tɪv/
protrusion /prəˈtruː.ʒən/
radiation /ˌreɪ.diˈeɪ.ʃən/
sickness /ˈsɪk.nəs/
rake /reɪk/
relate /rɪˈleɪt/
senile /ˈsiː.naɪl/
trip /trɪp/
use /juːz/
varicose vein /ˌvær.ɪ.kəʊsˈveɪn/
venous /ˈviː.nəs/ **capacitance**
/kəˈpæs.ɪ.tənts/
waste /weɪst/
yard /jɑːd/

Unit 22
Case study 1

You respond to a 63-year-old male who is complaining of sudden onset of extreme substernal chest pain that, he says, "feels like my insides are tearing." The patient states that the pain 1_____ to the middle of his back between his shoulder blades.

- What condition is this patient most likely suffering from? – Dissecting aortic aneurysm ◄

This patient is exhibiting classic signs and symptoms for a 2_____ _____
_____. The tearing sensation occurs as the intimal linings of the aorta are separated as blood collects between the tissues.

- What is a predisposing factor for this patient's condition? – Hypertension ◄

3_____ is present in 75-85% of dissecting aortic aneurysm cases.

- What medication may be ordered by medical control to treat this patient? – Morphine sulfate ◄

Morphine sulfate is the appropriate medication for this patient. Medications that increase cardiac rate, output, function, or contractile force are 4_____ while the dissection is occurring.

- Progression of this condition may cause: stroke, pericardial tamponade, acute myocardial infarction. ◄

These are all consequences of further dissection. Other 5_____ also include syncope, heart failure, and absent or reduced pulses and death.

a. Hypertension; b. radiates; c. conditions; d. contraindicated; e. dissecting aortic aneurysm

Case study 2

A 63-year-old male is complaining of substernal chest pain 1_____ to his left arm and jaw. He is 2_____ and cool to the touch. The cardiac monitor shows sinus tachycardia. The patient's vital signs are BP = 136/70, P = 118, and RR = 16. You have administered oxygen and established an IV.

- What should you do now? - Administer 3_____ nitroglycerin and evaluate the patient's response to the mediaction. ◄

The patient's heart rate is not fast enough to be the primary source of the chest pain. Therefore, administration of nitroglycerin may resolve the chief 4_____, which in turn may slow the heart rate down.

a. sublingual; b. complaint; c. radiating; d. diaphoretic

Case study 3

Which of the following conditions indicates the need for rapid transport?

a) Isolated 1_____ trauma by a knife in the upper forearm
b) A pedestrian struck by a motor vehicle travelling about 10 mph (16km per hour)
c) First-degree and second-degree 2_____ to the anterior chest
d) A pulse rate, 130; blood pressure, 90/60; and respiratory rate, 36/min ◄

The vital signs listed in the choice d). indicate the 3_____ __ _____. An isolated injury of penetrating trauma to the upper arm is not generally 4____ _____. A 10-mile-per-hour 5_____ to a pedestrian is not generally a significant MOI. Burns to the entire

chest cover a body surface area of approximately 9%; this would not in itself require rapid transport unless other problems existed.

a. impact; b. presence of shock; c. life threatening; d. penetrating; e. burns

Case study 4

These activities are performed by the EMT- Paramedic in the field:

- Maintaining and 1_____ of emergency-care equipment and supplies. ◄
- Directing and coordinating patient transport by 2_____ the best methods ◄
- Assigning 3_____ of emergency treatment ◄
- Initiating and continuing 4_____ _____ ◄

All of the activities are related to the practice of the paramedic.

a. emergency treatment; b. priorities; c. preparing; d. selecting

Case study 5

What is the 1_____ of a safety officer at a multi-casualty incident?

- to teach the Unit members to work together
- to decide when a scene is safe enough to enter ◄

- to stand in for the transportation officer as necessary
- to ensure patient safety before BLS Unit arrives

The function of the safety officer is to 2_____ the scene and make the "go/no go" 3_____ for the operation. The safety officer is also responsible for continuing to monitor 4_____ _____ during the operation.

a. evaluate; b. scene safety; c. decision; d. function

Case study 6

A tiered response system is one that: dispatches responders at various levels, depending on the incident.◄

In 1_____ _____, responders are 2_____ to calls depending upon the nature of the 3_____ as stated by the 112 caller and 4_____ by the dispatcher.

a. a tiered system; b. incident; c. evaluated; d. dispatched

Case study 7

In a motor vehicle 1_____, which of the following would be most important to understand in relation to the 2_____ ___ _____ and the potential for injury?

- speed and time of impact ◄
- weight of the vehicle
- road conditions at the scene
- condition of the vehicle's tyres

3_____ plays a greater role in the force changes during a motor vehicle crash. While the other items are important when evaluating an 4_____ _____, speed has the greatest influence on the potential for 5_____ ___ _____.

a. Speed; b. damage and injury; c. force of collision; d. crash; e. accident scene

Case study 8

Which statement about motorcycle crashes is correct?

- They seldom result in severe trauma, unless the motorcycle is operated at high speeds.
- Helmet use can reduce the incidence and severity of head injury.
- Helmet use can reduce the incidence and severity of spinal injury. ◄
- Leather clothing cannot protect the rider against soft-tissue injury.

Use of a 1_____ can protect the rider against head injury but not against 2_____ _____. Leather clothing is helpful in reducing the amount of 3____ _____ injury. Because the energy of the accident is mostly absorbed into the rider, 4_____ _____ is noted even in low-speed crashes

a. severe trauma; b. helmet; c. soft tissue; d. spinal injury

Case study 9

Asymetrical movement during respiration typically suggests which condition?

- COPD
- flail chest ◄
- 1_____ damage
- haemothorax

2_____ movement during respiration typically suggests injury to the 3_____ ____.

a. chest wall; b. Asymetrical; c. brain

Case study 10

Which patient is likely to need rapid transport to a trauma centre rather than assessment and stabilization on the scene?

a) Male, age 56, ejected from a crashed vehicle with a flail chest ◄
b) Female, age 60, burns to 10% BSI on her chest and abdomen
c) Male, age 28, fell 10 feet (3 m) from a 1_____ onto a pile of mulch
d) Female, age 46, 2_____ by car travelling 10 mph (16 km/h), no 3_____ injuries.

a) is correct. All the others do not have 4_____ mechanisms, so they should not receive 5_____ transportation.

a. penetrating; b. critical; c. platform; d. struck; e. rapid

Case study 11

This statement describes a tiered EMS system: 1_____ _____ of resources are dispatched to calls, depending on the nature of the incident. ◄

A tiered EMS system is one in which varying levels of 2_____ are dispatched to calls depending upon the 3_____ if the incident as determined by the 112 4_____.

a. resources; b. Varying levels; c. dispatcher; d. nature

Case study 12

A critically traumatized 18-year-old male is 1_____. It will be at least 15 minutes before he is freed. The community hospital is 20 minutes away by ground. A medical helicopter can be to the scene in eight minutes. A Level I trauma centre is one hour away by ground.

- Given the situation which is the best mode of transport for this patient? – Fly the patient from the scene to the Level I trauma centre. ◄

2_____ _____ offers the advantage of rapid transport to specialized facilities such as the Level I trauma centre. The amount of time needed to 3_____ the patient, coupled with the time to transport the patient to either the closest hospital or the trauma centre by ground, is too much. Flying the patient directly to the trauma centre is 4_____ _____.

> a. Most appropriate; b. Aeromedical
> transport; c. extricate; d. entrapped

Case study 13

Starting an IV on an 1_____
_____ who refuses one could
result in your being held liable
for which of the following?

- assault
- battery ◄
- libel
- slander

2_____ is the unlawful
touching of an individual without
consent. 3_____ is the threat
of bodily harm. 4_____ is saying
something that is not true.

> a. Libel; b. Assault; c. Battery; d. alert patient

Case study 14

A 5-year-old male has multiple
injuries in various stages of healing,
including 1_____ ____ and
a new suspected broken leg. On
questioning, his mother states that
he fell out of his bunk bed, but his
sister, age 9, says "Daddy beat him".

The mother insists that her
husband will take the child to the
hospital when he gets home from work.

- How should you 2_____?
  – Document your findings
  3_____ the mother that
  transport to the hospital
  is necessary, and report
  your 4_____
  of child abuse. ◄

In cases of suspected child abuse,
your responsibility is to ensure that the
patient 5_____ _____ ____
immediately and report your findings.

> a. proceed; b. convince; c. raccoon eyes;
> d. suspicions; e. receives necessary care

Case study 15

What should you do in
order to preserve 1_____
_____ in cases of suspected
sexual assault? – Avoid cleaning
wounds and handling clothing ◄

To preserve physical evidence,
avoid 2_____ clothing and
cleaning or bandaging wounds, unless
there is haemorrhage. 3__ ____ _____
the victim to bathe, comb her hair, or
change her clothing. Do not subject
the patient to any 4_____
physical examinations.

> a. unnecessary; b. Do not allow; c. handling;
> d. physical evidence

Case study 16

With whom does ultimate
responsibility for patient care
in the field always rest? – The
medical control physician. ◄

No matter who is actually
1_____ care or giving
2_____ to the responder,
ultimate responsibility always rests with
the 3_____ _____ physician.

> a. medical control; b. directions; c. providing

Case study 17

What situation represents
expressed consent? – The patient
says "Help me, my chest hurts". ◄

1_____ consent means that the patient gives you 2_____ to treat him or her, either 3_____ or in writing.

a. verbally; b. permission; c. Expressed

Case study 18

Your radio report to the hospital about the patient's medical condition should include which of the following?

- the complete medical history
- name, age, race, sex, and weight
- the chief complaint ◄
- estimated time of arrival on the scene

Although some details of the medical history, such as allergies, surgeries, and 1_____, are 2_____, a detailed history is not. Do not say the patient's name over the 3_____. Estimated 4_____ at the hospital is important, but the time of your arrival on the scene is generally not important.

a. radio; b. arrival; c. relevant; d. medications

Case study 19

A person with a serious illness can delegate the right to make medical decisions to someone else by enacting which of the following legal documents?

a) Living will
b) Durable power of attorney for healthcare ◄
c) Do Not Resuscitate order
d) Right To Die order

A durable power of attorney for healthcare 1_____ the right to make medical 2_____ to someone else in the event that the patient becomes 3_____ __ _____.

Choices a), b) and c) are all examples of advanced directives, stating one's 4____ regarding medical interventions.

a. delegates; b. disabled or incompetent; c. will; d. decisions

Case study 20

What is the legal term for an 1_____ deviation from the accepted 2_____ of care that results in harm to a patient?

- Negligence ◄
- Liability
- Res ipsa loquitur
- 3_____

a. standard; b. abandonment; c. intentional

Case study 21

The ideal helicopter landing zone should:

- contain a slope of no more than 15°
- be an area of at least 100 feet by 100 feet ◄
- be an area of at least 90 feet by 90 feet
- be in a fenced area for safety against onlookers

The ideal helicopter 1_____ _____ should be at least 100 feet by 100 feet square. Larger helicopters may require more room, so consult local air medical services if you are unsure of the size of 2_____ used in your area. The 3_____ _____ should be no more than 10° and the area should be clear of debris, fences, wires, or other 4_____.

---

a. landing zone; b. obstructions; c. ground slope; d. aircraft

---

Vocabulary 22

abandonment /əˈbæn.dən.mənt/
accepted /əkˈsep.tɪd/
advanced /ədˈvɑːnst/
directive /daɪˈrek.tɪv/
aeromedical /ˌeə.rəˈmed.ɪ.kəl/
service /sɜːvɪs/
beat /biːt/
BLS, Basic /ˈbeɪ.sɪk/ **Life Support** /ˈlaɪf.səˌpɔːt/
bunk /bʌŋk/ **bed** /bed/
by ground /graʊnd/
comb /koʊm/
consult /kənˈsʌlt/
convince /kənˈvɪns/
decision /dɪˈsɪʒ.ən/
disabled /dɪˈseɪbld/
EMT, Emergency /ɪˈmɜː.dʒənt .si/ **Medical** /ˈmed.ɪ.kəl/ **Technician** /tekˈnɪʃən/
enact /ɪˈnækt/
extricate /ˈek.strɪ.keɪt/
fence /fens/
generally /ˈdʒen.ə r.əl.i/
in writing /ˈraɪ.tɪŋ/
incompetent /ɪnˈkɒm.pɪ.tənt/
individual /ˌɪn.dɪˈvɪd.ju.əl/
leather /ˈleð.ər/
liability /ˌlaɪ.əˈbɪl.ɪ.ti/
liable /ˈlaɪ.ə.bl̩/
MO, Medical /ˈmed.ɪ.kəl/ **Officer** /ˈɒf.ɪ.sər/
mode /məʊd/

mulch /mʌltʃ/
multi /mʌl.ti-/
onlooker /ˈɒnˌlʊk.ər/
paramedic /ˌpærəˈmedɪk/
pedestrian /pɪˈdestrɪən/
permission /pəˈmɪʃ.ən/
pile /paɪl/
power /ˈpaʊə/
reduce /rɪˈdjuːs/
relation /rɪˈleɪ.ʃən/
Res ipsa loquitur
rider /ˈraɪ.dər/
seldom /ˈsel.dəm/
shoulder /ˈʃəʊl.dər/ **blade** /bleɪd/
slope /sləʊp/
speed /spiːd/
stand /stænd/ **in**
substernal /sʌbˈstɜː.nəl/
tiered /tɪəd/
tyre /taɪər/
ultimate /ˈʌl.tɪ.mət/
vary /ˈveə.ri/
weight /weɪt/

Unit 23
Case study 1

You have responded to a home for an unknown 1_____. Your patient, a 74-year-old male named George Evans, has been found at home with rigor mortis with dependent lividity.

- The best thing to tell his family initially is: "I'm sorry to tell you that Mr. Evans has died". ◀

Inform the family that the patient 2____ ____ in plain, simple language. This avoids any 3_____ and prevents any false hopes that may arise from a misunderstanding. Always deliver this news with 4_____ and respect.

> a. has died; b. compassion;
> c. misunderstanding; d. emergency

Case study 2

You are acting under the doctrine of implied consent when you treat which of the following patients?

- A person who is 1_____ and refuses treatment
- A 2_____ elderly man whose adult child is with him
- A small child whose parent is not present ◄
- A person who is 3_____ and mentally distraught

4_____ consent covers situations in which the patient is not capable of consenting to treatment but a reasonable person would do so.

> a. Implied; b. confused; c. upset; d. drunk

Case study 3

At what age is a person considered capable of giving consent to treatment? – 18.◄

In most states, 1 _____ for treatment must be obtained from all patients who are 18 years old or older. This can be 2_____ in situations of extenuating 3_____, such as when an underage minor is pregnant or has 4_____ _____ of a minor child in his or her care.

- In general, the court deems an emancipated minor to be

one who: is 5_____, is economically 6_____, maintains a separate home, is in the 7_____. ◄

> a. circumstances; b. consent; c. independent;
> d. legal custody; e. modified; f. married;
> g. military

Case study 4

What should you do when confronted with a patient whom you suspect to be a victim of elder abuse? – Report your suspicions to the appropriate authority. ◄

Report your suspicions promptly. Many states have 1_____ requiring you to report any suspicions of 2_____ _____, 3_____ _____, or 4_____ _____.

> a. domestic violence; b. laws; c. child abuse;
> d. elder abuse

Case study 5

An EMS crew attempts to resuscitate a 50-year-old male in cardiac arrest and is not successful. The family sues the EMS organization for 1_____.

- The crew will need to prove that its 2_____ during the resuscitation: were similar to the actions a reasonably prudent person would do under 3_____ circumstances. ◄

The "reasonable person" standard sets a minimum guideline for what similarly trained 4_____ would do under similar circumstances, in

286

this case, a cardiac arrest. As long as the crew could 5＿＿＿＿＿＿ that its actions were 6＿＿＿＿＿＿ and expected to be done by other 7＿＿＿＿＿＿-＿＿ providers in a similar situation, this would avoid a negligence allegation.

a. actions; b. personnel; c. negligence; d. prehospital-care; e. demonstrate; f. similar; g. reasonable

Case study 6

Which situation would constitute a moral dilemma for a paramedic?

a) A female rape victim who insists on being cared for only by a female paramedic or EMT.
b) A patient who has sustained a potentially serious head injury but refuses care or transport. ◄
c) A patient who signed a Do Not Resuscitate order who is now unconscious and dying
d) A patient who is found unconscious with no family member present to authorize care.

This b) situation constitutes a dilemma because the paramedic would have to choose between the duty to 1＿＿＿＿ ＿＿ and the duty to 2＿＿＿＿ ＿＿＿＿. If a patient has a signed DNR order, you should honour his or her 3＿＿＿. When a patient is unconscious, you treat him or her under the doctrine of 4＿＿＿＿ consent. The rape victim is simply requesting an

all-female crew, and you should try to 5＿＿＿＿＿＿ her wishes.

a. implied; b. obtain consent; c. provide care; d. order; e. accommodate

Case study 7

You are called to a physician's office to care for a patient who is 1＿＿＿＿＿＿ symptoms of a myocardial infarction. The physician tells you that she will 2＿＿＿＿＿ the patient herself and that she is assuming 3＿＿＿＿＿＿ for care. She does, however, wish for you to transport the patient to the hospital.

• How should you proceed?
  – Defer to the on-scene physician and take her to the hospital with you. ◄

4＿＿＿＿＿＿ should defer to a physician who is present on scene provided this individual is assuming responsibility for the continued care of this patient. Make sure you know the rules and regulations for your jurisdiction regarding 5＿＿-＿＿＿ physicians.

a. paramedic; b. responsibility; c. on-scene; d. experiencing; e. stabilize

Case study 8

What do you call a legal document that specifies what type of treatment a patient does and does not want to receive?
– An advanced directive. ◄

The living will and DNR order are both examples of 1＿＿＿＿ ＿＿＿＿＿＿ called advanced directives. They specify the kind of 2_____-____ a person does and does not want to receive in the event of their 3_____ _____.

a. legal documents; b. health-care; c. imminent death

Case study 9

Your patient is a 28-year-old man who is suffering a seizure. You monitor his condition during the seizure and throughout the postictal period, but when the patient recovers, he refuses transport or further treatment.

- What should you do next? – Consult with medical control, explain the risks of refusing care, and document the patient's refusal. ◄

If a 1_____ _____ patient refuses treatment and transport, you should 2_____ with medical control, explain to the patient the risks of refusal in detail, 3_____ the informed refusal, and, if possible, have the refusal 4_____ by someone who is not an EMS employee

a. competent adult; b. document; c. witnessed; d. consult

Case study 10

What is included in the management of a patient in a 1_____ state?

- placing the patient in a recumbent position

and 2_____ supplemental oxygen ◄

Place the patient in the lateral-recumbent position to prevent 3_____ and administer supplemental oxygen as needed; provide 4_____ and transport.

a. administering; b. aspiration; c. privacy; d. postictal

Case study 11

Your patient is age 7 and has a suspected broken arm and numerous bruises. The mother states that the child was hurt when he fell off his bike in the morning.

- What finding would lead you to suspect that the mother's account of the injuries is not true? – Purplish, yellowish, and greenish bruises ◄

Although children are often uncoordinated and subject to frequent falls, the presence of bruises in 1_____ _____ of healing would lead you to suspect that this child had been injured on more than one 2_____. Carefully note the 3_____ the child is living in and report your 4_____ of abuse or neglect to the proper 5_____.

a. environment; b. suspicions; c. occasion; d. various stages; e. authorities

Case study 12

What is the paramedic's primary goal in cases of suspected child

1_____? – Make sure that the child receives necessary treatment. ◄

In many states, medical personnel are 2_____ required to report all cases of suspected abuse and 3_____, but a paramedic's first 4_____ is to ensure that the child is transported to the hospital to 5_____ necessary treatment

---

a. receive; b. abuse; c. legally;
d. responsibility; e. neglect

Case study 13

You respond to a 56-year-old male who appears to be intoxicated. He is belligerent and disoriented and has a laceration on his forehead. You have made several attempts to convince him of the need for treatment, but he refuses treatment or transport.

- Given this situation, you should: call medical direction for advice and guidance. ◄

Medical direction should be sought if at all possible for any suspected 1_____-_____ patient refusing 2_____
__ _____. Because you are required to be an advocate for the patient, it is never advisable to simply transport someone against his or her 3_____, even if you 4_____ _____ due to drug or alcohol use.

It is also not advisable to allow him or her to 5_____ _ _____
_____ when it is obvious that they are in need of medical attention.

Treating the patient, then leaving the scene without transport, leaves you open to legal liability and a possible charge of 6_____.

The patient continues to insist he does not need medical attention.

- In this situation most important is: Properly 7_____ your advice to the patient and his continued refusal. ◄

Documentation should include the steps you took to convince him to seek medical attention, the potential 8_____ of his refusal, and your assessment findings.

---

a. consequences; b. substance-abuse;
c. suspect impairment; d. treatment or
transport; e. sign a refusal form; f. will;
g. document;◄ h. abandonment ◄

Case study 14

Which 1_____ can cause users to behave violently and aggressively? – PCP. ◄

PCP can cause 2_____ _____ as well as violent and uncontrollable 3_____.

---

a. bizarre delusions; b. behaviour; c. drug

Case study 15

In case a patient has been violently beaten: statements made by the patient should 1__ _____ in the report ◄

Managing the patient's injury is the 2_____ _____ of the EMS provider. Any statements made by

289

the patient should be recorded as possible 3_____ ___ ___ _____.

Regardless of any of the options considered in the previous question, the patient continues to insist he does not need medical attention.

- What is most important in this situation? – Properly 4_____ your advice to the patient and his continued refusal. ◄

It is important in this situation to make a complete documentation of the patient's 5_____ ___ _____ treatment. Documentation should include the steps you took to 6_____ him to seek medical attention, the potential 7_____ of his refusal, and your assessment findings.

a. evidence of the crime; b. be reported;
c. first priority; d. document; e. refusal to
accept; f. convince; g. consequences

Case study 16

An intoxicated person refuses treatment or transport. How should you proceed? – Try to 1_____ the person to accept your assistance. ◄

If a person who needs help refuses to 2_____ ___, you should try to persuade the person to accept aid and explain the 3_____ of refusing it. Only after doing so should you accept and document the 4_____ of care.

a. consequences; b. accept it; c. persuade;
d. refusal

Case study 17

Which patient may be legally placed in protective custody by the police if he or she refuses treatment? - A patient who is drunk and disorderly and who refuses treatment for a head wound ◄

1_____ _____ is used legally in cases of patients who are drunk, 2_____ ___ _____, or a 3_____ to themselves and others, when it is obvious that their condition is 4_____ their judgement.

a. Protective custody; b. impairing; c. danger;
d. high on drugs

Case study 18

You are the first paramedic Unit to arrive on the scene of a 1_____-_____ bus crash.

- What is your first responsibility? – Assume command of the incident and give 2_____ _____ to dispatch. ◄

The first paramedic Unit to arrive at the scene of a mass-casualty incident would immediately 3_____ _____ and transmit a report to dispatch, alerting them to the need for more 4_____. As other Units begin to arrive, they may be detailed to perform 5_____ or some other duty.

a. preliminary report; b. assume command;
c. units; d. multi-injury; e. triage

Case study 19

You respond to reports of a bus collision. Upon arrival, it appears that you have approximately 35 patients.

- What is your first priority?
  – Separate the 1_____
  _____ from the more severely injured. ◄

Using START triage, separating out the walking wounded from the 2____ _____ injured patients is the first step in triaging large numbers of patients.

- The first parameter to assess when using the START triage algorithm should be: breathing/airway. *

3_____/_____ is the first parameter that should be assessed, followed by pulse and mental status.

A male patient is found to have a respiratory rate of 38. This would place him in which of the following categories?

- Delayed
- Immediate ◄
- Nonsalvageable
- Critical

The 4_____ _____ acronym dictates that patients with respiratory rates above 30 be classified as immediate.

Another male patient is found to have a respiratory rate of 28 and a radial pulse of 84. He is confused about the incident. This patient would be placed in which of the following categories?

- Delayed
- Immediate ◄
- Nonsalvageable
- Critical

The 5_____ level of consciousness places the patient in the immediate category. Once he is moved to the 6_____ ____, he may be monitored for a while or transported quickly.

A female patient is found to have no spontaneous respirations.

- What should you do next?
  – Reposition the airway and check her again 7____ _____. ◄

Reposition the head and 8_____ ____ spontaneous respirations. If they are immediately present, 9_____ the patient s immediate. If they are absent, categorize the patient as 10____/_____ and move on to the next patient.

---

a. examine for; b. categorize; c. dead/
unsalvageable; d. for respirations;
e. decreased; f. START triage; g. walking
wounded; h. treatment area; i. more severely;
j. Breathing/airway

Case study 20

Your patient 1____ _____ a vehicle rollover in which another passenger in the vehicle died. He is 2_____

and not complaining of pain.
His vital signs are: pulse, 100;
systolic BP, 90; respirations, 28.

- What 3_____
  procedures are required
  prior to initiating transport?
  – Quickly immobilize him
  using the long backboard as a
  splint, and then transport. ◀

Even though the patient's
condition appears to be 4_____,
the mechanism of injury indicates
that 5_____ _____
injuries, such as internal bleeding,
may be present. 6_____
him quickly using the long board
as a full-body splint. 7_____
immediately in this case. You can
perform additional assessments
or treatments while en route.

---

a. serious underlying; b. stable; c. has
survived; d. alert; e. Transport; f. additional;
g. stable

Case study 21
Your Unit is the first to
arrive at the scene of a bombing
at a large office building.

- The purpose of your initial
  size-up of the incident
  is to: determine what
  1_____ _____
  will be needed. ◀

The purpose of the initial
scene 2____-__ at a mass-casualty
incident is to 3_____ what
additional resources will be needed.

---

a. determine; b. additional resources;
c. size-up

Vocabulary 23

accommodate /əˈkɒm.ə.deɪt/
acronym /ˈæk.rə.nɪm/
administer /ədˈmɪn.ɪ.stər/
advocate /ˈæd.və.keɪt/
algorithm /ˈæl.gə.rɪ.ðəm/
arise /əˈraɪz/ **(arose, arisen)**
attention /əˈten.ʃən/
authorize /ˈɔː.θər.aɪz/
beaten /ˈbiː.tən/
behave /bɪˈheɪv/
belligerent /bəˈlɪdʒ.ər.ənt/
bike /baɪk/
bombing /ˈbɒm.ɪŋ/
charge /tʃɑːdʒ/
consenting /kənˈsent.ɪŋ/ **adult** /əˈdʌlt/
consequence /ˈkɒn.sɪ.kwəns/
court /kɔːt/
deem /diːm/
defer /dɪˈfɜːr/
delusion /dɪˈluː.ʒən/
dilemma /daɪˈlem.ə/
disorderly /dɪˈsɔː.dəl.i/
doctrine /ˈdɒk.trɪn/
domestic /dəˈmes.tɪk/
drunk /drʌŋk/
emancipate /ɪˈmænsɪˌpeɪt/
employee /ɪmˈplɔɪ.iː/
extenuating /ɪkˈsten.ju.eɪ.tɪŋ/
greenish /ˈgriː.nɪʃ/
guidance /ˈgaɪ.dəns/
honour /ˈɑn.ər/
insist /ɪnˈsɪst/
jurisdiction /ˌdʒʊə.rɪsˈdɪk.ʃən/
lividity /lɪˈvɪd.ə.ti/
military /ˈmɪl.ɪ.tər.i/
misunderstanding /ˌmɪs.ʌn.dəˈstæn.dɪŋ/
nonsalvageable /ˌnɒn ˈsæl.vɪdʒə.bl̩/
occasion /əˈkeɪ.ʒən/
PCP, phencyclidine /fɛnˈsɪklɪˌdiːn/

persuade /pəˈsweɪd/
plain /pleɪn/
prehospital /ˌpriːˈhɒs.pɪ.təl/
preliminary /prɪˈlɪm.ɪ.nər.i/
prove /pruːv/
provided /prəˈvaɪ.dɪd/
prudent /ˈpruː.dənt/
resource /rɪˈzɔːs/
rigor mortis /ˌrɪg.əˈmɔː.tɪs/
rollover /ˈrəʊl.əʊ.vər/
seek /siːk/ (sought, sought)
similar /ˈsɪm.ɪ.lər/
size /saɪz/ up /ʌp/
specify /ˈspes.ɪ.faɪ/
survive /səˈvaɪv/
trained /treɪnd/
underage /ˌʌn.dəˈreɪdʒ/
violence /ˈvaɪə.ləns/
wounded /ˈwuːn.dɪd/
yellowish /ˈjel.əʊ.ɪʃ/

Unit 24

Case study 1

Your patient is a 26-year-old construction worker who has fallen approximately 35 feet (10.7 m) and suffered 1_____

_____. The Glasgow Coma Scale score is 9, respiratory rate is 32, respiratory expansion is normal, the blood pressure is 100/70, and capillary refill is 2_____.

- What 3_____ should this patient receive if you are using the Revised Trauma Score? – 13. ◄

The score on the Glasgow Coma Scale 4_____ ____ 4 points on the Revised Trauma Score; the patient receives 3 points

for respiratory rate, 1 point for respiratory expansion, 4 points for blood pressure, and 1 point for delayed 5_____ _____.

a. delayed; b. score; c. translates into;
d. capillary refill; e. multiple injuries

Case study 2

What is the process of transmitting 1_____ ____ from the field to the hospital over the 2_____ lines called?

- modulation
- biotelemetry ◄
- multiplexing
- trunking

3_____ physiological data over phone lines is called 4_____.

a. Transmitting; b. biotelemetry;
c. physiological data; d. phone

Case study 3

What sort of communication system would you need to be able to carry on a 1___-___ conversation with a 2_____ while also transmitting telemetry? - Multiplex transmission system ◄

A multiplex system allows for a two-way conversation and simultaneous transmission of 3_____ _____.

a. telemetry readings; b. physician;
c. two-way

Case study 4

What is the purpose of the START method? – To rapidly

293

1_____ large numbers of patients quickly and 2_____. ◄

3_____ stands for Simple Triage And Rapid Treatment and is designed to triage large 4_____ of patients as quickly as possible.

a. numbers; b. efficiently; c. triage; d. START

Case study 5

During a multi-casualty incident, the first two arriving paramedics should assume the roles of: medical group supervisor and triage officer ◄

The medical group supervisor will need to establish overall responsibility for the 1_____ _____ interacting with other lead officers such as police, fire, and public works. The triage officer will need to 2_____ the number of severity of victims as early as possible.

3_-____ is a mnemonic used to describe the components of an ICS system: command – finance, logistic, operations, planning.

a. medical section; b. C-FLOP; c. establish

Case study 6

At a mass-casualty incident (MCI), which sector should the incident commander establish first?

- triage sector ◄
- treatment sector
- supply sector
- transportation sector

Triage must be done before treatment can be properly 1_____. In many cases,

triage and scene-assessment 2_____ are in progress by the crew of the 3_____ _____ Unit. If it is not ongoing, triage should be established 4_____.

a. performed; b. first arriving; c. activities; d. first

Case study 7

The first step in triage at an MCI is to: 1_____ the walking wounded away from the scene. ◄

Regardless of the triage method utilized, the 2_____ _____ is to direct the walking wounded to a safe place where they can be 3_____ ___ and reassessed.

a. first step; b. cared for; c. direct

Case study 8

These are components of the START triage method: 1_____ assessment, 2_____ assessment, mentation/level of consciousness. ◄

Neuromuscular function is not part of the START algorithm. START assesses respiration, pulse, and 3_____ _____.

a. circulation; b. mental status; c. respiration

Case study 9

The three primary parameters assessed when using the START triage system are:

- airway, breathing, and circulation (ABC)
- respiration, perfusion, mentation (RPM) ◄

- appearance, respiration, mentation (ARM)
- pulse, perfusion perspiration (PPP)

Using the START triage system, the three primary parameters 1_____ are respiration, perfusion, and mentation (RPM). The parameters are a 2_____ _____ over or under 30 per minute, capillary refill under or over two seconds or presence of a 3_____ _____, and mentation (e.g. whether the patient is able to follow 4_____ _____).

> a. basic commands; b. respiratory rate; c. radial pulse; d. assessed

Case study 10

Which sector officer will coordinate with police to 1_____ _____ and provide access at an MCI?

- triage officer
- transportation officer
- supply officer
- staging officer ◄

The staging officer's responsibilities include coordinating with 2_____, ensuring access for vehicles, maintaining a log of available Units, and 3_____ requests for resources. The 4_____ _____ will establish the staging area if the incident commander has not already ordered one.

> a. coordinating; b. police; c. transportation officer; d. block streets

Case study 11

At a major incident response, what is the responsibility of the staging officer? – Maintain 1_ ____ __ _____ available and an inventory of special equipment. ◄

The staging officer is primarily responsible for assembling all 2_____ _____ to make sure they are 3_____ ____ deployment as needed

> a. a log of units; b. ready for; c. available vehicles

Case study 12

What is the major responsibility of the finance sector at a major incident? – To document the number of personnel and hours worked. ◄

Finance is responsible for the 1_____ _____ of the incident and may not be needed in a small-scale incident. In addition to tracking 2_____, finance approves rental and purchase of any additional 3_____ needed for the incident. Logistics is responsible for 4_____ resources, planning evaluates, and command sets 5____ ___ _____.

> a. acquiring; b. personnel; c. financial accounting; d. goals and objectives; e. equipment

Case study 13

This statement about the triage operation at a mass-casualty incident is correct. – Each patient's 1_____ and 2_____ _____ should take less than 60 seconds. ◄

START and METTAG, systems used at mass-casualty incidents, are designed to be 3_____ ___ very quickly by minimally trained personnel.

a. carried out; b. initial assessment; c. triage

Case study 14

During a multicasualty incident, a conscious patient presents with a fractured femur, a palpable radial pulse, and a respiratory rate of 24/ min.

- According to START, this patient would be placed into what triad category? – Delayed/yellow ◄

According to START triage principles, transport of this patient to definitive care can be 1_____. He is breathing 2_____, has a 3_____ _____, and is 4_____. The fractured femur is not factored into the evaluation of transport status.

a. conscious; b. radial pulse; c. delayed; d. spontaneously

Case study 15

You are conducting triage using the START system at a major incident. You encounter a patient who is not breathing. After you 1_____ the airway, the patient begins to breathe at a rate of 6 respirations per minute. Into which category would you now triage this patient?

- dead or dying
- immediate or critical. ◄
- delayed
- urgent or noncritical

When using the START triage system, you assess three parameters: respiration, pulse, and mental status (RPM). A patient with no respirations is considered 2___ __ _____; if the rate is under 10 or over 30, the patient is 3_____ __ _____. If the rate is between 10 and 30, 4_____ assessment is needed (so you would then assess pulse, and possibly also mental status, before deciding on a 5_____).

a. immediate or critical; b. category; c. position; d. dead or dying; e. additional

Case study 16

You are on the scene of a vehicle crash involving a bus. As triage officer, the first patient you encounter is sitting on the ground, conscious, confused, and breathing 1__ _____ per minute. She states that she was 2_____ ___ of her seat and 3_____ the side of her head.

- Your next action would be to: classify the patient as "Immediate" (red). ◄

A patient who is conscious and breathing over 30 times per minute is classified as "Immediate". There is no need to 4_____ ____ the presence or rate of the pulse. While she may need 5_____ _____, now is not the time to do so.

> a. oxygen therapy; b. struck; c. 40 times;
> d. thrown out; e. check for

Case study 17

Using the START triage method at a multiple-casualty accident scene, you encounter a patient who is making no spontaneous respiratory effort 1_____ _____ at repositioning.

- What should you do next? – 2____ the patient as unsalvageable and move on. ◄

If a patient continues to remain 3_____ following a second attempt to open the airway, he or she is considered 4_____.

> a. despite attempts; b. unsalvageable; c. Tag;
> d. apnoeic

Case study 18

Which of the following situations is most likely to be declared a major incident?

- an accident involving a school bus and car with five patients
- a fire at a 1_____ _____ during working hours ◄
- a 2_____ _____ on a state line with two people in the water
- a 3____ involving an isolated single-family residence

This incident has a 4_____-_____ component along with the potential for lots of patients. All the other incidents may be severe but should not 5_____ the normal resources for the area.

> a. overwhelm; b. fire; c. water accident;
> d. hazardous-materials; e. chemical plant

Case study 19

When responding to the scene of a hazardous-material incident, the EMS crew should 1_____ from: uphill and upwind. ◄

The patient should be 2_____ with the head elevated to enhance venous return. If congestive 3____ _____ is present, the patient should be positioned at least semi-Fowler's (4_____ ___ at least 45°).

> a. sitting up; b. supine; c. heart failure;
> d. approach

Case study 20

You respond to a 25- patient mass-casualty incident at a store. The 112 caller stated that she smelled something "funny" and then started to feel 1___ ___ _____. You are the second Unit on the scene. The initial Unit is nowhere to be seen, and they do not answer their radios.

- What should you determine first in this situation? - Whether this is a potential hazardous-material incident in progress.◄

This is a hazardous-material incident until proven

otherwise. Do not rush in after fallen rescuers because you may 2_____ _ _____, too.

- After you are instructed by the 3_____ ____ to begin treating decontaminated patients, you should: take universal 4_____ and wear protective 5_____. ◄

Always wear personal protective equipment to help avoid becoming personally contaminated. Unless you are trained to work in the hot zone, you should not treat anyone until they are properly 6_____.

a. weak and nauseous; b. precautions;
c. equipment; d. decontaminated; e. become a
victim; f. HAZMAT team

Case study 21

All of the following are correct statements about the care of patients who are contaminated by hazardous material.

- Trained personnel should immediately 1_____ non ambulatory patients from the "hot zone". ◄
- Decontamination activities should be 2_____ ____ while the patient is in the "warm zone". ◄
- Intravenous therapy and invasive procedures should begin only under specific 3_____ _____. ◄

An 4_____ assessment should be done while the patient is located within the "hot zone".

Only absolutely essential care, such as, 5_____ ____

_____ _____

should be done in the "hot zone".

a. initial; b. remove; c. carried out;
d. physician direction; e. ABCs and spinal
immobilization

Vocabulary 24

accounting /əˈkaʊn.tɪŋ/
assemble /əˈsem.bl̩/
available /əˈveɪ.lə.bl̩/
biotelemetry /ˌbaɪ.əʊ.təˈlem.ə.tri/
carry /ˈkær.i/ **on**
carry /ˈkær.i/ **st out** /aʊt/
commander /kəˈmæn.dər/
coordinate /kəʊˈɔː.dɪ.neɪt/
deployment /dɪˈplɔɪ.mənt/
enhance /ɪnˈhɑːns/
factor /ˈfæk.tər/
funny /ˈfʌn.i/
interact /ˌɪn.təˈrækt/
line /laɪn/
log /lɒg/
logistics /ləˈdʒɪs.tɪks/
modulation /ˌmɒd.jʊˈleɪ.ʃən/
multiplexing /ˈmʌl.tiˌpleksɪŋ/
plant /plɑːnt/
regardless /rɪˈgɑːd.ləs/
rush /rʌʃ/ **in**
seat /ˈsiː.t/
smell /smel/
unsalvageable /ʌnˈsæl.vɪdʒ.ə.bl̩/
urgent /ˈɜː.dʒənt/

Word Index

A

abandonment /əˈbæn.dən.mənt/
abbreviation /əˌbriː.viˈeɪ.ʃən/
ABCs /ˌeɪ.biːˈsiː/
abdomen /ˈæb.də.mən/
abdominal /æbˈdɒm.ɪ.nəl/
thrust /θrʌst/
abnormal /æbˈnɔː.məl/
abortion /əˈbɔː.ʃən/
above /əˈbʌv/
abrasion /əˈbreɪ.ʒən/
abrupt /əˈbrʌpt/
abruptio placentae /
æbˈrʌp.ʃi.əʊ.pləˈsen.tiː/
abruption / əˈbrʌp.ʃən/
abscess /ˈæb.ses/
absorb /əbˈzɔːb/
abuse /əˈbjuːz/
abuser /əˈbjuː.zər/
accelerate /ə kˈsel.ə.reɪt/
acceptable /əkˈsept.ə.bl̩/
accepted /əkˈsep.tɪd/
access /ˈæk.ses/
accessory /əkˈses.ər.i/
accident /ˈæksɪdənt/
accidental /ˌæk.sɪˈden.təl/
accommodate /əˈkɒm.ə.deɪt/
accomplish /əˈkʌm.plɪʃ/

accordance /əˈkɔː.dənt s/
accordingly /əˈkɔː.dɪŋ.li/
account /əˈkaʊnt/
accounting /əˈkaʊn.tɪŋ/
accumulate /əˈkjuː.mjʊ.leɪt/
accumulation /əˌkjuː.mjʊˈleɪ.ʃən/
accuracy /ˈæk.jʊ.rə.si/
accurate /ˈæk.jʊ.rət/
acetaminophen /əˌsiː.təˈmɪn.ə.fen/
achieve /əˈtʃiːv/
acid /ˈæs.ɪd/
acidosis /ˌæs.ɪˈdəʊ.sɪs/
acidotic /əˈsɪd.ə.tɪk/
acknowledge /əkˈnɒl.ɪdʒ/
acquire /əˈkwaɪər/
acronym /ˈæk.rə.nɪm/
acrylic /əˈkrɪl.ɪk/
act /ækt/
act /ækt/
ACTH, Adrenocorticotropic /
əˌdriː.nəʊˌkɔː.tɪ.kəʊˈtrɒf.
ɪk/ Hormone /ˈhɔː.məʊn/
activation /ˌæk.tɪˈveɪ.ʃən/
activity /ækˈtɪv.ɪ.ti/
actual /ˈæk.tʃu.əl/
acute /əˈkjuːt/
Addison's disease /ˈæd.ɪ.sənz.dɪˌziːz/
additional /əˈdɪʃ.ən.əl/
address /əˈdres/
Adenocard, adenosine /ə.denˈə.sin/
adequacy /ˈæd.ə.kwə.si/
adequate /ˈæd.ə.kwət/
adipose /ˈæd.ɪ.pəʊs/, /-pəʊz/
adjacent /əˈdʒeɪ.sənt/
adjoining /əˈdʒɔɪ.nɪŋ/
adjunct /ˈædʒ.ʌŋkt/
adjust /əˈdʒʌst/
administer /ədˈmɪn.ɪ.stər/
administration /ədˌmɪn.ɪˈstreɪ.ʃən/
admit /ədˈmɪt/
adult /ˈæd.ʌlt/,/əˈdʌlt/
advanced /ədˈvɑːnst/
directive /daɪˈrek.tɪv/
advanced /ədˈvɑːnst/
advantage /ədˈvɑː.n.tɪdʒ/

adventitious /ˌæd.vənˈtɪʃ.əs/
advice /ədˈvaɪs/
advisable /ədˈvaɪ.zə.bl̩/
advisory /ədˈvaɪ.zər.i/
advocate /ˈæd.və.keɪt/
AED, Automated /ˈɔː.tə.meɪ.
tɪd/ External /ɪkˈstɜː.nəl/
Defibrillator /ˌdiːˈfɪb.rɪ.leɪ.tər/
aeromedical /ˌeə.rəˈmed.ɪ.kəl/
service /sɜːvɪs/
affect /əˈfekt/
afterload /ˌɑː.f.tər.ˈləʊd/
age /eɪdʒ/
aggravate /ˈæg.rə.veɪt/
aggressively /əˈgres.ɪv.li/
agitated /ˈædʒ.ɪ.teɪ.tɪd/
agitation /ˌædʒ.ɪˈteɪ.ʃən/
agonal /ˈəg.əʊ.nəl/
aim /eɪm/ at /ət/
air /ˈeər/ embolism /ˈem.bə.lɪ.zəm/
air bag, airbag /ˈeə.bæg/
airborne /ˈeəˌbɔːn/
airflow /ˈeə.fləʊ/
airway /ˈeə.weɪ/
alarm /əˈlɑːm/
alcoholism /ˈæl.kə.hɒl.ɪ.zəm/
aldosterone /ˈɔːl.dəs.tər.əʊn/
alert /əˈlɜːt/
algorithm /ˈæl.gə.rɪ.ðəm/
align /əˈlaɪn/
alignment /əˈlaɪn.mənt/
alive /əˈlaɪv/
alkali /ˈæl.kəl.aɪ/
alkalize /ˈælkəˌlaɪz/
alkalosis /ˌælkəˈləʊ.sɪs/
all-terrain vehicle /ɔːl.tə.reɪnˈviː.ɪ.kl/
allegation /ˌæl.əˈgeɪ.ʃən/
allegiance /əˈliː.dʒəns/
alleviate /əˈliː.vi.eɪt/
alley /ˈæl.i/
allow /əˈlaʊ/
alpha /ˈæl.fə/
alteration /ˌɒl.təˈreɪ.ʃən/
altercation /ˌɔːltəˈkeɪʃən/
altered /ˈɔːltəd/

alternating /ˈɒl.tə.neɪ.tɪŋ/
alveolar /ˌæl.viˈəʊ.lər/
alveolus pl alveoli /ˌæl.viˈəʊ.ləs/
ambient /ˈæm.bi.ənt/
ambulance /ˈæm.bjʊ.ləns/
ambulation /ˈæm.bjʊ.lən.ʃən/
ambulatory /ˌæm.bjəˈleɪ.tər.i/
amenorrhoea /ˌeɪ.men.əˈriː.ə/
AMI, Acute /əˈkjuːt/
Myocardial /ˌmaɪ.əˈkɑː.di.əl/
Infarction /ɪnˈfɑːk.ʃən/
amniotic /ˌæm.niˈɒt.ɪk/
amniotic /ˌæm.niˈɒt.ɪk/ sac /sæk/
amniotic fluid /ˌæm.ni.ɒt.ɪkˈfluː.ɪd/
amount /əˈmaʊnt/
amputate /ˈæm.pjʊ.teɪt/
amputation /ˌæm.pjʊˈteɪ.ʃən/
amputee /ˌæm.pjʊˈtiː/
anaemia /əˈniː.mɪə/
anaesthetic /ˌæn.əsˈθet.ɪk/
anal /ˈeɪ.nəl/
anaphylactic /ˌæn.ə.frˈlæk.tɪk/
anaphylaxis /ˌæn.ə.frˈlæk.sɪs/
aneurysm /ˌæn.jʊə.rɪ.zəm/
angina /ænˌdʒaɪ.nə/
anginal /ænˌdʒaɪ.nəl/
angle /ˈæŋgəl/
angry /ˈæŋ.gri/
ankle /ˈæŋ.kl̩/
anniversary /ˌæn.ɪˈvɜː.sər.i/
anorexia nervosa /
æn.əˌrek.si.ə.nəˈvəʊ.sə/
antagonism /ænˈtæg.ə.nɪ.zəm/
anterior /ænˈtɪə.ri.ər/
anti-emetic /ˌæn.tɪ.ɪˈmet.ɪk/
antibody /ˈæn.tiˌbɒd.i/
anticonvulsant /ˌæn.tɪ.kən.ˈvʌl.sənt/
antidepressant /ˌæn.ti.dɪˈpres.ənt/
antidote /ˈæn.tɪ.dəʊt/
antigen /ˈæn.tɪ.dʒən/
anxiety /æŋˈzaɪ.ə.ti/
anxious /ˈæŋk.ʃəs/
aorta /eɪˈɔː.tə/
aortic /eɪˈɔː.tɪk/ aneurism /
ˌæn.jʊə.rɪ.zəm/

apart /əˈpɑːt/
Apgar /ˈæpgɑː/ score /skɔːr/
apical /ˈeɪ.pɪ.kəl/
apnoea /ˈæp.ni.ə/
apnoeic /æpˈniː.ɪk/
apparent /əˈpær.ənt/
appear /əˈpɪər/
appearance /əˈpɪə.rənt s/
appendicitis /ə‚pen.dɪˈsaɪ.tɪs/
appendix /əˈpen.dɪks/
applicable /əˈplɪk.ə.bl̩/
application /‚æp.lɪˈkeɪ.ʃən/
apply /əˈplaɪ/
appointment /əˈpɔɪnt.mənt/
apprehension /æp.rɪˈhen.ʃən/
apprehensive /‚æp.rɪˈhen.sɪv/
approach /əˈprəʊtʃ/
appropriate / əˈprəʊ.pri.ət/
appropriately /əˈprəʊ.pri.ət.li/
approximately /əˈprɒksɪmətlɪ/
argue /ˈɑːg.juː/
arise /əˈraɪz/ (arose, arisen)
arouse /əˈraʊz/
arrest /əˈrest/
arrhythmia /əˈrɪð.mi.ə/
arrow /ˈær.əʊ/
arsenic /ˈɑː.sən.ɪk/
arteria /aːˈtɪə.riə/ dorsalis /
dɔr.sə.lɪs/ pedis /ped.ɪs/
arterial /aːˈtɪə.ri.əl/
arterionecrosis /ɑː‚tɪə.rɪə.neˈkrəʊ.sɪs/
arteriosclerosis /ɑː‚tɪə.
ri.əʊ.sklə'rəʊ.sɪs/
arteriosum /ɑː‚tɪə.ri'ɒs.əm/
artery /ˈɑːtərɪ/
arthritis /ɑːˈθraɪ.tɪs/
articulation /ɑː‚tɪk.jʊ'leɪ.ʃən/
artificial /‚ɑː.tɪ'fɪʃ.əl/
ventilation /‚ven.tɪ'leɪ.ʃən/
ascent /əˈsent/
ascertain /‚æs.ə'teɪn/
ascites /æ'saɪ.tiːz/
asleep /əˈsliːp/
asphyxia /æsˈfɪksɪə/
aspirate /ˈæs.pɪ.rət/

aspiration /‚æspɪˈreɪʃən/
aspirator /æs.pə.reɪ.tər/
assault /əˈsɒlt/
assemble /əˈsem.bl̩/
assessment /əˈses.mənt/
assign /əˈsaɪn/
assist /əˈsɪst/
assistance /əˈsɪs.tənt s/
associated /əˈsəʊ.si.eɪ.tɪd/
assume /əˈsjuːm/
assumption /əˈsʌmp.ʃən/
assurance /əˈʃɔː.rəns/
assure /əˈʃɔːr/
asthma /ˈæs.mə/
asymmetrical /‚eɪ.sɪ'met.rɪk.əl/
asymptomatic /ə‚sɪmp.tə'mæt.ɪk/
asynchronous /eɪˈsɪŋ.krə.nəs/
asystole /ə.sɪs.tə.lɪ/
at /ət/ least /liːst/
at /ət/ rest /rest/
at /ət/ stake /steɪk/
ataxia /əˈtæk.si.ə/
ataxic /əˈtæk.sɪk/
atelectasis /‚ætə'lek.tə.sɪs/
atherosclerosis /‚æθ.ə.rəʊ.sklə'rəʊ.sɪs/
atmosphere / ˈæt.mə.sfɪər/
atrial /ˈeɪ.tri.əl/ fibrillation /
‚faɪ.brɪ'leɪ.ʃən/
atrial /ˈeɪ.tri.əl/
atrium pl atria /ˈeɪ.tri.əm/
atropine /ˈæt.rə.pɪn/ sulfate /ˈsʌl.feɪt/
attach /əˈtætʃ/
attack /əˈtæk/
attain /əˈteɪn/
attempt /əˈtemp t/
attend /əˈtend/
attention /əˈten.ʃən/
attentive /əˈten.tɪv/
attitude /ˈæt.ɪ.tjuːd/
attribute /ˈæt.rɪ.bjuːt/
atypical /‚eɪ'tɪp.ɪ.kəl/
audible /ˈɔː.dɪ.bl̩/
auditory / ˈɔːdɪtərɪ/
aura /ˈɔː.rə/
auscultation /‚ɔː.skəl'teɪ.ʃən/

authority /ɔːˈθɒr.ɪ.ti/
authorize /ˈɔː.θər.aɪz/
automacity /ɔːˈtɒm.ə.sɪt.i/
available /əˈveɪ.lə.bl̩/
average /ˈæv.ər.ɪdʒ/
awake /əˈweɪk/
aware /əˈweər/
awareness /əˈweə.nəs/
away /əˈweɪ/
awoke /əˈwəʊk/

B

back /bæk/ and forth /fɔːθ/
back /bæk/ out /aʊt/
back /bæk/
back-up /ˈbæk.ʌp/
backboard /ˈbæk.bɔːd/
backflow /ˈbæk.fləʊ/
backpressure /ˌbækˈpreʃ.ər/
backward /ˈbæk.wəd/
backyard /ˌbækˈjɑːd/
bag /bæg/ mask /mɑːsk/
bag /bæg/
bag /bæg/ valve /vælv/
bag-valve mask /mɑːsk/
balance /ˈbæl.əns/
ballistics /bəˈlɪs.tɪks/
balloon /bəˈluːn/
band /bænd/
bandage /ˈbæn.dɪdʒ/
bark /bɑːk/
barky /ˈbɑː.ki/
barrel /ˈbær.əl/
barrier /ˈbær.i.ər/
basal /beɪsəl/
base /beɪs/
based /beɪst/
basic /ˈbeɪ.sɪk/
basilar /ˈbæz.ɪ.lər/
bathe /beɪð/
battery /ˈbæt.ər.i/
Battle's /ˈbætəl/ sign /saɪn/
be /biː/ in charge /tʃɑːdʒ/ of
be /biː/ over /ˈəʊ.vər/
be /biː/ trapped /træpd/

bear /beər/ down /daʊn/
beat /biːt/
beaten /ˈbiː.tən/
Beck's triad /ˈtraɪ.æd/
bed /bed/
bedridden /ˈbed.rɪ.dən/
bee /biː/
behave /bɪˈheɪv/
behaviour /bɪˈheɪ.vjə/
belligerent /bəˈlɪdʒ.ər.ənt/
bend /bend/ (bent, bent)
beneficial /ˌben.ɪˈfɪʃ.əl/
benefit /ˈben.ɪ.fɪt/
benzodiazepines /benˈzɒ.dɪ.əˈzeˌpiːnz/
beta-2 /ˈbiː.tə.tuː/ agonists /ˈæg.ə.nɪsts/
bicuspid valve /baɪˈkʌs.pɪdˌvælv/
bike /baɪk/
bilateral /baɪˈlæt.ər.əl/
bilaterally /ˌbaɪˈlæt.ər.ə.li/
bilirubin /ˌbɪl.ɪˈruː.bɪn/
bin /bɪn/
bind /baɪnd/ (bound, bound)
binge eating /bɪndʒˌiː.tɪŋ/
biotelemetry /ˌbaɪ.əʊ.təˈlem.ə.tri/
bipolar disorder /baɪˈpəʊ.lə.dɪˌsɔː.dər/
birth /ˈbɜːθ/ canal /kəˈnæl/
birth /ˈbɜːθ/ control /kənˈtrəʊl/ pill /pɪl/
bite /baɪt/
bitterly /ˈbɪt.ə.li/
bizarre /bɪˈzɑːr/
black out /ˈblæk.aʊt/
bladder /ˈblæd.ər/
blade /bleɪd/
blast /blɑːst/
bleach /bliːtʃ/
bleb /bleb/
bleed /bliːd/
blind /blaɪnd/
blindly /ˈblaɪnd.li/
blister /ˈblɪs.tər/
blistering /ˈblɪs.tər.ɪŋ/
bloating /bləʊ.tɪŋ/
block /blɒk/
blockage /ˈblɒk.ɪdʒ/

blood /blʌd/ loss /lɒs/
blood /blʌd/ pressure /'preʃ.ər/
blood /blʌd/ sample /'sɑːm.pl̩/
blood /blʌd/ vessel /'ves.əl/
blood-borne /bɔːn/
bloodshot /'blʌd.ʃɒt/
blow /bləʊ/ (blew, blown)
blowing /ˌbləʊ.ɪŋ/
BLS, Basic /'beɪ.sɪk/ Life
Support /'laɪf.səˌpɔːt/
blue bloater /'bləʊ.tər/
blunt / blʌnt/
blurred /blɜːd/
board /bɔːd/
boardlike /bɔːd.laɪk/
bob /bɒb/
bodily /'bɒd.ɪ.li/
bolus /bəʊ.ləs/
bombing /'bɒm.ɪŋ/
bone /bəʊn/ marrow /'mær.əʊ/
border /bɔː.dər/
borderline /'bɔː.də.laɪn/
bound /baʊnd/
bowel /'baʊ.əl/ movement /
'muː.v.mənt/
bowel /'baʊ.əl/
bradycardia /ˌbræd.ɪ'kɑː.di.ə/
bradypnoea /ˌbræd.ɪ.'pni.ə/
brain /breɪn/
brainstem /'breɪn.stem/
breach /briːtʃ/
break /breɪk/ (broke broken)
break /breɪk/ down /daʊn/
breath /breθ/
breathing /'briː.ðɪŋ/
breech /briːtʃ/ presentation /
ˌprez.ən'teɪ.ʃən/
breech /briːtʃ/
brief /briːf/
bright /braɪt/
bring /brɪŋ/ about /ə'baʊt/
bronchial /'brɒŋ.ki.əl/ tree /triː/
bronchiole /'brɒŋ.ki.əʊl/
bronchiolitis /'brɒŋ.ki.ə'la.ɪ.tɪs/
bronchitis /brɒŋ'kaɪ.tɪs/

bronchoconstriction /
ˌbrɒŋ.kəʊ.kən'strɪk.ʃən/
bronchodilation /ˌbrɒŋ.kəʊ.'dɪleɪʃən/
bronchospasm /ˌbrɒŋ.kəʊ.'spæz.əm/
bronchus /'brɒŋ.kəs/ pl bronchi /-kaɪ/
Brown-Sequard's /braʊn-sei.
kahr/ syndrome /'sɪn.drəʊm/
brownie /'braʊ.ni/
bruise /bruːz/
bruising /'bruː.zɪŋ/
bruit /bruːt/
brush /brʌʃ/
BSA, Body /'bɒd.i/ Surface /
'sɜː.fɪs/ Area /'eərɪə/
BSI, British /'brɪt.ɪʃ/ Standards /
'stæn.dədz/ Institution /ˌɪnstɪ'tjuːʃən/
bubble /'bʌb.l̩/
bucket /bʌkɪt/
build /bɪld/ (built, built)
buildup /'bɪld.ʌp/
bulb /bʌlb/
bulge / bʌldʒ/
bulimia /bʊˌlɪm.i.ə/
bulky /'bʌl.ki/
bullet /'bʊl.ɪt/
bundle /'bʌn.dl̩/
bunk /bʌŋk/ bed /bed/
bunkroom /bʌŋk.rʊm/
burn /bɜːn/
burnout /'bɜːnaʊt/
bursitis /bɜː'saɪ.tɪs/
bury /'ber.i/
buttock /'bʌt.ək/
BVM, Bag Valve Mask
by ground /graʊnd/
bystander /'baɪˌstæn.dər/

C
C-spine, cervical /sə'vaɪ.
kəl/ spine /spaɪn/
caesarean section /sɪˌzeə.ri.ən'sek.ʃən/
cafeteria /ˌkæf.ə'tɪə.ri.ə/
caffeinated /'kæf.ɪ.neɪ.tɪd/
caffeine /'kæf.iːn/
calcaneus /kæl'keɪ.niəs/

calcium /'kæl.si.əm/

calculate /'kælkjʊˌleɪt/

calf /kɑːf/

call /kɔːl/

calm (sb) /kɑːm/ down /daʊn/

campus /'kæm.pəs/

canal / kə'næl/

cancer /'kænt.sər/

cancerous /'kæn.sər.əs/

cannula /kæn.jʊl.ə/

capable /'keɪ.pə.blˌ/

capacity /kə'pæs.ə.ti/

capillary /kə'pɪl.ər.i/ bed /bed/

capillary /kə'pɪl.ər.i/

capillary /kə'pɪl.ər.i/ refill /'riː.fɪl/

capnometer /kæp'ɒm.ɪ.tər/

capnometry /kæp'nɒm.ə.tri/

capture /'kæp.tʃər/

carbamate /'kɑːbəˌmeɪt/

carbohydrate /ˌkɑː.bəʊ'haɪ.dreɪt/

carbon /'kɑː.bən/ dioxide / daɪ'ɒk.saɪd/

carbon /'kɑː.bən/

carbon monoxide /ˌkɑː. bən.mə'nɒk.saɪd/

cardiac /'kɑː.di.æk/

cardiac /'kɑːdɪˌæk/ output /'aʊtˌpʊt/

cardiac arrest /'kɑr.diˌæk ə'rest/

cardiogenic /'kɑː.di.ə.'dʒen. ɪk/ shock /ʃɒk/

cardiopulmonary /ˌkɑː. di.əʊ'pʊl.mə.nə.ri/

cardioversion /ˌkɑː.di.ə.'vɜː.ʃən/

care /keə/ for / fɔː/

care /keə/

care /keə/ provider /prə'vaɪ.dər/

careful /'keə.fəl/

caregiver /'keəˌgɪv.ər/

caretaker /'keəˌteɪ.kər/

carina /kə'raɪn.ə/

caring /'keə.rɪŋ/

carotid artery /kəˌrɒt.ɪd'ɑː.tər.i/

carpopedal /ˌkɑː.pə'pɪː.d.əl/

carry /'kær.i/

carry /'kær.i/ on

carry /'kær.i/ st out /aʊt/

cartilage /'kɑː.təl.ɪdʒ/ chrupavka

cartilage /'kɑː.təl.ɪdʒ/ ring /rɪŋ/

case /keɪs/

catastrophic /ˌkæt.ə'strɒf.ɪk/

catching /'kætʃ.ɪŋ/

catecholamine /kat.ə.kəl.am.in/

catheter /'kæθɪtə/

Caucasian /kɔː'keɪ.ʒən/

causative /'kɔː.zə.tɪv/

cause /kɔːz/

caution /'kɔː.ʃən/

cautiously /'kɔː.ʃəs.li/

cavitation /ˌkæv.ɪ'teɪ.ʃən/

cavity /'kæv.ɪ.ti/

cease /siːs/

cell /sel/

cell, cellular /'sel.jʊ.lər /

telephone /'telɪˌfəʊn/

cellular /'sel.jʊ.lər/

center /'sen.tər/

central /'sen.trəl/

cerebral /'ser.ɪ.brəl/

cerebrospinal /ˌser.ɪ.brə'spaɪ.nəl/

cerebrovascular /ˌser.ɪ.brə'væskjʊlə/

cerebrum /sɪ'riː.brəm/

cervical /'sɜː.vɪkəl/ spine / spaɪn/

cervical /sə'vaɪ.kəl/

cervix /'sɜː.vɪks/ pl cervices /-vɪs.iːz/

cessation /ses'eɪ.ʃən/

chain /tʃeɪn/

challenge /'tʃæl.ɪndʒ/

chamber /'tʃeɪm.bə/

charcoal /'tʃɑː.r.kəʊl/

charge /tʃɑːdʒ/

charred /tʃɑːd/

chart /tʃɑːt/

check /tʃek/

chemical /'kem.ɪ.kəl/

chemistry /'kem.ɪ.stri/

chest /tʃest/

chest /tʃest/ wall /wɔːl/

CHF, Congestive /kən'dʒes.tɪv/ Heart /hɑːt/ Failure /'feɪ.ljər/

chickenpox /'tʃɪk.ɪn.pɒks/

chief /tʃiːf/
childbearing /ˈtʃaɪldˌbeə.rɪŋ/
childbirth /ˈtʃaɪld.bɜːθ/
chill /tʃɪl/
chin /tʃɪn/
chin-lift /tʃɪn/, /lɪft/
chlamydia /kləm.iˈde.ə/
choice /tʃɔɪs/
choke /tʃəʊk/
cholecystitis /ˌkəʊ.lɪ.sɪˈstaɪ.tɪs/
cholinergic /kɒ.lɪn.ə.dʒɪk/
chronic /ˈkrɒn.ɪk/
circle /ˈsɜː.kl̩/
circulate /ˈsɜː.kjʊ.leɪt/
circulation /ˌsɜː.kjʊˈleɪ.ʃən/
circumstance /ˈsɜː.kəm.stɑːnt s/
claim /kleɪm/
clammy /ˈklæm.i/
clamp /klæmp/
classify /ˈklæs.ɪ.faɪ/
clavicle /ˈklævɪkəl/
clavicular /kləˈvɪkjʊlə/
clear /klɪər/
clearly /ˈklɪə.li/
closure /ˈkləʊ.ʒə/
clot /klɒt/
clubbing /ˈklʌb.ɪŋ/
clump /klʌmp/
cluster /ˈklʌs.tər/
coach /kəʊtʃ/
coarse /kɔːs/
cocaine /kəʊˈkeɪn/
coccyx /ˈkɒk.sɪks/
coexist /ˌkəʊ.ɪɡˈzɪst/
cognitive /kɑɡ.nə.tɪv/
cold /kəʊld/
cold /kəʊld/ sore /sɔːr/
colicky /ˈkɒl.ɪ.ki/
colitis /kə.lɪ.tɪs/
collapse /kəˈlæps/
collar /ˈkɑl.ər/
collection /kəˈlekʃən/
collectively /kəˈlek.tɪv.li/
collision /kəˈlɪʒ.ən/
colon /ˈkoʊ.lən/

coma /ˈkəʊ.mə/
comb /koʊm/
Combi tube /komˈbi.tjuːb/
comfort /ˈkʌm.fət/
comfortable /ˈkʌmf.tər.bəl/
command /kəˈmɑːnd/
commander /kəˈmæn.dər/
commercial /kəˈmɜːʃəl/
commit /kəˈmɪt/
common /ˈkɒmən/
commonly /ˈkɒm.ən.lɪ/
communicable /kəˈmjuː.nɪ.kə.bl̩/
communicate /kəˈmjuː.nɪ.keɪt/
company /ˈkʌm.pə.ni/
compare /kəmˈpeər/
comparison /kəmˈpærɪsən/
compartment /kəmˈpɑːt.mənt/
compartment /kəmˈpɑːt.mənt/
syndrome /ˈsɪn.drəʊm/
compensate /ˈkɒm.pən.seɪt/
compensatory /ˌkɒm.pənˈseɪt.ə ri/
competency /ˈkɒmpɪtənsɪ/
complain /kəmˈpleɪn/
complaint /kəmˈpleɪnt/
complete /kəmˈpliːt/
completeness /kəmˈpliːt.nəs/
complex /kɒm.pleks/
compliance /kəmˈplaɪ.ənt s/
component /kəmˈpəʊnənt/
composed /kəmˈpəʊzd/ of
composition /ˌkɒm.pəˈzɪʃ.ən/
compress /kəmˈpres/
compression /kəmˈpreʃən/
compromise /ˈkɒmprəˌmaɪz/
concern /kənˈsɜːn/
concise /kənˈsaɪs/
conclude /kənˈkluːd/
conclusion /kənˈkluː.ʒən/
concussion /kənˈkʌʃ.ən/
condensation /ˌkɒn.denˈseɪ.ʃən/
condition /kənˈdɪʃ.ən/
conditioning /kənˈdɪʃ.ən.ɪŋ/
conduct /kənˈdʌkt/
conduction /kənˈdʌk.ʃən/
confidential /ˌkɒn.fɪˈden.t ʃəl/

confidentiality /ˌkɒn.fɪ.den.tʃiˈæl.ɪ.ti/
confined /kənˈfaɪnd/
confirmation /ˌkɒn.fəˈmeɪ.ʃən/
confirmed /kənˈfɜːmd/
confrontational /ˌkɒn.frʌnˈteɪ.ʃən.əl/
confused /kənˈfjuːzd/
confusion /kənˈfjuːʒən/
congestion /kənˈdʒes.tʃən/
congestive /kənˈdʒes.tɪv/ heart / haːt/ failure /ˈfeɪ.ljər/
congestive /kənˈdʒes.tɪv/
conjunction /kənˈdʒʌŋk.ʃən/
conjunctivitis /kənˌdʒʌŋk.tɪˈvaɪ.tɪs/
conscious /ˈkɒn.tʃəs/
consciously /ˈkɒn.ʃəs.li/
consciousness /ˈkɒn.ʃəs.nəs/
consent /kənˈsent/
consenting /kənˈsent.ɪŋ/ adult /əˈdʌlt/
consequence /ˈkɒn.sɪ.kwəns/
consideration /kənˌsɪd.əˈreɪ.ʃən/
considered /kənˈsɪd.əd/
consist /kənˈsɪst/
consistent /kənˈsɪs.tənt/ with /wɪð/
consolidation /kənˌsɒl.ɪˈdeɪ.ʃən/
constant /ˈkɒn.stənt/
constantly /ˈkɒn.stənt.li/
constitute /ˈkɒn.stɪ.tjuːt/
constricted /kənˈstrɪkt.ɪd/
constriction /kənˈstrɪk.ʃən/
consult /kənˈsʌlt/
consumption /kənˈsʌmp.ʃən/
contain /kənˈteɪn/
container /kənˈteɪ.nər/
containment /kənˈteɪn.mənt/
contaminant /kənˈtæm.ɪ.nənt/
contamination /kənˌtæm.ɪˈneɪ.ʃən/
content /kənˈtent/
continue /kənˈtɪn.juː/
continuous /kənˈtɪn.ju.əs/
continuously /kənˈtɪn.ju.əs.li/
contract /kənˈtrækt/
contractile /kənˈtræk.taɪl/
contractility /ˌkən.trækˈtɪ.lə.ti/
contraction /kənˈtræk.ʃən/
contraindicate /ˌkɒn.trəˈɪn.dɪ.keɪt/

contraindication /ˌkɒn.trə.ɪn.dɪˈkeɪ.ʃən/
contrecoup /ˈkɒn.trə.kuːp/
contribute /kənˈtrɪb.juːt/
contusion /kənˈtjuː.ʒən/
convert /kənˈvɜːt/
convince /kənˈvɪns/
cool /kuːl/
cooling /ˈkuː.lɪŋ/
cooperate /kəʊˈɒp.ər.eɪt/
cooperative /kəʊˈɒp.ər.ə.tɪv/
coordinate /kəʊˈɔː.dɪ.neɪt/
COPD, Chronic /ˈkrɒnɪk/ Obstructive /əbˈstrʌk.tɪv/ Pulmonary /ˈpʊl.mə.nə.ri/ Disease /dɪˈziːz/
cope /kəʊp/ with /wɪð/
copious /ˈkəʊ.pi.əs/
copper /ˈkɒp.ər/
copperhead /ˈkɒp.ər.hed/
cor /kɔːr/ pulmonale /ˈpʊl.mə.nə.l/
coral /ˈkɒr.əl/ snake /sneɪk/
cord /kɔːd/
core /kɔːr/
corneal /kɔːˈni.əl/
corner /ˈkɔː.nər/
coronary /ˈkɒr.ən.ər.i/
correct /kəˈrekt/
corrective /kəˈrek.tɪv/
correlate /ˈkɒrɪˌleɪt/
correlation /ˌkɒr.əˈleɪ.ʃən/
corresponding /ˌkɒr.ɪˈspɒn.dɪŋ/
cortisol /ˈkɔː.tɪ.sɒl/
costal /ˈkɒs.təl/
cotton /ˈkɒt.ən/
cottonmouth /ˈkɒt.ən.maʊθ/
cough /kɒf/
count /kaʊnt/ for
count /kaʊnt/
counteract /ˌkaʊn.tərˈækt/
counterproductive /ˌkaʊn.tə.prəˈdʌk.tɪv/
countertraction /ˌkaʊn.tərˈtræk.ʃən/
coup /kap/
couple /ˈkʌp.l/
courageous /kəˈreɪ.dʒəs/

course /kɔːs/
court /kɔːt/
covering /ˈkʌv.ər.ɪŋ/
CPAP, Continuous / kənˈtɪn.
ju.əs/ Positive /ˈpɒz.ə.tɪv/ Airway
/ˈeə.weɪ/ Pressure /ˈpreʃ.ər/
CPR, Cardiopulmonary /
ˌkɑː.di.əʊˈpʊl.mə.nə.ri/
Resuscitation /rɪˌsʌs.ɪˈteɪ.ʃən/
crack /kræk/
crackle /ˈkræk.l̩/
cramp /kræmp/
cranial /ˈkreɪ.ni.əl/
crash /kræʃ/
craving /ˈkreɪ.vɪŋ/
create /kriːˈeɪt/
crepitus /ˈkrep.ɪ.təs/
crew /kruː/
crib /krɪb/
cricoid /ˈkraɪ.kɔɪd/
cartilage /ˈkɑː.təl.ɪdʒ/
cricoid /ˈkraɪ.kɔɪd/
cricothyreotomy /ˈkraɪ.
kəˌθaɪəˈrɒ.tə.mɪ/
crime /kraɪm/
criterion /kraɪˈtɪə.ri.ən/
critical /ˈkrɪt.ɪ.kəl/
Crohn's disease /ˈkrəʊnz.dɪˌziːz/
crop /krɒp/
crossing /ˈkrɒs.ɪŋ/
crouch /kraʊtʃ/
croup /kruːp/
crow /krəʊ/
crowning /ˈkraʊ.nɪŋ/
crush /krʌʃ/
crush /krʌʃ/ syndrome /ˈsɪn.drəʊm/
crushing /ˈkrʌʃ.ɪŋ/
cuff /kʌf/
cumulative /ˈkjuː.mjʊ.lə.tɪv/
curl /kɜːl/
current /ˈkʌr.ənt/
curtain /ˈkɜː.tən/
curved /kɜːvd/
custody /ˈkʌs.tə.di/
cut st off /kʌt/

CVA, Cerebrovascular/
ˌser.ɪ.brəˈvæskjʊlə/
Accident /ˈæksɪdənt/
cyanide /ˈsaɪə.naɪd/
cyanosis /ˌsaɪəˈnəʊ.sɪs/
cycle /ˈsaɪ.kl̩/
cyst /sɪst/
cystitis /sɪˈstaɪ.tɪs/

D

dam /dæm/
damage /ˈdæm.ɪdʒ/
damaged /ˈdæm.ɪdʒd/
danger /ˈdeɪn.dʒər/
dangerous /ˈdeɪn.dʒər.əs/
dangerously /ˈdeɪn.dʒər.əs.li/
dashboard /ˈdæʃˌbɔːd/
daydream /ˈdeɪ.driːm/
dead /ded/
deadly /ˈded.li/
deal with /dɪəl/
debilitating /dɪˈbɪl.ɪ.teɪt.ɪŋ/
debrief /ˌdiːˈbriːf/
debriefing /ˌdiːˈbriː.f.ɪŋ/
debris /ˈdeb.riː/, /ˈdeɪ.briː/
deceased /dɪˈsiːst/
deceleration /diːˌseləˈreɪʃən/
decerebrate /diːˈser.əˈbreɪt/
posturing /ˈpɒs.tʃər.ɪŋ/
decision /dɪˈsɪʒ.ən/
decode /diːˈkəʊd/
decompensated /diːˈkɒmpenˌseɪt.əd/
decompensation /diːˌkɒm.pen'seɪ.ʃən/
decompress /ˌdiː.kəmˈpres/
decompression /ˌdiː.kəmˈpreʃ.ən/
decompression /ˌdiː.kəmˈpreʃ.
ən/ sickness /ˈsɪk.nəs/
decontamination /ˌdiː.
kən.tæm.ɪˈneɪ.ʃən/
decorticate /ˌdi.kɔːtiˈkeɪt/
posturing /ˈpɒs.tʃər.ɪŋ/
decrease /dɪˈkriːs/
deem /diːm/
deep /diːp/
deeply /ˈdiːp.li/

defamation /ˌdefəˈmeɪʃən/

defence /dɪˈfent s/

defer /dɪˈfɜːr/

defibrillate /ˌdiːˈfɪb.rɪ.leɪt/

defibrillation /diːˌfɪb.rɪˈleɪ.ʃən/

deficiency /dɪˈfɪʃ.ənt .si/

deficit /ˈdef.ɪ.sɪt/

definitive /dɪˈfɪn.ɪ.tɪv/

deflate /dɪˈfleɪt/

deflation /dɪˈfleɪ.ʃən/

deformity /dɪˈfɔː.mɪ.ti/

degenerative /dɪˈdʒen.ər.ə.tɪv/

degree /dɪˈgriː/

dehydrated /ˌdiː.haɪˈdreɪ.tɪd/

dehydration /ˌdiː.haɪˈdreɪ.ʃən/

delay / dɪˈleɪ/

delayed /dɪˈleɪd/

delegate /ˈdel.ɪ.gət/

delirium tremens / dɪˌlɪr.i.əmˈtrem.ənz/

deliver /dɪˈlɪv.ər/

delivery /dɪˈlɪv.ər.i/

delusion /dɪˈluː.ʒən/

delusional /dɪˈluː.ʒən.əl/

demand /dɪˈmɑːnd/

demented /dɪˈmen.tɪd/

dementia /dɪˈmen.ʃə/

demonstrate /ˈdem.ən.streɪt/

deny /dɪˈnaɪ/

department /dɪˈpɑːt.mənt/

dependence /dɪˈpen.dənt s/

dependent /dɪˈpen.dənt/

deploy /dɪˈplɔɪ/

deployment /dɪˈplɔɪ.mənt/

depressant /dɪˈpres.ənt/

depression /dɪˈpreʃ.ən/

deprive /dɪˈpraɪv/

depth /depθ/

derangement /dɪˈreɪndʒd.mənt/

dermis /ˈdɜː.mɪs/

descend /dɪˈsend/

despite /dɪˈspaɪt/

destination /ˌdes.tɪˈneɪ.ʃən/

destruction /dɪˈstrʌk.ʃən/

detached /dɪˈtætʃt/

detachment /dɪˈtætʃmənt/

detect /dɪˈtekt/

detector /dɪˈtek.tər/

deteriorate /dɪˈtɪə.ri.ə.reɪt/

deterioration /dɪˌtɪə.ri.əˈreɪ.ʃən/

determination /dɪˌtɜː.mɪˈneɪ.ʃən/

determine /dɪˈtɜː.mɪn/

detoxify /diːˈtɒk.sɪ.faɪ/

devastating /ˈdev.ə.steɪ.tɪŋ/

development /dɪˈvel.əp.mənt/

deviate /ˈdiː.vi.eɪt/

deviation /ˌdiː.vɪˈeɪʃən/

device /dɪˈvaɪs/

dextrose /ˈdek.strəʊs/

diabetic /ˌdaɪəˈbet.ɪk/

diabetic /ˌdaɪəˈbet.ɪk/ ketoacidosis /ˈkiː.təʊˌæs.ɪˈdəʊ.sɪs/

diagnose /ˈdaɪəgˌnəʊz/

diagnosis /ˌdaɪ.əgˈnəʊ.sɪs/

dialysis /daɪˈæl.ə.sɪs/

diameter /daɪˈæm.ɪ.tər/

diaphoresis /ˌdaɪ.ə.fəˈriː.sɪs/

diaphoretic /ˌdaɪ.ə.fəˈret.ɪk/

diaphragm /ˈdaɪ.ə.fræm/

diarrhoea /ˌdaɪ.əˈriː.ə/

diastole /daɪˈæs.tə.li/

diastolic /daɪˈæs.tə.lɪk/

differential /ˌdɪf.əˈren.t ʃəl/

diffuse /dɪˈfjuːz/

diffused /dɪˈfjuːst/

diffusion /dɪˈfjuː.ʒən/

digestion /daɪˈdʒes.tʃən/

digestive /da ɪˈdʒes.tɪv/

digit /ˈdɪdʒ.ɪt/

digital /ˈdɪdʒ.ɪ.təl/

digitalis /ˌdɪdʒ.ɪˈteɪ.lɪs/

dignity /ˈdɪg.nɪ.ti/

digoxin /dɪdʒ.ɒ k.sɪn/

dilatation /ˌdɪl.əˈteɪ.ʃən/

dilated /daɪˈleɪtɪd/

dilation /daɪˈleɪ.ʃən/

dilemma /daɪˈlem.ə/

diligent /ˈdɪl.ɪ.dʒənt/

dilute /daɪˈluːt/

dilution /daɪˈluː.ʃən/

diminish /dɪˈmɪnɪʃ/
diphenhydramine /di.fenˈhɪ.drə.mɪːn/
direct /daɪˈrekt/
direction /daɪˈrek.ʃən/
directive /daɪˈrek.tɪv/
directly /daɪˈrekt.li/
director /daɪˈrek.tər/
disable /dɪˈseɪbl/
disabled /dɪˈseɪbld/
disadvantage /ˌdɪs.ədˈvɑːn.tɪdʒ/
disappear /ˌdɪs.əˈpɪər/
disassemble /ˌdɪs.əˈsem.bl̩/
disaster /dɪˈzɑːstər/
disc /dɪsk/
discharge /dɪsˈtʃɑːdʒ/
discoloration /dɪˌskʌl.əˈreɪ.ʃən/
discomfort /dɪˈskʌmp.fət/
discontinuation /ˌdɪs.kənˌtɪn.juˈeɪ.ʃən/
discover /dɪˈskʌv.ər/
disease /dɪˈziːz/
disentanglement /ˌdɪs.ɪnˈtæŋ.ɡl̩.mənt/
disinfection /ˌdɪs.ɪnˈfek.ʃən/
dislocation /ˌdɪs.ləˈkeɪ.ʃən/
dislodge /dɪˈslɒdʒ/
disorder /dɪˈsɔː.dər/
disorderly /dɪˈsɔː.dəl.i/
dispatch /dɪˈspætʃ/
dispatcher /dɪˈspætʃər/
displace /dɪˈspleɪs/
displacement /dɪˈspleɪs.mənt/
dispose of /dɪˈspəʊz/
disposition /ˌdɪs.pəˈzɪʃ.ən/
disrupt /dɪsˈrʌpt/
disruption /dɪsˈrʌp.ʃən/
dissecting /daɪˈsekt.ɪŋ/ aortic /eɪˈɔː.
tɪk/ aneurysm /ˈæn.jʊə.rɪ.zəm/
dissipate /ˈdɪs.ɪ.peɪt/
distal /ˈdɪ.stəl/
distance /ˈdɪs.tənt s/
distant /ˈdɪs.tənt/
distend /dɪˈstend/
distension /dɪˈsten.t ʃən/
distinct /dɪˈstɪŋkt/
distinction /dɪˈstɪŋk.ʃən/
distinguish /dɪˈstɪŋ.ɡwɪʃ/

distorted /dɪˈstɔː.tɪd/
distraught /dɪˈstrɔːt/
distress /dɪˈstres/
distribute /dɪˈstrɪb.juːt/
distributive /dɪˈstrɪbjʊtɪv/
disturb /dɪˈstɜːb/
disturbance /dɪˈstɜː.bənt s/
diuretic /ˌdaɪ.jʊəˈret.ɪk/
dive /daɪv/
diverticulitis /ˌdaɪ.vəˌtɪk.jʊˈlaɪ.tɪs/
divide /dɪˈvaɪd/
diving /ˈdaɪ.vɪŋ/ reflex /ˈriː.fleks/
dizziness /ˈdɪz.ɪ.nəs/
Do Not Resuscitate /
rɪˈsʌs.ɪ.teɪt/ order /ˈɔː.dər/
doctrine /ˈdɒk.trɪn/
domestic /dəˈmes.tɪk/
doom /duːm/
dopamine /ˈdəʊ.pə.mɪːn/
dosage /ˈdəʊ.sɪdʒ/
dose /dəʊs/
down /daʊn/
downhill /ˌdaʊnˈhɪl/
downward /ˈdaʊn.wəd/
downwind /ˌdaʊnˈwɪnd/
drain /dreɪn/
drainage /ˈdreɪ.nɪdʒ/
draw /drɔː/
drawing /ˈdrɔː.ɪŋ/
dress /dres/
drip /drɪp/
drive /draɪv/
driveway /ˈdraɪv.weɪ/
drizzle /ˈdrɪz.əl/
drool /druːl/
droop /druːp/
drop /drɒp/
droplet /ˈdrɒp.lət/
drowning /ˈdraʊn.ɪŋ/
drowsiness /ˈdraʊ.zɪ.nəs/
drowsy /ˈdraʊ.zi/
drunk /drʌŋk/
due /djuː/ to /tʊ/
dig /dɪɡ/ out /aʊt/
dull /dʌl/

dullness /'dʌl.nəs/

duodenum /ˌdjuː.əˈdiː.nəm/

duplex /'djuː.pleks/

dura mater /ˌdjuə.rəˈmeɪ.tə/

durable /'djuərəbəl/

duration /djuəˈreɪ.ʃən/

dusky /'dʌs.ki/

duty /'djuːtɪ/

dysphasia /disˈfeɪ.zɪə/

dyspnoea /dɪs.pniː.ə/

dysrhythmia /dɪsˈrɪθ.mɪə/

E

earlobe /'ɪə.ləʊb/

easing /'iːz.ɪŋ/

eatery /'iːtərɪ/

ecchymosis /ˌekiˈməʊ.sɪs/

eclampsia /ɪˈklæmp.si.ə/

ectopic pregnancy / ek.tɒp.ɪkˈpreg.nən.si/

edge /edʒ/

effacement /ɪˈfeɪs.mənt/

effect /ɪˈfekt/

effective /ɪˈfek.tɪv/

effectiveness /ɪˈfek.tɪv.nəs/

efficiently /ɪˈfɪʃ.ənt.li/

effort /'ef.ət/

eject /ɪˈdʒekt/

ejection /ɪˈdʒekt.ʃən/

elasticity /ˌɪl.æsˈtɪs.ɪ.ti/

elder /'eldə/

elderly /'el.dəl.i/

electrical /ɪˈlek.trɪ.kəl/ line /laɪn/

electrocution /ɪˌlek.trəˈkjuː.ʃən/

electrolyte /ɪˈlek.trə.laɪt/

element /'elɪmənt/

elevate /'el.ɪ.veɪt/

elevated /'el.ɪ.veɪ.tɪd/

elevation /ˌel.ɪˈveɪ.ʃən/

eliminate /ɪˈlɪm.ɪ.neɪt/

elimination /ɪˌlɪm.ɪˈneɪ.ʃən/

emanate /'em.ə.neɪt/

emancipate /ɪˈmænsɪ.peɪt/

emancipated /ɪˈmæn.sɪ.peɪ.tɪd/

embedded /ɪmˈbed.ɪd/

embolism /'embəˌlɪzəm/

embolus pl emboli /'em.bə.ləs/

emerge /ɪˈmɜːdʒ/

emergency /ɪˈmɜː.dʒənt .si/

emesis /eˈmɪ.sɪs/

emotional /ɪˈməʊ.ʃən.əl/

emotionally /ɪˈməʊ.ʃən.əl.i/

emphysema /ˌemp.fəˈsiː.mə/

employee /ɪmˈplɔɪ.iː/

EMT, Emergency /ɪˈmɜː. dʒənt .si/ Medical /'med.ɪ.kəl/ Technician /tekˈnɪʃən/

en route, enroute /ˌɒnˈruːt/

enact /ɪˈnækt/

encephalopathy /enˌsef.əˈlɒp.ə.θi/

enclose /ɪnˈkləʊz/

encode /ɪnˈkəʊd/

encounter /ɪnˈkaʊntə/

encourage /ɪnˈkʌr.ɪdʒ/

end /end/ -tidal /'taɪ.d əl/

endocardium /ˌen.dəˈkɑː.di.əm/

endocrine /'en.də.krɪn/

endometriosis /ˌen.dəʊˌmiː.triˈəʊ.sɪs/

endometritis /ˌen.də.mɪˈtraɪ.tɪs/

endotracheal /en.dɒˈtrəˈkiː. əl/ tube /tjuːb/ (ET tube)

enforcement /ɪnˈfɔː.smənt/

engage /ɪnˈgeɪdʒ/

enhance /ɪnˈhɑːns/

enlist /ɪnˈlɪst/

ensure /ɪnˈʃɔːr/

entire /ɪnˈtaɪə/

entrap /ɪnˈtræp/

entrapment /ɪnˈtræp.mənt/

envenomation /ɪnˌven.əˈmeɪ.ʃən/

environment /ɪnˈvaɪ.rən.mənt/

epidural /ˌepɪˈdjuərəl/

epigastric /ˌepɪˈgæs.trɪk/

epigastrium /ˌepɪˈgæs.tri.əm/

epiglottis /ˌep.ɪˈglɒt.ɪs/

epiglottitis /ˌep.ɪ.gləˈtaɪ.tɪs/

epinephrine /ˌepɪˈnef.riːn/

episode /'ep.ɪ.səʊd/

equal /'iːkwəl/

equation /ɪˈkweɪ.ʒən/

equilibrium /ˌiːkwɪˈlɪbrɪəm/
equipment /ɪˈkwɪp.mənt/
equivalent /ɪˈkwɪv.əl.ənt/
erratic /ɪˈræt.ɪk/
error /ˈer.ər/
erythrocyte /ɪˈrɪθ.rəʊ.saɪt/
escape /ɪˈskeɪp/
essential /ɪˈsen.tʃəl/
establish /ɪˈstæb.lɪʃ/
estimate /ˈes.tɪ.meɪt/
ethanol /ˈeθ.ə.nɒl/
ethics /ˈeθɪk/
euphoria /juːˈfɔː.ri.ə/
eustress /juː.stres/
evacuate /ɪˈvæk.ju.eɪt/
evaluate /ɪˈvæl.ju.eɪt/
evaluation /ɪˌvæl.juˈeɪ.ʃən/
event /ɪˈvent/
evidence /ˈevɪdəns/
evident /ˈev.ɪ.dənt/
evisceration /ɪˌvɪs.əˈreɪ.ʃən/
exacerbation /ɪgˌzæsəˈbeɪʃən/
examination /ɪgˌzæm.ɪˈneɪ.ʃən/
examine /ɪgˈzæm.ɪn/
examiner /ɪgˈzæm.ɪ.nər/
exceed /ɪkˈsiːd/
excellent /ˈek.səl.ənt/
excess /ekˈses/
excessive /ekˈses.ɪv/
exchange /ɪksˈtʃeɪndʒ/
exclude /ɪkˈskluːd/
excluding /ɪkˈskluː.dɪŋ/
excretion /ɪkˈskriː.ʃən/
excruciating /ɪkˈskruː.ʃi.eɪ.tɪŋ/
exercise /ˈek.sə.saɪz/
exert /ɪgˈzɜːt/
exertion /ɪgˈzɜː.ʃən/
exhalation /ˌeks.h əˈleɪ.ʃən/
exhale /eksˈheɪl/
exhaustion /ɪgˈzɔːs.tʃən/
exhibit / ɪgˈzɪb.ɪt/
exophthalmos /ˌeks.ɒfˈθæl.məs/
expand /ɪkˈspænd/
expansion /ɪkˈspæn.tʃən/
expectorate /ɪkˈspek.tər.eɪt/

expedite /ˈek.spə.daɪt/
expel /ɪkˈspel/
expend /ɪkˈspend/
experience /ɪkˈspɪə.ri.ənt s/
experienced /ɪkˈspɪə.ri.ənst/
expiration /ˌek.spəˈreɪ.ʃən/
expiratory /ɪkˈspɪr.ə.tər.i/
explosion /ɪkˈspləʊ.ʒən/
explosive /ɪkˈspləʊ.sɪv/
explosive /ɪkˈspləʊ.sɪv/
delivery /dɪˈlɪv.ər.i/
exposed /ɪkˈspəʊzd/
exposure /ɪkˈspəʊ.ʒə/
express /ɪkˈspres/
expressed /ɪkˈspresd/
expression /ɪkˈspreʃ.ən/
expulsion /ɪkˈspʌl.ʃən/
extension /ɪkˈsten.tʃən/
extensive /ɪkˈsten.sɪv/
extenuating /ɪkˈsten.ju.eɪ.tɪŋ/
external /ɪkˈstɜː.nəl/
extraction /ɪkˈstræk.ʃən/
extravasation /eks.træ.vəˈseɪ.ʃən/
extreme /ɪkˈstriːm/
extremely /ɪkˈstriːm.li/
extremity /ɪkˈstrem.ɪ.ti/
extricate /ˈek.strɪ.keɪt/
extrication /ˌek.strɪˈkeɪ.ʃən/
extubate /eks.tjʊ.beɪt/
extubation /ˌeks.tjʊˈbeɪ.ʃən/
eyebrow /ˈaɪ.braʊ/
eyewear /ˈaɪweər/

F
face /feɪs/ **down** /daʊn/
facial /ˈfeɪ.ʃəl/
facilitate /fəˈsɪl.ɪ.teɪt/
factor /ˈfæk.tər/
faecal /ˈfiː.kəl/
faeces /ˈfiː.siːz/
fail /feɪl/
failure /ˈfeɪ.ljə/
faint /feɪnt/
faith /feɪθ/
fall /fɔːl/ **(fell, fallen)**

fallopian tube /fəˌləʊ.pi.ənˈtjuːb/
false /fɒls/ **imprisonment** /
ɪmˈprɪz.ən.mənt/
falsely /ˈfɒls.li/
familiar /fəˈmɪl.i.ər/ **with** /wɪð/
farther /ˈfɑː.ðər/
fast-moving /fɑːstˈmuː.vɪŋ/
fat-based /fæt.beɪst/
fatigue /fəˈtiːg/
favourably /ˈfeɪ.vər.ə.b̩i/
fear /fɪə/
febrile /ˈfiː.braɪl/
feedback /ˈfiːd.bæk/
feeding /ˌfiː.dɪŋ/
feeling /ˈfiː.lɪŋ/
female /ˈfiː.meɪl/
femoral /ˈfemərəl/
femur pl **femora** /ˈfiː.mər/
fence /fens/
fertilize /ˈfɜː.tɪ.laɪz/
fever /ˈfiː.vər/ horečka
fibrillate /ˈfaɪ.brɪ.leɪt/
fibrillation /ˌfaɪ.brɪˈleɪ.ʃən/
fibroserous /ˌfaɪ.brəˈsɪə.rəs/
fibula pl -**ae** /ˈfɪb.jʊ.lə/
field /fiːld/
fight or flight /ˌfaɪt.ɔːˈflaɪt/
fill /fɪl/
final /ˈfaɪ.nəl/
finding /ˈfaɪndɪŋ/
fingernail /ˈfɪŋ.gə.neɪl/
fingerstick /ˈfɪŋ.gə.stɪk/
fire fighter /ˈfaɪəˌfaɪ.tər/
fire-fighting /ˈfaɪəˌfaɪ.tɪŋ/
firewall /ˈfaɪə.wɔːl/
fireworks /ˈfaɪəˌwɜːk/
firm /fɜːm/
firmly /ˈfɜːm.li/
fist /fɪst/
fit /fɪt/
fixture /ˈfɪks.tʃər/
flaccid /ˈflæksɪd/
flail /fleɪl/ **chest** /tʃest/
flail /fleɪl/
flaming /ˈfleɪ.mɪŋ/

flank /flæŋk/
flare /fleər/
flash /flæʃ/
flat /flæt/
flavoured /fleɪ.vəd/
flexion /flek.ʃən/
flight /flaɪt/ **of stairs** /steərz/
flood /flʌd/
flotation /fləʊˈteɪ.ʃən/
equipment /ɪˈkwɪp.mənt/
flow /fləʊ/
flowing /ˈfləʊ.ɪŋ/
fluid /ˈfluː.ɪd/
flulike /fluː.laɪk/
flush /flʌʃ/
flushed /flʌʃt/
flutter /ˈflʌt.ər/
fly /flaɪ/ (**flew, flown**)
flying /ˈflaɪ.ɪŋ/
focused /ˈfəʊkəst/
foetal /ˈfiː.təl/
foetus /ˈfiː.təs/
fontanelle /ˌfɒn.təˈnel/
food /fuːd/ -**borne** /bɔːn/
footwear /ˈfʊt.weər/
force /fɔːs/
forced /fɔːst/
forcefully /ˈfɔːs.fəl.i/
forceps /ˈfɔː.seps/
forearm /ˈfɔː.rɑːm/
forehead /ˈfɒrɪd/, /ˈfɔːˌhed/
foreign /ˈfɒr.ən/ **body** /ˈbɒd.i/
foreshadow /fɔːˈʃæd.əʊ/
form /fɔːm/
formation /fɔːˈmeɪ.ʃən/
forward /ˈfɔː.wəd/
foul /faʊl/
found /faʊnd/
Fowler's /fow'ler/ **position** /pəˈzɪʃ.ən/
fracture /ˈfræk.tʃə/
frail /freɪl/
Frank-Starlings mechanism /ˈmekəˌnɪzəm/
fraternity /frəˈtɜː.nə.ti/
freak /friːk/

free /friː/
frequency /ˈfriː.kwən.si/
friction /ˈfrɪk.ʃən/
frostbite /ˈfrɒst.baɪt/
frostbitten /ˈfrɒst.bɪt.ən/
froth /frɒθ/
frown /fraʊn/
fruity /ˈfruː.tɪ/
fulcrum /ˈfʊl.krəm/
full /fʊl/
full-blown /ˌfʊlˈbləʊn/
full-term (infant) /fʊlˈtɜːm/
fundal /ˈfʌn.dəl/
fundus /ˈfʌn.dəs/ pl. -di
fungus /ˈfʌŋ.gəs/ (pl fungi)
funny /ˈfʌn.i/ zvláštní, podivný
furosemide /fjʊr.ɔsˈæm.aɪd/
furthermore /ˌfɜː.ðəˈmɔːr/

G
gag /gæg/
gag /gæg/ reflex /ˈriː.fleks/
gain /geɪn/
gall bladder, gallbladder /
ˈgɔːlˈblæd.ər/
gallon /ˈgæl.ən/
garbage /ˈgɑː.bɪdʒ/ can /kæn/
garbled /ˈgɑː.bl̩d/
garment /ˈgɑːmənt/
gas /gæs/
gaseous /ˈgeɪ.si.əs/
gasp /gɑːsp/
gastric /ˈgæs.trɪk/
gastric /ˈgæs.trɪk/ tube /tjuːb/
gastritis /gæsˈtraɪ.tɪs/
gather /ˈgæð.ər/
gauze /gɔːz/
gear /gɪə/
gel /dʒel/
general /ˈdʒen.ər.əl/
generalized /ˈdʒen.ə r.ə.laɪzd/
generally /ˈdʒen.ə r.əl.i/
generate /ˈdʒen.ər.eɪt/
genital /ˈdʒen.ɪ.təl/
genitourinary /ˌdʒen.ɪ.təʊˈjʊə.rɪ.nər,i/

gentle /ˈdʒen.tl̩/
gently /ˈdʒent.li/
geriatric /ˌdʒer.iˈæt.rɪk/
gestation /dʒesˈteɪ.ʃən/
get up /get.ʌp/
Glasgow /ˌglɑː.z.gəʊ/ Coma /
ˈkəʊ.mə/ Scale /skeɪl/
glottic /ˈglɒt.ɪk/
glottis /ˈglɒt.ɪs/ pl glotides
gloved /glʌvd/
glucometer /ˌgluː.kəˈm.ɪ.tər/
glucose /ˈgluː.kəʊs/
goal /gəʊl/
goblet /ˈgɒb.lət/
goggle /ˈgɒg.l̩/
golden /ˈgəʊl.dən/ rule/ ruːl/
gonorrhoea /ˌgɒn.əˈriː.ə/
goof /guːf/ around /əˈraʊnd/
govern /ˈgʌv.ən/
gown /gaʊn/
grab /græb/
grade /greɪd/
gradual /ˈgræd.jʊ.əl/
gradually /ˈgræd.jʊ.li/
grain /greɪn/
grand mal /ˌgrɑːndˈmæl/
grape /greɪp/
grave /greɪv/
Graves' /greɪvz/ disease /dɪˈziː.z/
gravida /ˌgræv.ɪ.də/
gravidity /grævˈɪd.ɪ.ti/
greenish /ˈgriː.nɪʃ/
greenstick /ˈgriːn.stɪk/
fracture / ˈfræktʃə/
grimace /ˈgrɪ.məs/
groin /grɔɪn/
gross /grəʊs/
ground /graʊnd/
grounded /graʊnd.ɪd/
growth /grəʊθ/
grunt /grʌnt/
guard /gɑːd/
guidance /ˈgaɪ.dəns/
guideline /ˈgaɪd.laɪn/
gunpowder /ˈgʌn.paʊ.dər/

313

gunshot /ˈgʌn.ʃɒt/
gutter /ˈgʌt.ər/
gynaecology /ˌgaɪ.nəˈkɒl.ə.dʒi/

H
haematoma pl haematomata /
ˌhiː.məˈtəʊ.mə/
haematuria /ˌhiː.məˈt jʊə.ri.ə/
haemodialysis /ˌhiːmə.daɪˈælɪsɪs/
haemodynamic /ˌhiːmə.daɪˈnæm.ɪk/
haemopneumothorax /ˈhiː.
mə.njuː.məˈθɔː.ræks/
haemoptysis /hiːˈmɒ.ptɪ.sɪs/
haemorrhage /ˈhem.ər.ɪdʒ/
haemostasis /ˌhiː.məˈsteɪ.sɪs/
haemothorax /ˈhiː.məˈθɔː.ræks/
hallmark /ˈhɔːl.maːk/
hallucination /həˌluː.sɪˈneɪ.ʃən/
hallucinogen /həˈluː.sɪ.nə.dʒen/
hand /hænd/ over /ˈəʊ.vər/
hand-held /ˈhændheld/
handgun /ˈhændˌgʌn/
handicapped /ˈhæn.dɪ.kæpt/
handle /ˈhæn.dl̩/
handlebar /ˌhæn.dl̩.baː/
handling /ˈhænd.lɪŋ/
hands-on /ˌhænd.ˈzɒn/
handwash /ˈhændˌwɒʃ/
hang /hæŋ/
hanging /ˈhæŋɪŋ/
hard /haːd/
harden /ˈhaː.dən/
harm /haːm/
harmful /ˈhaːm.fəl/
harsh /haːʃ/
hazard /ˈhæz.əd/
hazmat /ˈhæz.mæt/
head on, head-on /ˌhedˈɒn/
heal /hiːl/
health /helθ/ care, /keə/
health /helθ/ status /ˈsteɪ.təs/
hear /hɪər/ (heard, heard)
heart /haːt/ rate /reɪt/
heartbeat /ˈhaːt.biːt/
heat /hiːt/ cramp /kræmp/

heat /hiːt/ exhaustion /ɪgˈzɔːs.tʃən/
heat /hiːt/ stroke /strəʊk/
heave /hiːv/
Heimlich maneuver /
ˈhaɪm.lɪk.məˌnu.vər/
held /held/
helmet /ˈhel.mət/
helpless /ˈhelplɪs/
hemiparalysis /ˌhem.ɪ.pəˈræl.ə.sɪs/
hemiparesis /ˌhem.ɪ.pəˈriː.sɪs/
hepatic /hepˈæt.ɪk/
hepatitis /ˌhep.əˈtaɪ.tɪs/
herniation /ˌhɜː.niˈeɪ.ʃən/
herpes /ˈhɜː.piːz/
herpes /ˈhɜː.piːz/ simplex /ˈsɪm.pleks/
herpes /ˈhɜː.piːz/ zoster /zɒ.stər/
herpes-virus /ˈhɜː.piːzˈvaɪ.rəs/
HHNK, Hyperosmolar /ˌhaɪ.
pə.ɒz.mɒ.lər/ Hyperglycaemic /
ˌhaɪ.pə.glaɪ.ˈsiː.mɪk/ Nonketotic /
ˌnɒn.ke.tɒt.ɪk/ Coma /ˈkəʊmə/
hiatal /haɪˈeɪ.təl/ hernia /ˈhɜː.ni.ə/
hiatus /haɪˈeɪ.təs/
high-pitched /ˌhaɪˈpɪtʃt/
hip /hɪp/
histamine /ˈhɪs.tə.miːn/
history /ˈhɪs.tər.i/
hit /hɪt/ (hit, hit)
hives /haɪvz/
hoarse /hɔːs/
hoarseness /hɔːsnɪs/
hold /həʊld/
hole /həʊl/
hollow /ˈhɒl.əʊ/
Homans' /həʊ.mænz/ sign /saɪn/
homeless /ˈhəʊm.ləs/
homeostasis /ˌhəʊ.mi.əʊˈsteɪ.sɪs/
honour /ˈɑn.ər/
hopeless /ˈhəʊp.ləs/
host /həʊst/
humerus pl -ri /ˈhjuː.mə.rəs/
humid /ˈhjuː.mɪd/
humidified /hjuːˈmɪd.ɪ.faɪd/
humidity /hjuːˈmɪd.ɪ.ti/
humoral /ˈhjuː.mər.əl/

hunting /'hʌn.tɪŋ/ knife /naɪf/
hurt /hɜːt/ (hurt, hurt)
hydration /haɪ'dreɪ.ʃən/
hydrogen /'haɪ.drɪ.dʒən/
hyperactivity /ˌhaɪ.pər'æk'tɪv.ɪ.ti/
hyperadrenalism /ˌhaɪ.
pər.æd'riː.nəl.ɪzm/
hyperextension /ˌhaɪ.pər'ɪk'stenʃən/
hyperflexion /ˌhaɪ.pə'flæk.ʃən/
hyperglycaemia /ˌhaɪ.pə.glaɪ'siː.mi.ə/
hyperglycaemic /ˌhaɪ.pə.glaɪ.'siː.mɪk/
hyperkalaemia /ˌhaɪ.pə.kæ'liː.mi.ə/
hyperosmolar /ˌhaɪ.pə.ɒz.
mɒ.lər/ coma /'kəʊmə/
hyperresonance /ˌhaɪ.pə.'rez.ən.əns/
hyperresonant /ˌhaɪ.pə.'rez.ən.ənt/
hypersensitivity /ˌhaɪ.
pə.ˌsen.sɪ'tɪv.ɪ.ti/
hypertension /ˌhaɪ.pə'ten.ʃən/
hypertensive /ˌhaɪ.pə'ten.sɪv/
hyperthermia /ˌhaɪ.pə'θɜː.mɪ.ə/
hypertonia /ˌhaɪ.pə'təʊ.niə/
hypertrophy /haɪ'pɜː.trə.fi/
hyperventilate /haɪ.pə'ven.tɪ.leɪt/
hyperventilation /ˌhaɪ.
pə.ven.tɪ'leɪ.ʃən/
hypervolaemia /ˌhaɪ.pə.vɒ'liː.mi.ə/
hyphaema /haɪ.θe.mə/
hypocalcaemia /ˌhaɪ.pəʊ.kæl'siː.mi.ə/
hypoglycaemia /ˌhaɪ.pəʊ.glaɪ'siː.mi.ə/
hypokalaemia /ˌhaɪ.pəʊ.kæ'liː.mi.ə/
hypomagnesaemia /ˌhaɪ.
pəʊ.ˌmæg.nə'siː.mi.ə/
hypoperfusion /ˌhaɪ.pəʊ.pə'fjuː.ʒən/
hypotension /ˌhaɪ.pəʊ'ten.tʃən/
hypothermia /ˌhaɪ.pəʊ'θɜː.mi.ə/
hypothesize /haɪ'pɒθ.ə.saɪz/
hypotonia /ˌhaɪpəʊ'təʊ.niə/
hypoventilation /ˌhaɪpəʊˌven.tɪ'leɪ.ʃən/
hypovolaemia /ˌhaɪpəʊ.və'lː.mi.ə/
hypoxaemia /ˌhaɪ.pɒk'siː.mi.ə/
hypoxia /haɪ'pɒk.sɪə/
hypoxic /haɪ'pɒk.sɪk/ drive /draɪv/

I

ice /aɪs/ pack /pæk/
ICP, Intracranial /ɪn.trə'kreɪ.
ni.əl/ Pressure /'preʃ.ər/
identifiable /aɪ'den.tɪ.faɪ.ə.bļ/
identification /aɪˌden.tɪ.fɪ'keɪ.ʃən/
identify /aɪ'den.tɪ.faɪ/
idioventricular /ˌɪd.i.əʊ.ven'trɪk.jə.lər/
iliac /'ɪl.i.æk/ crest /krest/
illegal /ɪ'liː.gəl/
illegible /ɪ'ledʒ.ə.bļ/
illness /'ɪl.nəs/
image /'ɪm.ɪdʒ/
imbalance /ˌɪm'bæl.ənt s/
immediate /ɪ'miː.di.ət/
immediately /ɪ'miː.di.ət.li/
immerse /ɪ'mɜːs/
immersion /ɪ'mɜː.ʃən/
imminent /'ɪm.ɪ.nənt/
immobilization /ɪˌməʊ.bəl.aɪ'zeɪ.ʃən/
immunocompromised /ˌɪm.
jə.nəʊ'kɒm.prə.maɪzd/
impact /'ɪm.pækt/
impair /ɪm'peər/
impaired /ɪm'peəd/
impairment /ɪm'peər.mənt/
impale /ɪm'peɪl/
impending /ɪm'pen.dɪŋ/
imperative /ɪm'per.ə.tɪv/
implant /ɪm'plɑːnt/
implantation /ˌɪm.plæn'teɪ.ʃən/
implied /ɪm'plaɪd/
impression /ɪm'preʃ.ən/
improper /ɪm'prɒp.ər/
improperly /ɪm'prɒp.ər.li/
improve /ɪm'pruːv/
improvement /ɪm'pruːv.mənt/
impulse /'ɪm.pʌls/
in addition /ə'dɪʃ.ən/
in advance /əd'vɑːns/
in extremis /ˌɪn.ɪk'striː.mɪs/
in order to /'ɔː.dər/
in writing /'raɪ.tɪŋ/
inability /ˌɪn.ə'bɪl.ɪ.ti/
inaccurate /ɪ'næk.jʊ.rət/

IRENA BAUMRUKOVÁ

inactivity /ˌɪn.æk'tɪv.ɪ.ti/
inadequate /ɪ'næd.ɪ.kwət/
inadvertent /ˌɪn.əd'vɜː.tənt/
inappropriate /ˌɪn.ə'prəʊ.pri.ət/
inappropriately /ˌɪn.ə'prəʊ.pri.ət.li/
inattentiveness /ˌɪn.ə'ten.tɪv.nəs/
inch /ɪntʃ/
incidence /'ɪnt.sɪ.dənt s/
incident /'ɪnt.sɪ.dənt/
incline /ɪn'klaɪn/
incompatible /ˌɪn.kəm'pæt.ɪ.bl̩/
incompetent /ɪn'kɒm.pɪ.tənt/
incomplete /ˌɪn.kəm'pliːt/
incomprehensible /
ɪnˌkɒm.prɪ'hen.sɪ.bl̩/
incomprehensibly /
ɪnˌkɒm.prɪ'hen.sɪ.bl̩ i/
incontinent /ɪn'kɒn.tɪ.nənt/
increase /ɪn'kriːs/
increasingly /ɪn'kriː.sɪŋ.li/
indicate /'ɪn.dɪ.keɪt/
indication /ˌɪn.dɪ'keɪ.ʃən/
indicator /'ɪn.dɪ.keɪ.tər/
individual /ˌɪn.dɪ'vɪd.ju.əl/
indoors /ˌɪn'dɔːz/
infancy /'ɪn.fənt.si/
infant /'ɪnfənt/
infarction /ɪn'fɑːk.ʃən/
infectious /ɪn'fek.ʃəs/
inferior /ɪn'fɪə.ri.ər/
inferior /ɪn'fɪə.ri.ər/ vena
cava /ˌviː.nə'keɪ.və/
infiltration /ˌɪn.fɪl'treɪ.ʃən/
inflamed /ɪn'fleɪmd/
inflammation /ˌɪn.flə'meɪ.ʃən/
inflammatory /ɪn'flæm.ə.tər.i/
inflate /ɪn'fleɪt/
inflation /ɪn'fleɪ.ʃən/
influence /'ɪnfluəns/
influenza /ˌɪn.flu'en.zə/
informed /ɪn'fɔːmd/
infrapatellar /ˌɪn.frə.pə'tel.ər/
infrastructure /'ɪn.frəˌstrʌk.tʃər/
infusion /ɪn'fjuː.ʒən/
ingestion /ɪn'dʒes.tʃən/

inguinal /'ɪŋ.gwɪ.nəl/
inhalation /ˌɪn.hə'leɪ.ʃən/
inhale /ɪn'heɪl/
inhaler /ɪn'heɪ.lər/
inhibit /ɪn'hɪb.ɪt/
initial /ɪ'nɪʃ.əl/
initially /ɪ'nɪʃ.əl.i/
initiate /ɪ'nɪʃ.i.eɪt/
injury /'ɪndʒəri/
inner /'ɪn.ər/
innervate /'ɪn.ə.veɪt/
insatiable /ɪn'seɪ.ʃə.bl̩/
insect /'ɪn.sekt/
insert /ɪn'sɜːt/
insertion /ɪn'sɜː.ʃən/
insist /ɪn'sɪst/
insomnia /ɪn'sɒm.ni.ə/
inspect /ɪn'spekt/
inspection /ɪn'spek.ʃən/
inspiration /ˌɪn.spɪ'reɪ.ʃən/
inspiratory /ɪn'spaɪə.rə.tər.i/
instability /ˌɪn.stə'bɪl.ɪ.ti/
instead /ɪn'sted/
institute /'ɪn.stɪ.tjuːt/
institutionalization /ˌɪnt.
stɪˌtjuː.ʃən.əl.aɪ'zeɪ.ʃən/
instruct /ɪn'strʌkt/
instrument /'ɪn.strə.mənt/
insufficiency /ˌɪn.sə'fɪʃ.ən.si/
insulin /'ɪn.sjʊ.lɪn/
insult /'ɪn.sʌlt/
intact /ɪn'tækt/
intake /'ɪn.teɪk/
integral /'ɪn.tɪ.grəl/
integration /ˌɪn.tɪ'greɪ.ʃən/
integrity /ɪn'teg.rə.ti/
intense /ɪn'tens/
intensity /ɪn'ten.sɪ.ti/
intentional /ɪn'tenʃənəl/
interact /ˌɪn.tə'rækt/
intercostal /ˌɪn.tə'kɒs.təl/
intercostals /ˌɪn.tə'kɒs.təlz/
interfere /ˌɪn.tə'fɪər/
interference /ˌɪn.tə'fɪə.rəns/
interim /'ɪn.tər.ɪm/

interior /ɪnˈtɪə.ri.ər/
intermediate /ˌɪn.təˈmiː.di.ət/
intermittent /ˌɪn.təˈmɪt.ənt/
internal /ɪnˈtɜː.nəl/
interrupt /ˌɪn.təˈrʌpt/
interruption /ˌɪn.təˈrʌp.ʃən/
intervention /ˌɪn.təˈven.ʃən/
intestine /ɪnˈtes.tɪn/
intolerance /ɪnˈtɒl.ər.ənt s/
intoxication /ɪnˌtɒk.sɪˈkeɪ.ʃən/
intraabdominal /ɪn.trə.æbˈdɒm.ɪ.nəl/
intracerebral /ˌɪn.trəˈser.ə.brəl/
intracranial /ɪn.trəˈkreɪ.ni.əl/
intramuscular /ˌɪn.trəˈmʌs.kjʊ.lər/
intraosseous /ˌɪn.trəˈɒs.i.əs/
intrathoracic /ˌɪn.trə.θɔːˈræs.ɪk/
intravenous /ˌɪn.trəˈviː.nəs/
intravenous /ˌɪn.trəˈviː.nəs/ line /laɪn/
intravenously /ˌɪn.trəˈviː.nəs.li/
introduce /ˌɪn.trəˈdjuːs/
intubate /ɪnˈtjuː.beɪt/
intubation /ˌɪn.tjuːˈbeɪ.ʃən/
invasion /ɪnˈveɪ.ʒən/
invasive /ɪnˈveɪ.sɪv/
inverted/ ɪnˈvɜː.tɪd/
involuntary /ɪnˈvɒləntəri/
involvement /ɪnˈvɒlv.mənt/
inward /ˈɪn.wəd/
ion /ˈaɪ.ɒn/
ipecac /ˈɪp.ɪ.kæk/
iris /ˈaɪrɪs/
irregular /ɪˈreg.jə.lər/
irregularity /ɪˌreg.jəˈlær.ə.ti/
irreversible /ˌɪr.ɪˈvɜː.sɪ.bl̩/
irritability /ˌɪr.ɪ.təˈbɪl.ɪ.ti/
irritable /ˈɪr.ɪ.tə.bl̩/
irritant /ˈɪr.ɪ.tənt/
irritate /ˈɪr.ɪ.teɪt/
irritation /ˌɪr.ɪˈteɪ.ʃən/
ischaemia /ɪsˈkiː.mɪ.ə/
ischaemic /ɪsˈkiː.mɪk/
isolation /ˌaɪ.səl.eɪ.ʃən/
isotonic /aɪ.səʊˈtɒn.ɪk/
itching /ˈɪtʃ.ɪŋ/
itchy /ˈɪtʃ.i/

item /ˈaɪ.təm/
IV, intravenous /ˌɪn.trəˈviː.nəs/

J

jagged /ˈdʒæg.ɪd/
jaundice /ˈdʒɔːn.dɪs/
jaw /dʒɔː/
jaw /dʒɔː/ thrust /θrʌst/
jeopardize /ˈdʒep.ə.daɪz/
jerk /dʒɜːk/
judge /dʒʌdʒ/
judgment /ˈdʒʌdʒ.mənt/
jugular /ˈdʒʌg.jə.lər/
jugular /ˈdʒʌg.jə.lər/ vein /veɪn/
junction /ˈdʒʌŋk.ʃən/
junctional /ˈdʒʌŋk.ʃən.əl/
tachycardia /ˌtæk.ɪˈkɑː.di.ə/
jungle /ˈdʒʌŋ.gl̩/ gym /dʒɪm/
junky- /ˈdʒʌŋ.ki/ sounding /ˈsaʊndɪŋ/
jurisdiction /ˌdʒʊə.rɪsˈdɪk.ʃən/
JVD, Jugular /ˈdʒʌg.jə.lər/ Venous /
ˈviː.nəs/ Distension /dɪˈsten.tʃən/

K

Kaposi's /kæˈpəʊ.sɪz/
sarcoma /sɑːˈkəʊ.mə/
keep from /kiːp/ (kept, kept)
ketoacidosis /ˈkiː.təʊˌæ.ɪˈdəʊ.sɪs/
ketone /ˈkiː.təʊn/
kidney /ˈkɪd.ni/ stones /stəʊnz/
kidney /ˈkɪd.ni/
knee /niː/ -chest /tʃest/
position /pəˈzɪʃ.ən/
kneecap /ˈniː.kæp/
knife /naɪf/
knock /nɒk/

L

label /ˈleɪ.bəl/
labour /ˈleɪ.bər/
laboured /ˈleɪ.bəd/
lacerate /ˈlæs.ər.eɪt/
laceration /ˌlæsəˈreɪʃən/
lack /læk/
lacrimation /ˌlæk.riˈmeɪ.ʃən/

lactate /læk'teɪt/
lactic /'læk.tɪk/ acid /'æs.ɪd/
ladder /'læd.ər/
land /lænd/
landing /'lændɪŋ/ zone /zəʊn/
lapse /læps/
large /lɑːdʒ/ bore /bɔː/, large-bore
laryngeal /ləˈrɪn.dʒi.əl/
laryngectomy /ˌlær.ɪnˈdʒek.təm.i/
laryngoscope /ˌlærɪŋˈɡɒ.skəʊp/
laryngoscopy /ˌlærɪŋˈɡɒ.skə.pi/
laryngospasm /læˈrɪŋ.ɡə.spæz.əm/
larynx /'lær.ɪŋks/ (pl. larynges)
last /lɑːst/
lasting /'lɑːstɪŋ/
late /leɪt/
lateral /'læt.rəl/
law /lɔː/ -enforcement /ɪnˈfɔːs.mənt/ agency /'eɪ.dʒən.si/
law /lɔː/ enforcement /ɪnˈfɔːs.mənt/
law /lɔː/
lawn mower /'lɔːnˌməʊ.ər/
layer /'leɪ.ə/
lead /led/
lead /liːd/
lead /liːd/
leading /'liː.dɪŋ/
leaf /liːf/ pl leaves
leak /liːk/
leakage /'liː.kɪdʒ/
leaking /'liːk.ɪŋ/
lean /liːn/ forward /'fɔː.wəd/
leather /'leð.ər/
LeFort II fracture /'fræk.tʃə/
legal /'liːɡəl/
lengthy /'leŋ.θi/
lens /lenz/
lesion /'liː.ʒən/
lessen /'les.ən/
lethal /'liː.θəl/
lethargic /ləˈθɑː.dʒɪk/
lethargy /'leθ.ə.dʒi/
leukocyte /'ljuː.kə.saɪt/
levothyroxine /lev.ɒ.θaɪˈrɒk.sɪn/
liability /ˌlaɪ.əˈbɪl.ɪ.ti/

liable /'laɪ.ə.bl̩/
libel /'laɪ.bəl/
licensure /'laɪ.sənˌʃər/
lie /laɪ/
life support /'laɪf.səˌpɔːt/
life-saving /'laɪfˌseɪ.vɪŋ/
life-threatening /'laɪfˌθret.ən.ɪŋ/
lifeguard /'laɪf.ɡɑːd/
lift /lɪft/
lifting /lɪft.ɪŋ/
ligament /'lɪɡ.ə.mənt/
ligamentum /ˌlɪɡ.əˈmen.təm/
arteriosum /ɑːˌtɪə.riˈɒs.əm/
light /laɪt/
light-headed /ˌlaɪtˈhed.ɪd/
lightheadedness /ˌlaɪtˈhed.ɪd.nəs/
lightning /'laɪt.nɪŋ/
like /laɪk/
likelihood /'laɪ.kli.hʊd/
likely /'laɪklɪ/
limb /lɪm/
lime /laɪm/
limit /'lɪm.ɪt/
limited /'lɪm.ɪ.tɪd/
limp /lɪmp/
line /laɪn/-drive /draɪv/
line /laɪn/
lingual /'lɪŋɡwəl/
lip /lɪp/
liquefaction /ˌlɪkwɪˈfækʃən/
list /lɪst/
listening /'lɪs.ən.ɪŋ/
liver /'lɪv.ər/
lividity /lɪˈvɪd.ə.ti/
living /'lɪvɪŋ/ will /wɪl/
load /ləʊd/
lobe /ləʊb/
LOC, Level /'levəl/ of
consciousness /'kɒn.ʃəs.nɪs/
LOC, Loss /lɒs/ of
consciousness /'kɒn.ʃəs.nɪs/
localize /'ləʊ.kəl.aɪz/
localized /'ləʊ.kəl.aɪzd/
locate /ləʊˈkeɪt/
log /lɒɡ/ -roll /rəʊl/, logroll

log /lɒg/
logistics /lə'dʒɪs.tɪks/
lone /ləʊn/
look /lʊk/
looking /lʊk.ɪŋ/
loop /luːp/
loose /luːs/
loose /luːs/ weight /weɪt/
loss /lɒs/
lotion /'ləʊ.ʃən/
loudly /'laʊd.li/
low /ləʊ/
low-pitched /ˌləʊ'pɪtʃt/
lower /'ləʊ.ə/ airways /'eə.weɪz/
LPM, Liter /'liːtə/ Per /
pə/ Minute /'mɪnɪt/
lumbar /'lʌm.bər/
lumen /'luː.mən/ pl -mina
lung /lʌŋ/

M

magnesium /mæg'niː.zi.əm/
magnesium /mæg'niː.zi.əm/
sulphate /'sʌl.feɪt/
main /meɪn/
mainstem /meɪn.stəm/
bronchus /'brɒŋ.kəs/
maintain /meɪn'teɪn/
maintenance /'meɪntɪnəns/
major /'meɪ.dʒə/
majority /mə'dʒɒr.ə.ti/
malaise /mæl'eɪz/
malfeasance /mæl'fiː.zəns/
Mallory-Weis /'mæl.ər.i-vaɪs/
syndrome /'sɪn.drəʊm/
malocclusion /mæl.ə'kluː.ʒən/
mammalian /mə'meɪ.li.ən/
manage /'mæn.ɪdʒ/
management /'mænɪdʒmənt/
mandate /'mæn.deɪt/
manhole /'mæn.həʊl/
manic /'mæn.ɪk/
manifest /'mæn.ɪ.fest/
manipulation /mə.nɪp.jʊ'leɪ.ʃən/
manner /'mæn.ər/

manoeuvre /mə'nuː.və/
manual /'mæn.ju.əl/
margin /'mɑː.dʒɪn/
mark /mɑːk/
marked /mɑːkt/
markedly /'mɑː.kɪd.li/
maroon /mə'ruːn/
mask /mɑːsk/
mass /mæs/
massage /'mæs.ɑː.ʒ/ masáž, masírovat
MAST, Military Anti-
Shock Trousers
mastoid /'mæs.tɔɪd/
maternal /mə'tɜː.nəl/
matter /'mæt.ər/
mature /mə'tjʊər/
maxillary /mæk'sɪl.ər.i/
maximal /'mæk.sɪ.məl/
mean /miːn/
means /miːnz/
measure /'meʒ.ər/
measurement /'meʒ.ə.mənt/
mechanic /mɪ'kænɪk/
mechanics /mə'kæn.ɪks/
meconium /mɪ'kəʊ.nɪ.əm/
medial /'miː.di.əl/
mediastinal /ˌmiː.di.əs'taɪ.nəl/
medical /'med.ɪ.kəl/
medication /ˌmed.ɪ'keɪ.ʃən/
medium /miː.di.əm/ -sized /saɪzd/
medium /miː.di.əm/
melaena /mə'liː.n.ə/
membrane /'mem.breɪn/
meningitis /ˌmen.ɪn'dʒaɪ.tɪs/
mental /'men.təl/
mental /'men.təl/ status /'steɪtəs/
mentally /'men.təl.i/
mentation /men'teɪ.ʃən/
mercury /'mɜː.kjʊ.ri/
messy /'mes.i/
metabolize /mɪ'tæbə.laɪz/
metallic /mə'tæl.ɪk/
metastatic /ˌmet.ə'stæt.ɪk/
methamphetamine /
ˌmeθ.æm'fet.ə.miːn/

method /'meθ.əd/

meticulous /mə'tɪk.jʊ.ləs/

METTAG, Medical /'med.ɪ.kəl/
Emergency /ɪ'mɜ:.dʒənt .si/
Triage /'traɪ.ɪdʒ/ Tag /tæg/

MI, Myocardial /maɪ.ə‚kɑ:.
di.əl/ Infarction /ɪn'fɑ:k‚ʃən/

mid /mɪd/

midaxillary /mɪd.æk'sɪl.ər.i/

midclavicular /mɪd.klə'vɪk.jʊ.lər/

middle /'mɪd.l̩/ age /eɪdʒ/

middle /'mɪd.l̩/

midline /'mɪd.laɪn/

migrate /maɪ'greɪt/

mild /maɪld/

military /'mɪl.ɪ.tər.i/

mimic /'mɪm.ɪk/

mind /maɪnd/

minimise / 'mɪn.ɪ.maɪz/

minor / 'maɪ.nə/

miosis /maɪ'əʊ.sɪs/

miscarriage /'mɪs‚kær.ɪdʒ/

misinterpret /‚mɪs.ɪn'tɜ:.prɪt/

misleading /‚mɪs'li:.dɪŋ/

misperception /‚mɪs.pə'sep.ʃən/

mist /mɪst/

mistaken /mɪ'steɪ.kən/

misunderstanding /‚mɪs.
ʌn.də'stæn.dɪŋ/

mitral valve /'maɪ.trəl‚vælv/

mittelschmerz /mɪtl‚ʃmərθ/

mnemonic /nɪ'mɒn.ɪk/

MO, Medical /'med.ɪ.kəl/
Officer /'ɒf.ɪ.sər/

modality /məʊ'dæl.ə.ti/

mode /məʊd/

moderate /'mɒd.ər.ət/

moderately /'mɒd.ər.ət.li/

modify /'mɒdɪ‚faɪ/

modulation /‚mɒd.jʊ'leɪ.ʃən/

moist /mɔɪst/

moisten /'mɔɪsən/

molecule /'mɒl.ɪ.kju:l/

mood /mu:d/ disorder /dɪ'sɔ:..dər/

mood /mu:d/

mood /mu:d/ swing /swɪŋ/

moral /'mɒrəl/

morbidly /‚mɔ:'bɪd.ɪ.ti/

morgue /mɔ:g/

morphine /'mɔ:..fi:n/

morphine /'mɔ:..fi:n/

sulphate /'sʌl.feɪt/

mortality /mɔ:'tæl.ə.ti/

motion /'məʊʃən/

motionless /'məʊ.ʃən.ləs/

motor /'məʊ.tər/

mottled /'mɒt.l̩d/

mouth /maʊθ/

move /mu:v/

movement /'mu:v.mənt/

moving /'mu:vɪŋ/

MPH, Miles /maɪlz/ Per /
pə/ Hour /aʊə/

mucosa /mju:'kəʊ.sə/

mucous membrane /
‚mju:.kəs'mem.breɪn/

mucus /'mju:..kəs/

muffle /'mʌf.l̩/

mulch /mʌltʃ/

multi /mʌl.ti-/

multifocal /mʌl.ti'fəʊ.kəl/

multigravida /mʌl.ti'græv.ɪ.də/

multipara /mʌl.ti'pær.ə/

multiparity /mʌl.ti'pær.ɪt.ɪ/

multiple /'mʌl.tɪ.pl̩/

multiplex /'mʌl.tɪ.pleks/

multiplexing /'mʌlti‚pleksɪŋ/

multiply /'mʌltɪplaɪ/

multisystem /'mʌl.tɪ'sɪs.təm/

murmur /'mɜ:..mər/

Murphy's /'mɜ:.fiz/ sign /saɪn/

muscle /'mʌsəl/

muscle /'mʌsəl/ tone /təʊn/

muscular /'mʌs.kjʊ.lər/

mustard /'mʌs.təd/

MVC, Motor /'məʊtə/ Vehicle /
'vi:.ɪ.kl̩/ Collision /kə'lɪʒ.ən/

mydriasis /maɪ'draɪ.ə.sɪs/

myocardial /maɪ.ə‚kɑ:..di.əl/

myocardium /‚maɪ.ə'kɑ:.di.əm/

N

NaCl, sodium /ˈsəʊ.di.əm/
chloride /ˈklɔːraɪd/
nail /neɪl/ **bed** /bed/
nail /neɪl/ **polish** /ˈpɒl.ɪʃ/
Naloxone /nəˈlɒksəʊn/
narcotic /nɑːˈkɒt.ɪk/
narrative /ˈnærətɪv/
narrow /ˈnær.əʊ/
nasal /ˈneɪ.zəl/ **flaring** / fleər.ɪŋ/
nasal /ˈneɪ.zəl/
nasopharyngeal /ˌneɪ.zə.fəˈrɪn.dʒi.əl/
nasopharynx /ˌneɪ.zəˈfær.ɪŋks/
nasotracheal /ˌneɪ.zə.trəˈkiː.əl/
nature /ˈneɪ.tʃər/
nausea /ˈnɔː.zi.ə/
near /nɪər/
nebulized /ˈneb.jə.laɪzd/
nebulizer /ˈneb.jə.laɪz.ər/
necessitate /nəˈses.ɪ.teɪt/
necrosis /neˈkrəʊsɪs/
need /niːd/
needle /ˈniː.dl̩/
needle /ˈniː.dl̩/ **stick** /stɪk/
negative /ˈneg.ə.tɪv/
neglect /nɪˈglekt/
negligence /ˈneglɪdʒəns/
negligent /ˈneg.lɪ.dʒənt/
neonate /ˈniː.əʊˈneɪ.t/
neoplasm /ˈniː.əʊˈplæz.əm/
nerve /nɜːv/
nest /nest/
neural /ˈnjʊə.rəl/
neurogenic /ˌnjʊə.rəˈdʒen.ɪk/
neurological /ˌnjʊə.rəˈlɒdʒ.ɪ.kəl/
neuropathy /ˌnjʊəˈrɒp.ə.θi/
neurosis /njʊəˈrəʊ.sɪs/
neurotoxicity /ˌnjʊər.ə.tɒkˈsɪs.ɪ.ti/
neutral /ˈnjuː.trəl/
newborn /ˈnjuː.bɔːn/
nightmare /ˈnaɪt.meər/
niple /ˈnɪp.l̩/
nitrogen /ˈnaɪ.trə.dʒən/
nitroglycerin /ˌnaɪ.trəʊˈglɪs.ər.iːn/
Nitronox /ˌnaɪ.trə.nɒks/

nitrous oxide /ˌnaɪ.trəsˈɒk.saɪd/
no matter /ˈmætə/
nocturnal /nɒkˈtɜː.nəl/
noise /nɔɪz/
non-judgemental /ˌnɒn.dʒʌdʒˈmen.təl/
non-productive /ˌnɒn.prəˈdʌk.tɪv/
nonadherent /ˌnɒn.ədˈhɪə.rənt/
noncompliance /ˌnɒn.kəmˈplaɪəns/
nondeliverable /ˌnɒn.dɪˈlɪv.ər.ə.bl̩/
nondiscernible /ˌnɒn.dɪˈsɜː.nɪ.bl̩/
nonintact /ˌnɒn.ɪnˈtækt/
nonketotic /ˌnɒn.ke.tɒt.ɪk/
nonperfusing /ˌnɒn.pər.fjuː.z.ɪŋ/
nonrebreather /ˌnɒn.rəbrə.
ðər/ **mask** / mɑːsk/
nonsalvageable /ˌnɒn ˈsæl.vɪdʒə.bl̩/
norepinephrine /nɔrˌep.əˈnef.rɪn/
normal /ˈnɔː.məl/
note /nəʊt/
notice /ˈnəʊtɪs/
noticeable /ˈnəʊ.tɪ.sə.bl̩/
noticeably /ˈnəʊ.tɪ.sə.bli/
notify /ˈnəʊtɪˌfaɪ/
nucha /njuːkə/
nuchal /nuːkəl/
nullipara /nʌˈlɪp.ər.ə/
numbness /ˈnʌm.nəs/
numerous /ˈnjuː.mə.rəs/
nurse /nɜːs/
nursing /ˈnɜː.sɪŋ/
nutrient /ˈnjuː.tri.ənt/

O

obesity /əʊ ˈbiː.sɪ.ti/
object /ˈɒb.dʒɪkt/
obscenity /əbˈsen.ɪ.ti/
observable /əbˈzɜː.vəbəl/
observation /ˌɒb.zəˈveɪ.ʃən/
observe /əbˈzɜː.v/
obstetrics /ɒbˈstetrɪks/
obstruct /əbˈstrʌkt/
obstruction /əbˈstrʌk.ʃən/
obstructive /əbˈstrʌk.tɪv/
obtain /əbˈteɪn/
obtrude /əbˈtruːd/

obvious /ˈɒb.vi.əs/

occasion /əˈkeɪ.ʒən/

occasional / əˈkeɪʒənəl/

occasionally /əˈkeɪ.ʒən/

occipital /ɒkˈsɪp.ɪ.təl/

occlusion /əˈkluː.ʒən/

occlusive /ɒˈkluː.sɪv/

dressing /ˈdres.ɪŋ/

occlusive /ɒˈkluː.sɪv/

occupational /ˌɒk.juˈpeɪ.ʃən.əl/

occur /əˈkɜːr/

occurrence /əˈkʌr.ənt s/

odour /ˈəʊ.dər/

oedema /ɪˈdiː.mə/

oedematous /ɪˈdiː.mə.təs/

oesophageal /iːˌsɒfəˈdʒiːəl/

oesophagus /ɪˈsɒf.ə.gəs/

officer /ˈɒf.ɪ.sər/

official /əˈfɪʃəl/

ominous /ˈɒmɪnəs/

oncoming /ˈɒnˌkʌmɪŋ/

oncotic /ɒŋ.kɒ.tɪk/ **pressure** /ˈpreʃ.ər/

ongoing /ˈɒŋˌgəʊ.ɪŋ/

onion /ˈʌn.jən/

online /ˈɒn.laɪn/

onlooker /ˈɒnˌlʊk.ər/

onset /ˈɒnˌset/

OPA, Oropharyngeal /ˈɔː.rə .fəˈrɪn.dʒi.əl/ **Airway** /ˈeə.weɪ/

opening / ˈəʊ.pən.ɪŋ/

operation /ˌɒp.ərˈeɪ.ʃən/

ophthalmologist /ˌɒf.θælˈmɒl.ə.dʒɪst/

opiate /ˈəʊ.pi.ət/

opinion /əˈpɪn.jən/

opponent /əˈpəʊ.nənt/

opportunistic /ˌɒp.ə.tjuːˈnɪs.tɪk/

opposite /ˈɒp.ə.zɪt/

OPQRST, Onset, Provocation, Quality, Radiation, Severity, Time

opt /ɒpt/

option /ˈɒpʃən/

orally /ˈɔː.rə.li/

order /ˈɔː.dər/

order /ˈɔːdə/

ordered /ˈɔː.dəd/

organophosphates / ɔːˌgæn.əʊˈfɒs.feɪts/

oriented /ˈɔːriəntɪd/

original /əˈrɪdʒ.ɪ.nəl/

originate /əˈrɪdʒ.ɪ.neɪt/

oropharyngeal /ˈɔː.rə .fəˈrɪn.dʒi.əl/

oropharynx /ˈɔː.rə ˈfær.ɪŋks/

orthostatic /ˌɔː.θəˈstæt.ɪk/

os /ɒs/ *pl.* ossa

osmolarity /ɒz.məˈlær.ə.ti/

osmosis /ɒzˈməʊ.sɪs/

osmotic /ɒzˈmɒt.ɪk/ **pressure** /ˈpreʃ.ər/

osteomyelitis /ɒs.ti.əʊ.maɪ.əlˈaɪ.tɪs/

osteoporosis /ɒs.ti.əʊ.pəˈrəʊ.sɪs/

otherwise /ˈʌð.ə.waɪz/

outcome /ˈaʊtˌkʌm/

outermost /ˈaʊ.tə.məʊst/

outpatient /ˈaʊt.peɪ.ʃənt/

outpouching /ˈaʊt.paʊtʃ.ɪŋ/

output /ˈaʊtˌpʊt/

outset /ˈaʊt.set/

outside /ˌaʊtˈsaɪd/

outstretched /ˌaʊtˈstretʃt/

outward /ˈaʊt.wəd/

ovarian /əʊˈveə.ri.ən/

ovary /ˈəʊ.vər.i/

overactive /ˈəʊ.vərˈæk.tɪv/

overall /ˌəʊ.vəˈrɔːl/

overcooling /ˌəʊ.vəˈkuː.lɪŋ/

overdose /ˈəʊ.və.dəʊs/

overhear /ˌəʊvəˈhɪə/

overhydration /ˌəʊvə.haɪˈdreɪ.ʃən/

overinflation /ˌəʊvə.ɪnˈfleɪʃ.ən/

overload /ˌəʊ.vəˈləʊd/

overly /ˈəʊ.vəl.i/

overpressure /ˌəʊ.vəˈpreʃ.ər/

overuse /ˌəʊ.vəˈjuːz/

overweight /ˌəʊ.vəˈweɪt/

overwhelm /ˌəʊ.vəˈwelm/

ovum /ˈəʊ.vəm/ pl ova

oxygen /ˈɒk.sɪ.dʒən/

oxygenate /ˈɒk.sɪ.dʒə.neɪt/

oxygenation /ˈɒk.sɪ.dʒə.neɪ.ʃən/

oxytocin /ˌɒk.sɪˈtəʊ.sɪn/

P

pace /peɪs/
pack /pæk/
packing /'pæk.ɪŋ/
PaCO₂, partial /'paːʃəl/ pressure
/'preʃ.ər/ of carbon /'kaː.bən/
dioxide /daɪ'ɒk.saɪd/ in arterial /
aː'tɪərɪəl/ blood /blʌd/
padded /'pæd.ɪd/
padding /'pæd.ɪŋ/
paediatric /ˌpiː.di'æt.rɪk/
paediatrics /ˌpiː.diː'æt.rɪks/
pain /peɪn/
painful /'peɪn.fəl/
painless /'peɪn.ləs/
pale /peɪl/
palliative /'pæl.i.ə.tɪv/
pallor /'pæl.ər/
palm /paːm/
palpable /'pæl.pə.bl̩/
palpate /'pæl.peɪt/
palpation /pæl'peɪ.ʃən/
palpitations /ˌpæl.pɪ'teɪ.ʃənz/
palsy /'pɔːl.zi/
pancreas /'pæŋ.kri.əs/
pancreatic /ˌpæŋ.krɪ'æ.tɪk/
pancreatitis /ˌpæŋ.kri.ə'taɪ.tɪs/
pant /pænt/
paradoxical /ˌpær.ə'dɒk.sɪ.kəl/
paradoxically /ˌpær.ə'dɒk.sɪ.kəl.i/
paradoxus /'pær.ə.dɒk.səs/
paralyse /'pær.əl.aɪz/
paralysis /pə'ræl.ə.sɪs/
paramedic /ˌpærə'medɪk/
paramount /'pær.ə.maʊnt/
parasympathetic /'pær.ə.sɪm.pə'θet.ɪk/
parental /pə'ren.təl/
parenteral /pə'ren.tə.rəl/
parietal /pə'raɪə.təl/
parity /'pærɪti/
paroxysm /'pær.ɒk.sɪ.zəm/
paroxysmal /ˌpær.ɒk.'sɪz.məl/
part /paːt/
partial /'paː.ʃəl/

partial /'paː.ʃəl/ pressure /'preʃ.ər/
partially /'paː.ʃəl.i/
particle /'paː.tɪ.kl̩/
particularly /pə'tɪk.jʊ.lə.li/
particulate /pə'tɪ.kjuː.lət/
PASG, Pneumatic /
njʊ'mætɪk/ Antishock /'æn.
tɪ.ʃɒk/ Garment /'gaːmənt/
pass /paːs/ out /aʊt/
pass /paːs/
passage /'pæsɪdʒ/
past /paːst/
pasty /'pæs.ti/
patency /'peɪ.tənt.si/
patent /'peɪ.tənt/
path /paːθ/
pathogen /'pæθ.ə.dʒən/
pathogenic /ˌpæθ.ə'dʒen.ɪk/
pathology /pə'θɒl.ə.dʒi/
pathophysiology /ˌpæθ.ə.fɪz.i'ɒl.ə.dʒi/
pathway /'paːθ.weɪ/
pattern /'pæt.ən/
PCP, phencyclidine /fen'sɪklɪˌdiːn/
PEA, Pulseless /pʌls.ləs/ Electrical
/ɪ'lek.trɪ.kəl/ Activity /æk'tɪv.ɪ.ti/
peak /piːk/ flow /fləʊ/ meter /m.ɪ.tər/
peak /piːk/ flow /fləʊ/
peak /piːk/
pearly /'pɜː.li/
pedal /'ped.əl/
pedestrian /pɪ'destrɪən/
peers /pɪərz/
pelvic /'pel.vɪk/ inflammatory /
ɪn'flæm.ə.tər.i/ disease /dɪ'ziː.z/
pelvis /'pel.vɪs/
pending /'pen.dɪŋ/
penetrate /'pen.ɪ.treɪt/
penetrating /'pen.ɪ.treɪ.tɪŋ/
percentage /pə'sen.tɪdʒ/
perception /pə'sep.ʃən/
percuss /pə'kʌs/
percussion /pə'kʌʃ.ən/
perfect /'pɜː.fekt/
perforate /'pɜː.fər.eɪ.t/
perforation /ˌpɜː.fər'eɪ.ʃən/

perform /pəˈfɔːm/
perfuse /pəˈfjuːz/
perfusion /pəˈfjuː.ʒən/
pericardial /ˌper.ɪˈkɑ:di.əl/
pericardium /ˌper.ɪˈkɑ:di.əm/
perineum /ˌper.ɪˈniː.əm/
period /ˈpɪə.ri.əd/
periorbital /ˌper.ɪ.ˈɔːbɪtəl/
peripheral /pəˈrɪf.ər.əl/
peritoneal /ˌper.ɪ.təˈni.əl/
peritonitis /ˌper.ɪ.təˈnaɪ.tɪs/
periumbilical /ˌper.ɪ.ʌmˈbɪl.ɪ.kəl/
permissible /pəˈmɪs.ə.bļ/
permission /pəˈmɪʃ.ən/
permit /pəˈmɪt/
persist /pəˈsɪst/
persistent /pəˈsɪs.tənt/
personnel /ˌpɜːsəˈnel/
persuade /pəˈsweɪd/
pertinent /ˈpɜːtɪnənt/
pertussis /pəˈtʌ.sɪs/
petechia /piˈtiː.ki.ə/ pl petechiae
petechial /piˈtiː.ki.əl/
petit mal /ˌpəˈtiˈmæl/
pH /ˌpiːˈeɪtʃ/
phase /feɪz/
phenomenon /fəˈnɒm.ɪ.nən/
pl phenomena
phlegm /flem/
phobia /ˈfəʊ.bi.ə/
physical /ˈfɪz.ɪ.kəl/
physician /fɪˈzɪʃ.ən/
physiological /ˌfɪz.i.ˈɒl.ə.dʒi.kəl/
pickup /pɪkʌp/
Pickwickian /pɪkˈwɪk.i.ən/
syndrome /ˈsɪndrəʊm/
PID, Pelvic /ˈpel.vɪk/ Inflammatory
/ɪnˈflæm.ə.tər.i/ Disease /dɪˈziːz/
pierce /pɪəs/
pigmentation /ˌpɪg.mənˈteɪ.ʃən/
pile /paɪl/
pill /pɪl/
pill-rolling /ˈpɪl.rəʊ.
lɪŋ/ tremor /ˈtrem.ər/
pin /pɪn/

pin-point, pinpoint /ˈpɪn.pɔɪnt/
pinch /pɪntʃ/
pinna /pin.ə/
pipe /paɪp/
pit /pɪt/ viper /ˈvaɪ.pər/
pitch /pɪtʃ/
pitting /pɪt.ɪŋ/ oedema /ɪˈdiː.mə/
pituitary gland /pɪˈtjuː.ɪ.tər.iˌglænd/
place /pleɪs/
placement /ˈpleɪs.mənt/
placenta /pləˈsen.tə/ praevia /priː.vi.ə/
plain /pleɪn/
plant /plɑːnt/
plaque /plɑːk/, /plæk/
plasma /ˈplæz.mə/
platelet /ˈpleɪt.lət/
pledge /pledʒ/
pleura /ˈplʊə.rə/
pleural /ˈplʊə.rəl/
pleuric /ˈplʊə.rɪk/ disease /dɪˌziːz/
plug /plʌg/
PND, Paroxysmal /ˌpær.
ɒk.ˈsɪz.məl/ Nocturnal /nɒkˈtɜː.
nəl/ Dyspnea /dɪs.pniː.ə/
pneumatic /njʊˈmætɪk/
pneumonia /njuːˈməʊ.ni.ə/
pneumothorax /ˌnjuːməʊˈθɔːræks/
poikilothermy /ˌpɔɪ.kɪl.əˈθɜːm.i/
point /pɔɪnt/
point /pɔɪnt/ to /tə/
poison /ˈpɔɪ.zən/
poisoning /ˈpɔɪ.zən.ɪŋ/
pole /pəʊl/
polite /pəˈlaɪt/
polycythaemia /ˌpɒl.ɪ.saɪˈθiːm.ɪ.ə/
polydipsia /ˌpɒl.ɪˈdɪp.sɪ.ə/
polyphagia /ˌpɒl.ɪˈfeɪ.dʒə/
polyuria /ˌpɒl.ɪˈjʊə.rɪ.ə/
pool /puːl/
pool /puːl/ hall /hɔːl/
pool /puːl/ stick /stɪk/, pool cue /kjuː/
pooling /puːl.ɪŋ/
poorly /ˈpɔː.li/
pop /pɒp/
popliteal /ˌpɒp.lɪˈtiː.əl/

portion /ˈpɔː.ʃən/
position /pəˈzɪʃ.ən/
positive /ˈpɒz.ə.tɪv/
possession /pəˈzeʃ.ən/
posterior /pɒsˈtɪə.ri.ər/
postictal /ˈpəʊstˈɪkt.əl/
postpartum /ˌpəʊstˈpɑː.təm/
posttraumatic /ˌpəʊst.trɔːˌmæt.ɪk/
postural /ˈpɒst.ʃər.əl/
posture /ˈpɒs.tʃər/
potassium /pəˈtæs.i.əm/
potent /ˈpəʊ.tənt/
potential /pəˈten.ʃəl/
power /ˈpaʊə/ line /laɪn/
power /ˈpaʊə/
power /paʊər/ company /ˈkʌm.pə.ni/
power /paʊər/ of attorney /əˈtɜː.ni/
practice /ˈpræk.tɪs/
pre-existing /ˌpriː.ɪgˈzɪs.tɪŋ/
prearrival /ˌpriː.əˈraɪ.vəl/
precaution /prɪˈkɔː.ʃən/
precede /prɪˈsiːd/
precipitous /prɪˈsɪp.ɪ.təs/
predispose /ˌpriː.dɪˈspəʊz/
preeclampsia /ˌpri.ɪˈklæmp.si.ə/
pregnancy /ˈpreg.nən.si/
pregnant /ˈpregnənt/
prehospital /ˌpriːˈhɒs.pɪ.təl/
preliminary /prɪˈlɪm.ɪ.nər.i/
preload /ˌpriːˈləʊd/
premature /ˈprem.ə.tʃər/
prerespiratory /ˌpriːˈres.pər.əˌtɔr.i/
prescribe /prɪˈskraɪb/
presence /ˈprez.ənt s/
present /ˈprez.ənt/
presentation /ˌprez.ənˈteɪ.ʃən/
presenting /prɪˈzent.ɪŋ/ part /pɑːt/
preserve /prɪˈzɜːv/
press /pres/
pressure /ˈpreʃ.ə/ dressing /ˈdres.ɪŋ/
pressure /ˈpreʃ.ə/
pressurized /ˈpreʃ.ər.aɪzd/
presume /prɪˈzjuːm/
pretend /prɪˈtend/
preventable /prɪˈven.tə.bl̩/

previous /ˈpriː.vi.əs/
primarily /praɪˈmer.ɪ.li/
primary /ˈpraɪ.mə.ri/
prior /ˈpraɪə/ to /tʊ/
priority /praɪˈɒr.ɪ.ti/
privacy /ˈpraɪvəsɪ/
procedure /prəˈsiː.dʒə/
proceed /prəˈsiːd/
produce /prəˈdjuːs/
product /ˈprɒd.ʌkt/
production /prəˈdʌk.ʃən/
productive /prəˈdʌk.tɪv/
profound /prəˈfaʊnd/
profoundly /prəˈfaʊnd.li/
profusely /prəˈfjuːs.li/
profusion /prəˈfjuːˌʒən/
prognostic /prɒgˈnɒs.tɪk/
progress /ˈprəʊ.gres/
progressively /prəˈgres.ɪv.li/
projected /prəˈdʒek.tɪd/
projectile /prəˈdʒek.taɪl/
prolapsed /prəʊˈlæpst/
prolonged /prəˈlɒŋd/
promote /prəˈməʊt/
prompt /prɒmp t/
promptly /ˈprɒmptlɪ/
pronation /prəʊˈneɪ.ʃən/
prone /prəʊn/ to /tə/
prone /prəʊn/
pronounced /prəˈnaʊnst/
propelled /prəˈpeld/
proper /ˈprɒpə/
properly /ˈprɒp.əl.i/
property /ˈprɒp.ə.ti/
proportionally /prəˈpɔːˌʃən.əli/
protection /prəˈtekʃən/
protective /prəˈtek.tɪv/
protein /ˈprəʊ.tiːn/ a
proteinuria /ˈprəʊ.tiːn.jʊəˈriː.ə/
protrude /prəˈtruːd/
protrusion /prəˈtruːˌʒən/
prove /pruːv/
proven /ˈpruː.vən/
provide /prəˈvaɪd/
provided /prəˈvaɪ.dɪd/

provider /prə'vaɪ.dər/
provocation /ˌprɒvə'keɪʃən/
provoke /prə'vəʊk/
proximal /'prɒk.sɪ.məl/
proximate /'prɒk.sɪ.mət/
proxy /'prɒk.sɪ/
prudent /'pruː.dənt/
pruritus /prʊə'raɪ.təs/
pseudoseizure /'sjuː.dəʊ.'siː.ʒər/
psychiatric /ˌsaɪ.ki'æt.rɪk/
psychogenic /ˌsaɪ.kəʊ'dʒɛ.nɪk/
psychosis /saɪ'kəʊ.sɪs/
puffy /'pʌf.i/
pull /pʊl/
pulmonary /'pʊl.mə.nə.ri/
congestion /kən'dʒes.tʃən/
pulmonary /'pʊl.mə.nə.ri/
pulsate /pʌl'seɪ.t/
pulzovat, tepat, bušit
pulsatile /'pʌlsəˌtaɪl/ mass /mæs/
pulsation /pʌl'seɪ.ʃən/
pulse /pʌls/ oximeter /'ɒk.sɪ.m.ɪ.tər/
pulse /pʌls/ oximetry /'ɒk.sɪ.m.ə.tri/
pulse /pʌls/
pulseless /pʌls.ləs/
pulselessness /pʌls.ləs.nəs/
pulsus /pʌls.əs/ paradoxus /
'pær.ə.dɒks.əs/
pump /pʌmp/
puncture / 'pʌŋk.tʃə/
pupil /'pjuː.pəl/
pupillary /pjuː.pɪl.ər.i/
pure /pjʊər/
purplish /'pɜː.pl̩.ɪʃ/
purpose /'pɜː.pəs/
purse /pɜːs/
pursed /pɜːsd/-lip /lɪp/
push /pʊʃ/
put /pʊt/ pressure /'preʃ.ər/
PVCs, Premature /'premə.tjʊə/
Ventricular /ven'trɪk.jə.lər/
Contractions /kən'trækʃəns/

Q
quadrant /'kwɒd.rənt/

quality /kwɒlɪtɪ/
quantity /'kwɒn.tɪ.ti/
questionable /'kwes.tʃə.nə.bl̩/

R
rabies /'reɪ.biːz/
raccoon /rə'kuːn/ eyes /aɪz/
radial /'reɪ.di.əl/
radiate /'reɪ.di.eɪt/
radiation /ˌreɪ.di'eɪ.ʃən/
sickness /'sɪk.nəs/
radiation /ˌreɪ.di'eɪ.ʃən/
radius /'reɪ.di.əs/
railing /'reɪ.lɪŋ/
railroad /'reɪl.rəʊd/
raise /reɪz/
rake /reɪk/
rale /raːl/
rambling /'ræm.blɪŋ/
range /reɪndʒ/
rape /reɪp/
rapid /'ræp.ɪd/
rapport /ræ'pɔːr/
rarely /'reə.li/
rash /ræʃ/
rate /reɪt/
ratio /'reɪ.ʃi.əʊ/
rattle /'ræt.l̩/
reach /riːtʃ/
reactive /ri'æk.tɪv/
reading /'riː.dɪŋ/
rear-end /'rɪə.rend/
reasonable /'riː.zən.ə.bl̩/
reassess /ˌriː.ə'ses/
reassessment /ˌriː.ə'ses.mənt/
reassure /ˌriː.ə'ʃɔːr/
rebound /ˌriː'baʊnd/
rebound /ˌriː'baʊnd/
tenderness /'ten.dər.nəs/
receive /rɪ'siː.v/
recent /'riː.sənt/
recheck /riː.tʃek/
recirculate /riː'sɜː.kjʊ.leɪt/
recliner /rɪ'klaɪ.nər/
recognition /ˌrek.əg'nɪʃ.ən/

recognize /'rekəg͵naɪz/
recoil /rɪ'kɔɪl/
recommended /͵rekə'mendɪd/
recompression /͵riː.kəm'preʃ.
ən/ chamber /'tʃeɪm.bər/
record /'rekɔːd/
recording /rɪ'kɔː.dɪŋ/
recover /rɪ'kʌv.ər/
recumbent /rɪ'kʌm.bənt/
recurrence /rɪ'kʌr.əns/
red /red/ blood /blʌd/ cell /sel/
redden /'red.ən/
reduce /rɪ'djuːs/
reevaluate /͵riː.ɪ'væljueɪt/
reexperience /͵riː.ɪk'spɪə.ri.əns/
refer /rɪ'fɜːr/
reference /'ref.ər.ənt s/
referral /rɪ'fɜː.rəl/
referred /rɪ'fɜːd/ pain /peɪn/
refill /'riː.fɪl/
reflect /rɪ'flekt/
reflux /'riː͵flʌks/
refreeze /͵riː.'friː.z/
refusal /rɪ'fjuːzəl/
refuse /rɪ'fjuːz/
regain /rɪ'geɪn/
regarding /rɪ'gɑː.dɪŋ/
regardless /rɪ'gɑːd.ləs/
regimen /'redʒ.ɪ.mən/
region /'riː.dʒən/
regional /'riː.dʒən.əl/
regular /'reg.jʊ.lər/
regularity /͵reg.jʊ'lær.ə.ti/
regulate /'regjʊ͵leɪt/
regulation /͵reg.jʊ'leɪ.ʃən/
reinflate /͵riː.ɪn'fleɪt/
reinsert /͵riː.ɪn'sɜːt/
relate /rɪ'leɪt/
relation /rɪ'leɪ͵ʃən/
relationship /rɪ'leɪ͵ʃən͵ʃɪp/
relaxation /͵riː.læk'seɪ͵ʃən/
relaxed /rɪ'lækst/
relay /'riː͵leɪ/
release /rɪ'liːs/
relief /rɪ'liːf/

relieve /rɪ'liːv/
rely /rɪ'laɪ/ upon /ə͵pɒn/
remain /rɪ'meɪn/
remove /rɪ'muːv/
renal /'riː.nəl/ calculi /'kæl.kjʊ.laɪ/
renal /'riː.nəl/
reorient /riː.'ɔː.ri.ənt/
repeatedly /rɪ'piː.tɪd.li/
replacement / rɪ'pleɪs.mənt/
report /rɪ'pɔːt/
reportable /rɪ'pɔːt'ebəl/
reposition /͵riː.pə'zɪʃən/
reproducible /͵riː.prə.djuːsɪ.bḷ/
require /rɪ'kwaɪər/
requirement /rɪ'kwaɪə.mənt/
Res ipsa loquitur
rescue /'reskjuː/
rescuer /'res.kjuː.ər/
reserve /rɪ'zɜːv/
reservoir /'rez.ə.vwɑːr/
residence /'rez.ɪ.dəns/
residual /rɪ'zɪd.ju.əl/
residue /'rez.ɪ.djuː/
resistance /rɪ'zɪs.tənt s/
resolve /rɪ'zɒlv/
resource /rɪ'zɔːs/
respiratory /rɪ'spɪr.ə.tər.i/
pattern /'pæt.ən/
respond /rɪ'spɒnd/
responder /rɪ'spɒnd.ər/
response /rɪ'spɒns/
responsibility /rɪ͵spɒn.sə'bɪ.lɪ.tɪ/
responsible /rɪ'spɒnt.sɪ.bḷ/
responsive /rɪ'spɒnt.sɪv/
responsiveness /rɪ'spɒn.sɪv.nəs/
rest /rest/
restate /͵riː'steɪt/
restless /'rest ͵ləs/
restlessness /'rest.ləs.nəs/
restore /rɪ'stɔːr/
restrain /rɪ'streɪn/
restraint /rɪ'streɪnt/
restricted /rɪ'strɪk.tɪd/
result /rɪ'zʌlt/
resume /rɪ'zjuːm/

resuscitate /rɪˈsʌs.ɪ.teɪt/
retain /rɪˈteɪn/
retinal /ˈret.ɪ.nəl/
retraction /rɪˈtræk.ʃən/
retroperitoneal /ˌret.rəʊˌper.ɪ.təʊ.ˈniː.əl/
reveal /rɪˈviːl/
reverse /rɪˈvɜːs/
revise /rɪˈvaɪz/
revision /rɪˈvɪʒ.ən/
revolve /rɪˈvɒlv/
rewarm /ˌriːˌwɔːm/
rhonchus /rongˈkəs/ pl. -chi
rib /rɪb/ cage /keɪdʒ/
rib /rɪb/
rider /ˈraɪ.dər/
rifle /ˈraɪ.fl̩/
right /raɪt/
rigid /ˈrɪdʒ.ɪd/
rigidity /rɪˈdʒɪd.ɪ.ti/
rigor mortis /ˌrɪg.əˈmɔː.tɪs/
ring /rɪŋ/
Ringer's lactate /lækˈteɪt/
ringing /rɪŋ.ɪŋ/
rip /rɪp/
rise /raɪz/
rock /rɒk/
roll /rəʊl/ over /ˈəʊ.vər/
roll /rəʊl/
roller /ˈrəʊ.lər/ bandage /ˈbæn.dɪdʒ/
rollover /ˈrəʊl.əʊ.vər/
rooftop /ˈruːf.tɒp/
room /ruːm/
roommate /ˈrʊm.meɪt/
rotate /rəʊˈteɪt/
rotation /rəʊˈteɪ.ʃən/
rotator /rəʊˈteɪt.ər/ cuff /kʌf/
rotator /rəʊˈteɪt.ər/
rotor /ˈrəʊtə/
rough /rʌf/
round /raʊnd/
route /ruːt/
routine /ruːˈtiːn/

RSV, Human /hjuːmən/ Respiratory /rɪˈspɪr.ə.tər.i/ Syncytial /sɪnˈsɪ.ʃi.əl/ Virus /ˈvaɪrəs/
rub /rʌb/
rubivirus /ruːbɪˈvaɪ.rəs/
rule /ruːl/ out /aʊt/
rule /ruːl/ of nines /naɪnz/
runny /ˈrʌn.i/
rupture /ˈrʌp.tʃər/
rush /rʌʃ/ in
rush /rʌʃ/

S
sac /sæk/
sacral /ˈseɪ.krəl/
safety /ˈseɪftɪ/
Salicylates /səˈlɪs.ɪˌleɪts/
saline /ˈseɪ.laɪn/
salivation /ˈsæl.ɪ.veɪ.ʃən/
salvageable /ˈsæl.vɪdʒə.bl̩/
sample /sɑːmpl/
SAMPLE, Signs and Symptoms, Allergies, Medications, Past medical history, Last oral intake
sarcoma /sɑːˈkəʊ.mə/
saturate /ˈsæt.jʊ.reɪt/
saturation /ˌsæt.jʊˈreɪ.ʃən/
saw /sɔː/
scale /skeɪl/
scalp /skælp/
scalpel /ˈskæl.pəl/
scapula /ˈskæp.jʊ.lə/ pl -ae
scar /skɑːr/
scenario /sɪˈnɑːˌri.əʊ/
schizophrenic /ˌskɪt.səˈfren.ɪk/
scissors /ˈsɪz.əz/
sclera /ˈsklɪə.rə/
scold /skəʊld/
scope /skəʊp/
score /skɔː/
scream /skriːm/
scuba diving /ˈskuːˌbəˌdaɪ.vɪŋ/
seal /siːl/
seal /siːl/
search /sɜːtʃ/ for /fɔː/

seat /ˈsiː.t/

seat /siːt/ belt /belt/

seated /ˈsiː.tɪd/

secondary /ˈsek.ən.dri/

secretion /sɪˈkriː.ʃən/

section /ˈsek.ʃən/

secure /sɪˈkjʊə/

security /sɪˈkjʊə.rɪ.ti/

sedation /sɪˈdeɪ.ʃən/

sedative /ˈsed.ə.tɪv/

seek /siːk/ (sought, sought)

segment /ˈseg.mənt/

seize /siːz/

seizure /ˈsiː.ʒə/ disorder /dɪˌsɔː.dər/

seizure /ˈsiː.ʒə/

seldom /ˈsel.dəm/

self-induced /ˌself.ɪnˈdjuːst/

semi /ˌsem.i/ -seated /ˈsiː.tɪd/

semiconscious /ˌsem.iˈkɒn.ʃəs/

sender /ˈsen.dər/

senile /ˈsiː.naɪl/

sensation /senˈseɪ.ʃən/

sense /sens/

sensory / ˈsent.sər.i/

sentence /ˈsen.təns/

separate /ˈsep.ər.ət/

separation /ˌsepəˈreɪʃən/

sepsis /ˈsep.sɪs/

septic /ˈsep.tɪk/

septum /ˈsep.təm/

serious /ˈsɪə.ri.əs/

seriously /ˈsɪə.ri.əs.li/

setting /ˈset.ɪŋ/

sever /ˈsev.ər/

severe /sɪˈvɪə/

severity /sɪˈver.ɪ.ti/

sexual /ˈsek.sjʊəl/

intercourse /ˈɪn.tə.kɔːs/

shaft /ʃɑːft/

shake /ʃeɪk/ (shook, shaken)

shaken /ˈʃeɪkən/ baby /ˈbeɪ. bi/ syndrome /ˈsɪn.drəʊm/

shallow /ˈʃæl.əʊ/

shaped /ʃeɪpt/

sharp /ʃɑːp/

shear /ˈʃɪə.r/

sheet /ʃiːt/

shellfish /ˈʃel.fɪʃ/

shelter /ˈʃel.tər/

shield /ʃiːld/

shift /ʃɪft/

shine /ʃaɪn/

shiver /ˈʃɪv.ər/

shock /ʃɒk/

shockable /ˈʃɒk.ə.bl̩/

shopping /ˈʃɒp.ɪŋ/ mall /mɔːl/

short /ʃɔːt/ of st

shorten /ˈʃɔː.tən/

shortness /ˈʃɔːt.nəs/

shortness /ˈʃɔːt.nəs/ of breath /breθ/

shoulder /ˈʃəʊl.dər/ blade /bleɪd/

shoulder /ˈʃəʊl.dər/

shouting /ˈʃaʊ.tɪŋ/

show /ˈʃəʊ/

showing /ˈʃəʊ.ɪŋ/

shuffle /ˈʃʌf.l̩/

shunt /ʃʌnt/

shut /ʃʌt/ off /ɒf/ v

sick-looking /sɪkˈlʊk.ɪŋ/

side /saɪd/ effect /ɪˈfekt/

side /saɪd/

sigh /saɪ/

sign /saɪn/

signal /ˈsɪg.nəl/

significance /sɪgˈnɪf.ɪ.kəns/

significant /sɪgˈnɪf.ɪ.kənt/

silence /ˈsaɪ.ləns/

silo /ˈsaɪ.ləʊ/

similar /ˈsɪm.ɪ.lər/

simple /ˈsɪm.pl̩/

simplex /ˈsɪm.pleks/

simultaneous /ˌsɪm.əlˈteɪ.ni.əs/

singe /sɪndʒ/

single /ˈsɪŋgəl/

sinus /ˈsaɪ.nəs/

siren /ˈsaɪərən/

site /saɪt/

size /saɪz/ up /ʌp/

size /saɪz/

skate /ˈskeɪ.t/

skeletal /'skel.ı.təl/
skid /skɪd/
skill /skɪl/
skull /skʌl/
slander /'slɑːndə/
slang /slæŋ/
slap /slæp/
slight /slaɪt/
slightly /'slaɪt.li/
slip /slɪp/
slipper /'slɪp.ər/
slippery /'slɪp.ər.i/
slope /sləʊp/
slowdown /'sləʊ.daʊn/
sludge /slʌdʒ/
SLUDGE, Salivation, Lacrimation, Urination, Diarrhoea, Gastrointestinal distress, Emesis
slump /slʌmp/
slur /slɜːr/
slurred /'slɜːd/
small /smɔːl/ bowel /'baʊ.əl/
smell /smel/
smooth /smuːð/
snake /sneɪk/
snap /snæp/
sneeze /sniːz/
sniffing /snɪf.ɪŋ/
snore /snɔːr/
soaked /səʊkt/
sob /sɒb/
soccer /'sɒk.ər/
sodium /'səʊ.di.əm/
chloride /'klɔːraɪd/
sodium /'səʊ.di.əm/
sodium bicarbonate /ˌsəʊ. di.əm.baɪˈkɑː.bən.ət/
soft /sɒft/
softly /'sɒft.li/
sole /səʊl/
solid /'sɒl.ɪd/
solution /səˈluː.ʃən/
solvent /'sɒl.vənt/
somatic /səˈmæt.ɪk/
somewhat /'sʌm.wɒt/

sore /sɔː/ throat /θrəʊt/
sore /sɔːr/
sorting /sɔːt.ɪŋ/
sound /saʊnd/
source /sɔːrs/
space /speɪs/
spasm /'spæz.əm/
spasmodic /spæzˈmɒd.ɪk/
specific /spəˈsɪf.ɪk/
specify /'spes.ɪ.faɪ/
speck /spek/
speech /spiːtʃ/
speed /spiːd/
speed up /'spiːd.ʌp/
spell /spel/
sphincter /'sfɪŋk.tər/
spider /'spaɪ.dər/
spiderweb /'spaɪ.dəz.web/
spill /spɪl/
spinal /'spaɪ.nəl/ cord /kɔːd/
spinal /'spaɪ.nəl/
spine /spaɪn/ board /bɔːd/
splash /splæʃ/
spleen /spliːn/
splenic /spliːn.ɪk/
splint /splɪnt/
sponge /spʌndʒ/
spontaneous /spɒnˈteɪ.ni.əs/
spot /spɒt/
spotting /spɒt.ɪŋ/
spousal /'spaʊzəl/
spouse /spaʊs/
sprain /spreɪn/
spray /spreɪ/
spurt /spɜːt/
sputum /'spjuː.təm/
squad /skwɒd/
squeeze /skwiːz/
stab /stæb/
stabilization /ˌsteɪ.bɪ.laɪˈzeɪ.ʃən/
stable /'steɪ.bl̩/
stage /steɪdʒ/
stagnate /stægˈneɪt/
stain /steɪn/
stand /stænd/ for /fə/

stand /stænd/ in
standard /'stæn.dəd/
standing /stænd.ɪŋ/ order /'ɔːdə/
state /steɪt/
statement /'steɪt.mənt/
station /'steɪ.ʃən/
status /'steɪ.təs/ asthmaticus / æsθ'mæt.ɪk.əs/
status /'steɪ.təs/
statute /'stætjuːt/
steadily /'sted.ɪ.li/
steady /'sted.i/
steering /'stɪər.ɪŋ/ wheel /wiːl/
sternal /'stɔː.nəl/
sternum /'stɜː.nəm/
stethoscope /'steθ.ə.skəʊp/
stick /stɪk/ (stuck, stuck)
stick /stɪk/
stiff /stɪf/
stiffness /'stɪf.nəs/
stimulant /'stɪm.jʊ.lənt/
stimulus /'stɪm.jʊ.ləs/ pl stimuli
sting /stɪŋ/
stingray /'stɪŋ.reɪ/
stoma /'stəʊ.mə/
stomach /'stʌm.ək/
stonelike /'stəʊn.laɪk/
stool /stuːl/
storage /'stɔː.rɪdʒ/
storm /stɔːm/
straight /streɪt/
strain /streɪn/
streak /striːk/
stream /striːm/
strenuous /'stren.ju.əs/
stressor /'stres.ə/
stretch /stretʃ/
stretcher /'stretʃə/
stridor /straɪd.ər/
strike /straɪk/ (struck, struck)
strike /straɪk/
striking /'straɪ.kɪŋ/
stroke /strəʊk/
stroke /strəʊk/ volume /'vɒl.juːm/
structural /'strʌktʃərəl/

structure /'strʌk.tʃər/
stupor /'stjuː.pər/
subarachnoid /ˌsʌb.ə'ræk.nɔɪd/
subclavian /sʌb'kleɪv.ɪ.ən/
subconjunctival /ˌsʌbˌkɒn.dʒʌŋk.'tɪ.vəl/
subcutaneous /ˌsʌb.kjʊ'teɪ.ni.əs/
subdiaphragmatic / ˌsʌbˌdaɪə.fræg'mæt.ɪk/
subdural /sʌb'djʊ.ə.rəl/
subglottic /sʌb'glɒt.ɪk/
sublingual /sʌb'lɪŋ.gwəl/
subluxation /ˌsʌb.lʌk'seɪ.ʃən/
subsequent /'sʌb.sɪ.kwənt/
subside /səb'saɪd/
substance /'sʌb.stənts/
substantial /səb'stæn.ʃəl/
substernal /sʌb'stɜː.nəl/
successfully /sək'ses.fə.li/
succession /sək'seʃ.ən/
suck /sʌk/
suction /'sʌk.ʃən/
sudden /'sʌd.ən/
suddenly /'sʌd.ən.li/
sue /sjuː/
suffer /'sʌf.ər/
suffering /'sʌf.ər.ɪŋ/ from /frəm/
suggestive /sə'dʒes.tɪv/
suicidal /ˌsuː.ɪ'saɪdəl/
suit /sjuːt/
suitable /'sjuː.tə.bl̩/
sulphate /'sʌl.feɪt/
superheat /'suː.pəˌhiːt/
superior /suː'pɪə.ri.ər/
supervise /'suː.pəˌvaɪz/
supervisor /'suː.pə.vaɪ.zər/
supination /'suː.pɪn.eɪ.ʃən/
supine /'suː.paɪn/
supplement /'sʌp.lɪ.mənt/
supplemental /ˌsʌp.lɪ'men.təl/
supply /sə'plaɪ/
support /'səˌpɔːt/
supportive /sə'pɔː.tɪv/
suppress /sə'pres/
suppression /sə'preʃ.ən/

suppressive /səˈpres.ɪv/
supraventricular /ˈsuːprə.venˈtrɪk.jə.lər/
surface /ˈsɜː.fɪs/
surfactant /sərˈfakˈtənt/
surgery /ˈsɜː.dʒər.i/
surround /səˈraʊnd/
surroundings /səˈraʊn.dɪŋz/
survey /ˈsɜː.veɪ/
survivability /səˈvaɪv.ə.ˈbɪl.ə.ti/
survival /səˈvaɪ.vəl/
survive /səˈvaɪv/
survivor /səˈvaɪ.vər/
susceptible /səˈsep.tɪ.bl̩/
suspect /səˈspekt/
suspected /səˈspek.tɪd/
suspicion /səˈspɪʃən/
suspicious /səˈspɪʃ.əs/
sustain /səˈsteɪn/
swallow / ˈswɒl.əʊ/
sweat /swet/
sweep /swiːp/ (swept, swept)
swelling /ˈswelɪŋ/
swiftly /ˈswɪft.li/
swing /swɪŋ/
switch /swɪtʃ/
swollen /ˈswəʊ.lən/
sympathetic /ˌsɪm.pəˈθet.ɪk/
sympathomimetic /ˌsɪm.pə.θə.mɪˈmet.ɪk/ syndrome /ˈsɪn.drəʊm/
symptom /ˈsɪmp.təm/
syncope /ˈsɪŋ.kə.pɪ/
syncytial /sɪnˈsɪ.ʃi.əl/ virus /ˈvaɪrəs/
syndrome /ˈsɪn.drəʊm/
syphilis /ˈsɪf.ɪ.lɪs/
syringe /sɪˈrɪndʒ/
systemic /sɪˈstem.ɪk/
systolic /sɪsˈtɑl.ɪk/

T
tachycardia /ˌtæk.ɪˈkɑː.di.ə/
tachydysrhythmia /ˌtæk.ɪ.dɪsˈrɪθ.mɪə/
tachypnoea /ˌtæk.ɪp.ˈniː.ə/
tackle /ˈtæk.l̩/
tag /tæg/

tail /teɪl/
take /teɪk/ breath /breθ/
take /teɪk/ care /keər/
take /teɪk/ time /taɪm/
tamponade /ˌtæm.pəˈneɪd/
tan /tæn/
tank /tæŋk/
tap /tæp/
tape /teɪp/
target /ˈtɑː.gɪt/
tarry /ˈtær.i/
task /tɑːsk/
teammate /ˈtiːm.meɪt/
tear /teər/
tearing /ˈteər.ɪŋ/
tearing /ˈtɪer.ɪŋ/
teary /ˈtɪə.r.i/
telephone /ˈtel.ɪ.fəʊn/
temporal /ˈtem.pər.əl/
temporary /ˈtempərəri/
tend /tend/ to the needs of sb
tendency /ˈten.dən.si/
tender /ˈten.dər/
tenderness /ˈten.də.nəs/
tendon pl. tendines /ˈten.dən/
tension /ˈtent.ʃən/ pneumothorax /ˌnjuːməˈθɔː.ræks/
tension /ˈtent.ʃən/
tepid /ˈtep.ɪd/
teres /ˈtiː.riːz/ pl teretes
term /tɜːm/
terminal /ˈtɜː.mɪ.nəl/
terminate /ˈtɜː.mɪ.neɪt/
termination /ˌtɜː.mɪˈneɪ.ʃən/
tertiary /ˈtɜː.ʃər.i/
therapy /ˈθer.ə.pi/
thereby /ˌðeəˈbaɪ/
therefore /ˈðeə.fɔːr/
thermal /ˈθɜː.məl/
thiamine /ˈθaɪ.ə.miːn/
thick /θɪk/
thicken /ˈθɪk.ən/
thickness /ˈθɪknɪs/
thigh /θaɪ/
thin /θɪn/

thoracic /θɔːˈræs.ɪk/ **cavity** /ˈkæv.ɪ.ti/
thorax /ˈθɔː.ræks/
thorough /ˈθʌr.ə/
thought /θɔːt/
thrash /θræʃ/
thready /ˈθred.i/
threat /θret/
threaten /ˈθret.ən/
threshold /ˈθreʃ.h əʊld/
thrombolytic /θrɒm.bɒˈlit.
ɪk/ **therapy** /ˈθer.ə.pi/
thrombolytic /θrɒm.bəˈlɪt.ɪk/
thrombosis /θrɒmˈbəʊ.sɪs/
through /θruː/
throughout /θruːˈaʊt/
throw /θrəʊ/ **(threw, thrown)**
thrust /θrʌst/
thumb / θʌm/
thyroid /ˈθaɪə .rɔɪd/ **storm** /stɔːm/
thyroid gland /ˈθaɪə .rɔɪd ˌglænd/
thyrotoxicosis /ˌθaɪˈrəˌtɒksiˈkəʊ.sɪs/
tibia /ˈtɪb.i.ə/ pl -ae
tidal /ˈtaɪ.dəl/
tidal /ˈtaɪdəl/ **volume** /ˈvɒljuːm/
tiered /tɪəd/
tight /taɪt/
tightly /ˈtaɪt.li/
tightness /ˈtaɪt.nəs/
tilt /tɪlt/
time /taɪm/
times /taɪmz/
timing /ˈtaɪ.mɪŋ/
tip /tɪp/
tired /ˈtaɪəd/
tiring /ˈtaɪə.rɪŋ/
tissue /ˈtɪʃ.uː/, /ˈtɪs.juː/
titrate /ˈtaɪ.treɪt/
TKO, To Keep (venous /
ˈviː.nəs/ infusion / ɪnˈfjuː.
ʒən/ line /laɪn/) Open
toddler /ˈtɒd.lər/
toe /təʊ/
tolerance /ˈtɒl.ər.əns/
tolerate /ˈtɒl.ər.eɪt/
tone /təʊn/

tongue /tʌŋ/
tool /tuːl/
top /tɒp/
topical /ˈtɒp.ɪ.kəl/
total /ˈtəʊ.təl/
touch /tʌtʃ/
touching /ˈtʌtʃ.ɪŋ/
tourniquet /ˈtʊə.nɪ.keɪ/
toward /təˈwɔːd/
towel /taʊəl/
toxaemia /tɒkˈsiː.mi.ə/
toxicity /tɒkˈsɪs.ɪ.ti/
toxin /ˈtɒk.sɪn/
trachea /trəˈkiː..ə/
tracheal /trəˈkiː.əl/
tracheobronchial /trə.kiː.əˈbrɒŋ.ki.əl/
tracheostomy /ˌtræk.iˈɒst.ə.mi/
track /træk/
traction /ˈtræk.ʃən/
trained /treɪnd/
transection /ˌtrænˈsek.ʃən/
transfer /trænsˈfɜːr/
transient /ˈtræn.zi.ənt/
transition /trænˈzɪʃ.ən/
transmit /trænzˈmɪt/
transparent /trænˈspær.ənt/
transport /ˈtræn.spɔːt/
trap /træp/
trauma /ˈtrɔː.mə/
traumatic /trɔːˈmæt.ɪk/
travel /ˈtræv.əl/
treat /triːt/
treatable /triːt.ə.bļ/
treatment /ˈtriːt.mənt/
tremendous /trɪˈmen.dəs/
tremor /ˈtrem.ər/
trench /trentʃ/
Trendelenburg /tren.del.ˈen.
berg/ **position** /pəˈzɪʃ.ən/
triad /ˈtraɪ.æd/
triage /ˈtraɪ.ɪdʒ/
tricuspid valve /traɪˈkʌs.pɪd ˌvælv/
trigger /ˈtrɪg.ər/
trim /trɪm/
trimester /trɪˈmes.tər/

trip /trɪp/
tripod /'traɪ.pɒd/
troubleshoot /'trʌb.l̩.ʃuːt/
truck /trʌk/
trunk /trʌŋk/
trunking /'trʌŋkɪŋ/
trust /trʌst/
tube /tjuːb/
tug /tʌg/
tumour /'tjuː.mər/
turn /tɜːn/ blue /bluː/
turn /tɜːn/ off /ɒf/
turn out /'tɜːn͵aʊt/
twist/͵twɪst/
twitch /twɪtʃ/
tympanic /'tɪm.pə.nik/
membrane /mem.breɪn/
tympanic /'tɪm.pə.nik/
tyre /taɪər/

U
ulcer /'ʌl.sər/
ultimate /'ʌl.tɪ.mət/
umbilical /ʌm'bɪl.ɪ.kəl/
umbilical cord /ʌm'bɪl.ɪ.kəl͵kɔːd/
umbilicus /ʌm'bɪl.ɪ.kəs/
unaffected /͵ʌn.ə'fek.tɪd/
unambiguous /͵ʌnæm'bɪgjʊəs/
unattended /͵ʌn.ə'ten.dɪd/
unaware /͵ʌn.ə'weər/
uncomfortable /ʌn'kʌmp f.tə.bl̩/
uncompensated /͵ʌn'kɒmpənseɪtɪd/
unconscious /ʌn'kɒnʃəs/
unconsciousness /ʌn'kɒn.ʃəs.nəs/
uncontrollably /͵ʌn.kən'trəʊ.lə.bli/
uncontrolled /͵ʌn.kən'trəʊld/
under /'ʌn.dər/
underage /͵ʌn.də'reɪdʒ/
underground /͵ʌn.də'graʊnd/
underlying /͵ʌndə'laɪ.ɪŋ/
underneath /͵ʌn.də'niːθ/
undernourished /͵ʌn.də'nʌr.ɪʃt/
undetected /͵ʌn.dɪ'tekt.əd/
uneasiness /ʌn'iː.zi.nəs/
unequal /ʌn'iː.kwəl/

unevenly /ʌn'iː.vən.li/
unfamiliar /͵ʌn.fə'mɪl.i.ər/
unilateral /͵juː.nɪ'læt.ər.əl/
unilaterally /͵juː.nɪ'læt.ər.əl.i/
unintentional /͵ʌn.ɪn'ten.ʃən.əl/
unlawful /ʌn'lɔːfʊl/
unlike /ʌn'laɪk/
unlikely /ʌn'laɪ.kli/
unnoticed /ʌn'nəʊ.tɪst/
unprovoked /͵ʌn.prə'vəʊkt/
unrecognized /ʌn'rek.əg.naɪzd/
unrelated /͵ʌn.rɪ'leɪ.tɪd/
unremarkable /͵ʌn.rɪ'mɑː.kə.bl̩/
unresponsive /͵ʌn.rɪ'spɒnt .sɪv/
unrestrained /͵ʌn.rɪ'streɪnd/
unsafe /ʌn'seɪf/
unsalvageable /ʌn'sæl.vɪdʒ.ə.bl̩/
unseen /ʌn'siːn/
unstable /ʌn'steɪ.bl̩/
unsure /ʌn'ʃɔːr/
untreated /ʌn'triː.tɪd/
unwanted /ʌn'wɒn.tɪd/
upgrade /ʌp'greɪd/
uphill /͵ʌp'hɪl/
upon /ə'pɒn/
upper /'ʌp.ər/
upright /'ʌp.raɪt/
upset /ʌp'set/
upwind /͵ʌp'wɪnd/
uraemia /jʊə'riː.mɪ.ə/
uraemic /jʊə'riː.mɪk/
urea /jʊə'riː.ə/ frost /frɒst/
urethra /jʊə'riː.θrə/
urge /ɜːdʒ/
urgent /'ɜː.dʒənt/
urinate /'jʊə.rɪ.neɪt/
urination /͵jʊə.rɪ'neɪ.ʃən/
urticaria /͵ɔː.tɪ'keə.ri.ə/
use /juːz/
uterine /'juː.tər.aɪn/ wall /wɔːl/
uterus /'juː.tər.əs/
utility /juː'tɪl.ɪ.ti/
utilize /'juː.tɪ.laɪz/

V
vagal /ˈveɪ gəl/ **tone** /təʊn/
vagal /ˈveɪ gəl/
vague /veɪg/
vagus /vəɪ.gəs/ pl -gi
valid /ˈvælɪd/
Valium /ˈvæl.i.əm/
vallecula /vəˈlek.jʊl.ə/
Valsalva /vælˈsæl.və/
manoeuvre /məˈnuː.vər/
valuable /ˈvæl.jʊ.bl̩/
value /ˈvæl.juː/
valve /vælv/
varicella /ˌvær.ɪˈsel.ə/
varicose vein /ˌvær.ɪ.kəʊsˈveɪn/
varied /ˈveə.rɪd/
variety /vəˈraɪə.ti/
varix /ˌveə.rɪks/ pl varices /ˈvær.ɪ.siːz/
vary /ˈveə.ri/
vascular /ˈvæs.kjʊ.lər/
vasculature /ˈvæs.kjʊ.lə.tʃər/
vasoconstriction /ˌveɪ.zə.kənˈstrɪk.ʃən/
vasodilatation /ˌveɪ.zə.daɪ.ləˈteɪ.ʃən/
vasodilator /ˌveɪ.zə.daɪˈleɪ.tər/
vasospasm /ˌveɪ.zəʊˈspæzm/
vasovagal /ˌveɪ.zəʊˈvæg.əl/
vault /vɔːlt/
vein /veɪn/
velocity /vɪˈlɒsɪtɪ/
vena cava /ˌviː.nəˈkeɪ.və/
venipuncture /ˌve.niˈpʌŋk.tʃər/
venom /ˈvenəm/
venous /ˈviː.nəs/ **return** /rɪˈtɜːn/
venous /ˈviː.nəs/ **capacitance**
/kəˈpæs.ɪ.tənts/
vent /vent/
ventilate /ˈven.tɪ.leɪt/
ventilation /ˌven.tɪˈleɪ.ʃən/
ventilatory /ˈventɪˌleɪtə.rɪ/
ventricle /ˈven.trɪ.kl̩/
ventricular /venˈtrɪk.jə.lər/
fibrillation /ˌfaɪ.brɪˈleɪ.
ʃən/, /ˌfɪb.rɪˈleɪ.ʃən/
ventricular /venˈtrɪk.jə.lər/
verification /ˌver.ɪ.fɪˈkeɪ.ʃən/

verify /ˈver.ɪ.faɪ/
vertebral /ˈvɜː.tɪ.brəl/
vessel /ˈves.əl/ céva
vestibular /vesˈtɪb.jə.lər/
via /ˈvaɪə/
viable /ˈvaɪ.ə.bl̩/
victim /ˈvɪk.tɪm/
violate /ˈvaɪəˌleɪt/
violence /ˈvaɪə.ləns/
violent /ˈvaɪələnt/
violently /ˈvaɪə.lənt.li/
visceral /ˈvɪs.ər.əl/
visibility /ˌvɪz.ɪˈbɪl.ɪ.ti/
visible /ˈvɪz.ɪ.bl̩/
visibly /ˈvɪz.ɪ.bli/
vision /ˈvɪʒ.ən/
visualization /ˌvɪʒ.u.əl.aɪˈzeɪˌʃən/
visualize /ˈvɪʒ.u.əl.aɪz/
vital /ˈvaɪ.təl/ **signs** /saɪnz/
vitals /ˈvaɪ.təlz/
vocal /ˈvəʊkəl/ **cords** /kɔːdz/
voice /vɔɪs/
volume /ˈvɒl.juːm/
voluntary /ˈvɒləntərɪ/
vomit /ˈvɒm.ɪt/
vomitus /ˈvɒm.ɪ.təs/

W
waist /weɪst/
wander /ˈwɒn.dər/
warmed /ˌwɔːmd/
warning /ˈwɔː.nɪŋ/ **sign** /saɪn/
warning /ˈwɔː.nɪŋ/
warrant /ˈwɒr.ənt/
waste /weɪst/
waste /weɪst/ **product** /ˈprɒdʌkt/
watch /wɒtʃ/
wave /weɪv/
weak /wiːk/
weakly /ˈwiːk.li/
weakness /ˈwiːk.nəs/
wear /weər/
weight /weɪt/ **loss** /lɒs/
weight /weɪt/
well /wel/

welt /welt/
wheal /wiːl/
wheeze /wiːz/
whereas /weərˈæz/
whimper /ˈwɪmpə/
whisper /ˈwɪs.pər/
whistle /ˈwɪs.l/
white /waɪt/
widen /ˈwaɪ.dən/
will /wɪl/
windshield /ˈwɪnd.ʃiːld/
wipe /waɪp/
wiper /ˈwaɪp.ər/
wire /waɪər/
wire /waɪər/ ladder /ˈlæd.ər/
wish /wɪʃ/
withdraw /wɪðˈdrɔː/
withdrawal /wɪðˈdrɔː.əl/
withdrawn /wɪðˈdrɔːn/
withhold /wɪðˈhəʊld/
within /wɪˈðɪn/
witness /ˈwɪt.nəs/
worker /ˈwɜː.kər/

workout /ˈwɜːkˌaʊt/
worsen /ˈwɜː.sən/
wounded /ˈwuːn.dɪd/
wrap /ræp/
wreck /rek/
wrestler /ˈres.lər/
wrinkle /ˈrɪŋkəl/
wrist /rɪst/

X
X-ray /ˈeks.reɪ/
xiphoid /zi.foid/ **process** /ˈproʊ.ses/

Y
yard /jɑːd/
yell /jel/
yellow jacket /ˈjel.oʊˌdʒæk.ɪt/
yellowish /ˈjel.əʊ.ɪʃ/

Z
zone /zəʊn/
zoster /zɒ.stər/

Key to Casuistics
Volume 1
Part 1
Airway and breathing

Unit 1
Case study 1
1h; 2f; 3g; 4e; 5d; 6a; 7c; 8b
Case study 2
1b; 2a; 3c; 4d
Case study 3
1a; 2b
Case study 4
1a; 2c; 3b
Case study 5
1c; 2e; 3a; 4d; 5b
Case study 6
1a; 2b; 3c
Case study 7
1c; 2b; 3d; 4a
Case study 8
1c; 2a; 3d; 4b
Case study 9
1b; 2c; 3e; 4a
Case study 10
1a; 2c; 3d; 4b
Case study 11
1b; 2a; 3b

Case study 12
1d; 2a; 3c; 4b
Case study 13
1c; 2b; 3d; 4a
Case study 14
1d; 2e; 3c; 4a; 5b
Case study 15
1a; 2b; 3c
Case study 16
1c; 2b; 3a
Case study 17
1a; 2b; 3c
Case study 18
1c; 2a; 3b
Case study 19
1a; 2d; 3e; 4b; 5c
Case study 20
1c; 2d; 3a; 4b
Case study 21
1b; 2d; 3c; 4a
Case study 22
1c; 2d; 3a; 4b

Unit 2
Case study 1
1c; 2b; 3d; 4a
Case study 2
1c; 2a; 3b
Case study 3
1b; 2c; 3a
Case study 4
1c; 2b; 3a
Case study 5
1c; 2a; 3b
Case study 6
1c; 2b; 3a
Case study 7
1c; 2a; 3b
Case study 8
1d; 2a; 3b; 4e; 5c
Case study 9
1c; 2d; 3a; 4b
Case study 10
1c; 2b; 3a

Case study 11
1e; 2b; 3a; 4f; 5d; 6c; 7g
Case study 12
1a; 2c; 3b
Case study 13
1b; 2c; 3a
Case study 14
1d; 2a; 3c; 4b; 5e
Case study 15
1c; 2a; 3d; 4b
Case study 16
1c; 2a; 3b
Case study 17
1c; 2d; 3a; 4b
Case study 18
1c; 2a; 3b
Case study 19
1b; 2a; 3d; 4c; 5e
Case study 20
1c; 2a; 3e; 4b; 5d; 6f
Case study 21
1a; 2c; 3b
Case study 22
1d; 2c; 3a; 4b

Unit 3
Case study 1
1a; 2d; 3e; 4b; 5c
Case study 2
1c; 2a; 3d; 4b
Case study 3
1d; 2a; 3c; 4e; 5b
Case study 4
1c; 2a; 3d; 4b
Case study 5
1c; 2a; 3b
Case study 6
1c; 2d; 3a; 4b
Case study 7
1b; 2c; 3a
Case study 8
1c; 2b; 3a; 4d
Case study 9
1b; 2c; 3a
Case study 10

1d; 2b; 3c; 4a
Case study 11
1a; 2c; 3b
Case study 12
1d; 2e; 3c; 4b; 5a
Case study 13
1c; 2a; 3b
Case study 14
1c; 2b; 3a
Case study 15
1c; 2a; 3b
Case study 16
1b; 2c; 3a
Case study 17
1c; 2a; 3b
Case study 18
1c; 2d; 3a; 4b
Case study 19
1c; 2a; 3b
Case study 20
1d; 2a; 3e; 4c; 5b
Case study 21
1c; 2a; 3c; 4b
Case study 22
1b; 2c; 3a
Case study 23
1a; 2c; 3b

Part 2
Cardiology
Unit 1
Case study 1
1a; 2c; 3b
Case study 2
1c; 2a; 3b
Case study 3
1a; 2d; 3b; 4e; 5f; 6c
Case study 4
1d; 2b; 3a; 4c
Case study 5
1a; 2c; 3d; 4b
Case study 6
1a; 2b; 3e; 4c; 5d
Case study 7
1c; 2a; 3b

Case study 8
1a; 2c; 3b

Case study 9
1c; 2a; 3b

Case study 10
1b; 2a; 3c

Case study 11
1c; 2a; 3b

Case study 12
1d; 2b; 3a; 4c

Case study 13
1a; 2c; 3b

Case study 14
1c; 2a; 3d; 4b

Case study 15
1d; 2e; 3c; 4f; 5b; 6a

Case study 16
1b; 2c; 3a

Case study 17
1a; 2b; 3a

Case study 18
1b; 2c; 3a; 4d

Case study 19
1c; 2a; 3b

Case study 20
1c; 2b; 3a

Case study 21
1b; 2d; 3c; 4a

Unit 2
Case study 1
1c; 2a; 3d; 4b

Case study 2
1d; 2a; 3b; 4c

Case study 3
1a; 2b; 3c

Case study 4
1b; 2a; 3c

Case study 5
1a; 2b; 3c

Case study 6
1a; 2d; 3b; 4c

Case study 7
1d; 2a; 3b; 4c

Case study 8
1c; 2a; 3b

Case study 9
1a; 2b; 3d; 4c

Case study 10
1d; 2b; 3e; 4c; 5a

Case study 11
1c; 2a; 3b

Case study 12
1d; 2e; 3c; 4b; 5a

Case study 13
1a; 2d; 3b; 4c

Case study 14
1d; 2b; 3c; 4a

Case study 15
1d; 2b; 3c; 4a

Case study 16
1c; 2b; 3a

Case study 17
1b; 2d; 3c; 4e; 5a

Case study 18
1c; 2b; 3a

Case study 19
1d; 2e; 3c; 4b; 5a

Case study 20
1b; 2d; 3a; 4c

Case study 21
1d; 2c; 3a; 4b

Part 3
Medical emergencies
Unit 1
Case study 1
1a; 2c; 3b

Case study 2
1e; 2d; 3a; 4c; 5b

Case study 3
1d; 2b; 3a; 4c; 5e

Case study 4
1c; 2b; 3a

Case study 5
1c; 2a; 3b

Case study 6
1a; 2d; 3c; 4b

Case study 7
1d; 2a; 3b; 4c
Case study 8
1c; 2a; 3b
Case study 9
1b; 2c; 3a
Case study 10
1c; 2a; 3b
Case study 11
1c; 2a; 3b
Case study 12
1c; 2b; 3d; 4a
Case study 13
1b; 2c; 3d; 4a
Case study 14
1c; 2b; 3a
Case study 15
1c; 2a; 3b
Case study 16
1c; 2b; 3a
Case study 17
1a; 2c; 3b
Case study 18
1d; 2c; 3b; 4a
Case study 19
1f; 2h; 3e; 4a; 5n; 6i; 7g; 8m;
9c; 10k; 11j; 12l; 13b; 14d
Case study 20
1c; 2b; 3a

Unit 2
Case study 1
1e; 2c; 3b; 4d; 5a
Case study 2
1e; 2g; 3l; 4k; 5b; 6j; 7h;
8a; 9i; 10d; 11f; 12c
Case study 3
1g; 2a; 3f; 4e; 5d; 6b; 7c
Case study 4
1m; 2f; 3i; 4g; 5a; 6b; 7j; 8c;
9k; 10h; 11d; 12l; 13e
Case study 5
1c; 2d; 3a; 4b
Case study 6
1a; 2c; 3b

Case study 7
1c; 2b; 3a
Case study 8
1a; 2k; 3d; 4j; 5h; 6i; 7g;
8c; 9e; 10b; 11f
Case study 9
1c; 2d; 3a; 4b
Case study 10
1e; 2b; 3a; 4d; 5c
Case study 11
1a; 2c; 3b
Case study 12
1c; 2e; 3b; 4f; 5d; 6a
Case study 13
1d; 2e; 3f; 4b; 5a; 6c
Case study 14
1a; 2e; 3d; 4b; 5f; 6g; 7c
Case study 15
1d; 2c; 3a; 4b
Case study 16
1c; 2b; 3d; 4a
Case study 17
1c; 2b; 3d; 4a
Case study 18
1b; 2c; 3a
Case study 19
1c; 2b; 3a
Case study 20
1a; 2d; 3c; 4b

Unit 3
Case study 1
1b; 2c; 3a
Case study 2
1c; 2b; 3d; 4a; 5e
Case study 3
1c; 2d; 3a; 4b
Case study 4
1c; 2b; 3a
Case study 5
1f; 2h; 3c; 4e; 5g; 6a; 7b; 8d
Case study 6
1c; 2e; 3f; 4a; 5d; 6b
Case study 7
1b; 2f; 3c; 4a; 5d; 6g; 7h; 8e

Case study 8
1c; 2d; 3b; 4e; 5a
Case study 9
1d; 2e; 3a; 4c; 5b
Case study 10
1d; 2g; 3h; 4b; 5a; 6f; 7i; 8e; 9c
Case study 11
1b; 2d; 3a; 4f; 5c; 6e
Case study 12
1b; 2c; 3d; 4a
Case study 13
1c; 2d; 3b; 4a
Case study 14
1e; 2b; 3c; 4a; 5d
Case study 15
1c; 2a; 3d; 4b
Case study 16
1g; 2b; 3a; 4f; 5h; 6e; 7c; 8d
Case study 17
1d; 2c; 3b; 4a
Case study 18
1c; 2d; 3b; 4a
Case study 19
1a; 2g; 3f; 4d; 5e; 6h; 7c; 8b
Case study 20
1c; 2d; 3a; 4e; 5b

Unit 4
Case study 1
1b; 2c; 3d; 4a
Case study 2
1d; 2b; 3f; 4e; 5a; 6c
Case study 3
1c; 2m; 3n; 4a; 5k; 6l; 7b; 8g;
9d; 10f; 11h; 12e; 13j; 14i
Case study 4
1c; 2a; 3b
Case study 5
1b; 2c; 3a
Case study 6
1b; 2d; 3f; 4a; 5e; 6c
Case study 7
1e; 2f; 3c; 4a; 5b; 6d; 7g
Case study 8
1c; 2b; 3a

Case study 9
1g; 2f; 3b; 4d; 5c; 6e; 7a
Case study 10
1c; 2b; 3a
Case study 11
1c; 2b; 3d; 4a
Case study 12
1c; 2d; 3b; 4a
Case study 13
1a; 2f; 3d; 4i; 5j; 6b; 7g; 8h; 9e; 10c
Case study 14
1c; 2c; 3b; 4a
Case study 15
1b; 2f; 3e; 4d; 5g; 6a
Case study 16
1b; 2c; 3a
Case study 17
1c; 2a; 3b
Case study 18
1b; 2c; 3a
Case study 19
1c; 2d; 3b; 4a
Case study 20
1d; 2e; 3c; 4b; 5a
Case study 21
1d; 2a; 3b; 4c

Part 4
Trauma
Unit 1
Case study 1
1b; 2d; 3c; 4a
Case study 2
1d; 2e; 3c; 4b; 5a
Case study 3
1h; 2c; 3a; 4g; 5d; 6f; 7b; 8e
Case study 4
1h; 2e; 3f; 4g; 5i; 6d; 7a; 8c; 9b
Case study 5
1d; 2c; 3b; 4a
Case study 6
1b; 2c; 3d; 4e; 5a
Case study 7
1e; 2b; 3f; 4a; 5d; 6g; 7c

Case study 8
1a; 2c; 3b
Case study 9
1e; 2g; 3d; 4f; 5k; 6a; 7m;
8j; 9l; 10c; 11b; 12i
Case study 10
1b; 2c; 3a
Case study 11
1c; 2b; 3a; 4e; 5d; 6f
Case study 12
1h; 2e; 3b; 4g; 5f; 6a; 7c; 8d
Case study 13
1g; 2h; 3a; 4b; 5d; 6c; 7f; 8e
Case study 14
1b; 2c; 3d; 4f; 5g; 6e; 7i; 8a; 9h
Case study 15
1b; 2h; 3g; 4i; 5d; 6f; 7e; 8a; 9c
Case study 16
1e; 2a; 3f; 4b; 5c; 6d
Case study 17
1c; 2b; 3d; 4e; 5a; 6f

Unit 2
Case study 1
1e; 2f; 3h; 4c; 5g; 6d; 7a; 8i; 9b
Case study 2
1c; 2d; 3b; 4a
Case study 3
1c; 2d; 3b; 4e; 5a
Case study 4
1d; 2e; 3a; 4c; 5b
Case study 5
1c; 2a; 3b
Case study 6
1a; 2b; 3d; 4c
Case study 7
1f; 2e; 3c; 4a; 5d; 6b
Case study 8
1c; 2d; 3b; 4a
Case study 9
1e; 2b; 3c; 4a; 5d
Case study 10
1d; 2c; 3e; 4b; 5a
Case study 11
1b; 2a; 3c

Case study 12
1d; 2f; 3b; 4a; 5g; 6c; 7h; 8i; 9e
Case study 13
1d; 2c; 3b; 4a
Case study 14
1d; 2e; 3f; 4a; 5b; 6c
Case study 15
1d; 2e; 3a; 4b; 5c
Case study 16
1c; 2d; 3e; 4b; 5f; 6a

Unit 3
Case study 1
1d; 2e; 3f; 4a; 5b; 6g; 7c
Case study 2
1c; 2a; 3b
Case study 3
1a; 2c; 3b; 4d; 5e
Case study 4
1c; 2a; 3b; 4d
Case study 5
1b; 2c; 3d; 4a; 5e
Case study 6
1d; 2b; 3c; 4a
Case study 7
1d; 2b; 3c; 4a
Case study 8
1c; 2d; 3b; 4a; 5e
Case study 9
1e; 2d; 3b; 4a; 5c
Case study 10
1e; 2f; 3c; 4a; 5b; 6d
Case study 11
1c; 2b; 3a
Case study 12
1b; 2c; 3a
Case study 13
1a; 2e; 3b; 4c; 5d
Case study 14
1d; 2e; 3b; 4c; 5a
Case study 15
1a; 2b; 3c

Case study 16
1p; 2t; 3s; 4r; 5u; 6o; 7n; 8j;
9i; 10m; 11l; 12k; 13b; 14d;
15e; 16t; 17g; 18a; 19h; 20c
Case study 17
1c; 2b; 3a

Part 5
Gynaecology, obstetrics, paediatrics
Unit 1
Case study 1
1a; 2e; 3c; 4d; 5b
Case study 2
1c; 2a; 3b; 4d
Case study 3
1c; 2a; 3b
Case study 4
1c; 2a; 3b
Case study 5
1a; 2f; 3e; 4b; 5c; 6d
Case study 6
1b; 2e; 3d; 4c; 5a
Case study 7
1b; 2d; 3e; 4c; 5a
Case study 8
1a; 2c; 3b
Case study 9
1c; 2a; 3d; 4b; 5g; 6h; 7f; 8i
Case study 10
1b; 2c; 3a
Case study 11
1c; 2a; 3c
Case study 12
1a; 2c; 3d; 4b
Case study 13
1c; 2h; 3b; 4d; 5e; 6g; 7f; 8a
Case study 14
1e; 2d; 3f; 4b; 5c; 6a
Case study 15
1b; 2a; 3c
Case study 16
1c; 2d; 3a; 4b
Case study 17
1d; 2a; 3b; 4c

Case study 18
1c; 2a; 3e; 4b; 5d; 6f
Case study 19
1c; 2a; 3b
Case study 20
1b; 2c; 3a

Unit 2
Case study 1
1a; 2c; 3d; 4a
Case study 2
1b; 2c; 3e; 4d; 5a
Case study 3
1d; 2b; 3c; 4f; 5a; 6e
Case study 4
1c; 2a; 3d; 4b
Case study 5
1c; 2b; 3d; 4a
Case study 6
1b; 2a; 3c; 4d
Case study 7
1a; 2c; 3b
Case study 8
1a; 2c; 3b
Case study 9
1b; 2a; 3d; 4c; 5e
Case study 10
1a; 2d; 3c; 4e; 5e; 6f
Case study 11
1c; 2b; 3d; 4a
Case study 12
1a; 2e; 3d; 4c; 5b
Case study 13
1c; 2a; 3b
Case study 14
1a; 2d; 3b; 4g; 5e; 6f; 7c; 8h
Case study 15
1a; 2e; 3b; 4d; 5c
Case study 16
1c; 2a; 3b
Case study 17
1e; 2a; 3b; 4d; 5c
Case study 18
1b; 2d; 3a; 4c

Case study 19
1e; 2b; 3d; 4c; 5a
Case study 20
1e; 2b; 3d; 4f; 5a; 6c
Case study 21
1d; 2e; 3f; 4g; 5c; 6a; 7b

Unit 3
Case study 1
1c; 2b; 3a
Case study 2
1b; 2c; 3a; 4e; 5d
Case study 3
1a; 2d; 3c; 4b
Case study 4
1a; 2c; 3b; 4d
Case study 5
1a; 2d; 3c; 4b
Case study 6
1d; 2c; 3a; 4b
Case study 7
1b; 2c; 3a
Case study 8
1c; 2b; 3b; 4a
Case study 9
1d; 2c; 3a; 4b
Case study 10
1a; 2d; 3c; 4b
Case study 11
1c; 2d; 3b; 4a
Case study 12
1d; 2a; 3e; 4b; 5c
Case study 13
1b; 2a; 3c; 4e; 5d
Case study 14
1b; 2d; 3c; 4a; 5e
Case study 15
1b; 2c; 3a
Case study 16
1a; 2f; 3e; 4d; 5b; 6c
Case study 17
1c; 2d; 3e; 4f; 5a; 6b
Case study 18
1b; 2a; 3d; 4c

Case study 19
1b; 2c; 3d; 4a
Case study 20
1c; 2d; 3b; 4a; 5e
Case study 21
1d; 2a; 3c; 4b

Unit 4
Case study 1
1c; 2d; 3b; 4a
Case study 2
1b; 2a; 3c
Case study 3
1d; 2b; 3a; 4c
Case study 4
1b; 2c; 3a
Case study 5
1b; 2d; 3c; 4a
Case study 6
1d; 2c; 3a; 4b
Case study 7
1a; 2b; 3c; 4d
Case study 8
1a; 2c; 3b
Case study 9
1b; 2a; 3d; 4c
Case study 10
1c; 2b; 3d; 4a
Case study 11
1a; 2d; 3b; 4e; 5c; 6f
Case study 12
1d; 2a; 3c; 4b
Case study 13
1b; 2a; 3c
Case study 14
1d; 2b; 3c; 4a
Case study 15
1c; 2d; 3b; 4a
Case study 16
1c; 2b; 3d; 4a
Case study 17
1d; 2c; 3a; 4b
Case study 18
1d; 2e; 3a; 4c; 5b

Case study 19
1c; 2d; 3a; 4b
Case study 20
1e; 2c; 3b; 4d; 5a
Case study 21
1e; 2c; 3a; 4d; 5b

Unit 5
Case study 1
1c; 2b; 3a
Case study 2
1d; 2e; 3c; 4a; 5b
Case study 3
1g; 2e; 3c; 4a; 5b; 6f; 7d
Case study 4
1b; 2a; 3d; 4c
Case study 5
1b; 2d; 3c; 4a
Case study 6
1c; 2a; 3b
Case study 7
1b; 2d; 3c; 4e; 5a
Case study 8
1d; 2b; 3c; 4a
Case study 9
1e; 2b; 3a; 4c; 5d
Case study 10
1c; 2d; 3a; 4b
Case study 11
1b; 2c; 3a
Case study 12
1c; 2b; 3a
Case study 13
1c; 2a; 3b
Case study 14
1c; 2b; 3a
Case study 15
1c; 2b; 3a
Case study 16
1b; 2c; 3d; 4e; 5a
Case study 17
1f; 2b; 3d; 5e; 6g; 7a
Case study 18
1d; 2g; 3a; 4b; 5c; 6e; 7f

Case study 19
1a; 2d; 3c; 4b
Case study 20
1f; 2b; 3e; 4c; 5d; 6g; 7a
Case study 21
1d; 2e; 3c; 4a; 5b
Part 6
Operations
Unit 1
Case study 1
1c; 2b; 3a
Case study 2
1b; 2c; 3a
Case study 3
1b; 2d; 3c; 4e; 5a
Case study 4
1b; 2d; 3c; 4a
Case study 5
1c; 2a; 3b
Case study 6
1c; 2a; 3b
Case study 7
1b; 2a; 3c
Case study 8
1c; 2b; 3a
Case study 9
1c; 2b; 3a
Case study 10
1a; 2c; 3b
Case study 11
1c; 2a; 3b
Case study 12
1c; 2b; 3a
Case study 13
1c; 2b; 3a
Case study 14
1d; 2c; 3a; 4b
Case study 15
1c; 2b; 3a
Case study 16
1b; 2c; 3a
Case study 17
1b; 2c; 3a
Case study 18
1c; 2d; 3b; 4a

Case study 19
1a; 2b; 3c
Case study 20
1c; 2b; 3a

Unit 2
Case study 1
1c; 2a; 3b
Case study 2
1c; 2a; 3d; 4b
Case study 3
1a; 2b; 3c
Case study 4
1a; 2c; 3b
Case study 5
1a; 2c; 3b
Case study 6
1c; 2a; 3b
Case study 7
1a; 2b; 3c
Case study 8
1b; 2a; 3c
Case study 9
1a; 2c; 3b
Case study 10
1c; 2a; 3b
Case study 11
1c; 2d; 3a; 4b
Case study 12
1b; 2c; 3a
Case study 13
1d; 2c; 3b; 4a
Case study 14
1c; 2d; 3b; 4a
Case study 15
1b; 2c; 3a
Case study 16
1c; 2b; 3a
Case study 17
1c; 2a; 3b
Case study 18
1c; 2a; 3b
Case study 19
1a; 2d; 3c; 4b

Case study 20
1c; 2a; 3b

Unit 3
Case study 1
1c; 2b; 3a
Case study 2
1d; 2b; 3a; 4e; 5c
Case study 3
1a; 2c; 3b
Case study 4
1c; 2a; 3d; 4b
Case study 5
1b; 2a; 3c
Case study 6
1c; 2b; 3a
Case study 7
1b; 2a; 3c; 4d
Case study 8
1b; 2c; 3a
Case study 9
1c; 2d; 3a; 4b
Case study 10
1a; 2c; 3b
Case study 11
1b; 2a; 3c
Case study 12
1c; 2d; 3e; 4a; 5b
Case study 13
1a; 2b; 3c
Case study 14
1a; 2b; 3d; 4c
Case study 15
1c; 2b; 3a
Case study 16
1b; 2d; 3c; 4a
Case study 17
1e; 2d; 3a; 4b; 5c
Case study 18
1c; 2a; 3b
Case study 19
1h; 2b; 3a; 4d; 5c; 6f; 7e; 8g
Case study 20
1a; 2c; 3b

Unit 4

Case study 1
1c; 2b; 3a

Case study 2
1c; 2b; 3a

Case study 3
1c; 2a; 3b; 4d

Case study 4
1c; 2b; 3c; 4a

Case study 5
1a; 2b; 3c

Case study 6
1b; 2a; 3c

Case study 7
1b; 2c; 3d; 4a

Case study 8
1b; 2c; 3d; 4a

Case study 9
1c; 2b; 3a

Case study 10
1c; 2a; 3b

Case study 11
1c; 2b; 3a

Case study 12
1d; 2c; 3a; 4b

Case study 13
1c; 2a; 3b

Case study 14
1b; 2d; 3a; 4c

Case study 15
1c; 2b; 3a; 4d

Case study 16
1c; 2a; 3b

Case study 17
1c; 2f; 3g; 4e; 5d; 6a; 7b

Case study 18
1a; 2b; 3c

Case study 19
1d; 2a; 3b; 4c; 5e

Case study 20
1d; 2b; 3a; 4c

Case study 21
1c; 2d; 3e; 4a; 5b

Volume 2

Unit 1

Case study 1
1b; 2d; 3c; 4a

Case study 2
1e; 2a; 3d; 4f; 5c; 6b

Case study 3
1c; 2e; 3b; 4d; 5a; 6f

Case study 4
1a; 2d; 3b; 4c

Case study 5
1a; 2d; 3b; 4c

Case study 6
1b; 2c; 3a; 4g; 5h; 6i; 7f; 8d

Case study 7
1a; 2c; 3g; 4d; 5e; 6b; 7f

Case study 8
1a; 2b; 3c

Case study 9
1c; 2d; 3b; 4a

Case study 10
1e; 2d; 3c; 4b; 5a

Case study 11
1a; 2c; 3d; 4b; 5e; 6f

Case study 12
1b; 2c; 3e; 4d; 5a

Case study 13
1a; 2c; 3b

Case study 14
1c; 2b; 3a

Case study 15
1f; 2c; 3b; 4d; 5e; 6a

Case study 16
1c; 2b; 3e; 4d; 5f; 6a

Case study 17
1c; 2a; 3b; 4d

Case study 18
1c; 2a; 3b; 4d

Case study 19
1b; 2d; 3a; 4c

Case study 20
1e; 2i; 3d; 4f; 5a; 6h; 7g; 8b; 9c

Unit 2
Case study 1
1d; 2a; 3b; 4c
Case study 2
1d; 2e; 3b; 4c; 5a
Case study 3
1d; 2a; 3b; 4c
Case study 4
1d; 2c; 3b; 4a
Case study 5
1d; 2c; 3b; 4a
Case study 6
1a; 2c; 3b; 4d
Case study 7
1c; 2a; 3b
Case study 8
1b; 2d; 3c; 4a
Case study 9
1b; 2a; 3d; 4e; 5c
Case study 10
1c; 2a; 3b
Case study 11
1c; 2e; 3b; 4f; 5a; 6d
Case study 12
1b; 2e; 3d; 4e; 5c; 6f; 7a
Case study 13
1d; 2b; 3e; 4c; 5a
Case study 14
1a; 2c; 3b
Case study 15
1b; 2c; 3a
Case study 16
1e; 2b; 3c; 4d; 5a
Case study 17
1b; 2a; 3c; 4 d
Case study 18
1b; 2e; 3c; 4a; 5f; 6d
Case study 19
1c; 2d; 3b; 4e; 5a
Case study 20
1b; 2c; 3d; 4a

Unit 3
Case study 1
1c; 2d; 3b; 4a

Case study 2
1c; 2a; 3d; 4b
Case study 3
1b; 2c; 3a
Case study 4
1c; 2a; 3b
Case study 5
1b; 2d; 3c; 4a
Case study 6
1c; 2a; 3b
Case study 7
1b; 2e; 3a; 4d; 5c
Case study 8
1e; 2a; 3d; 4c; 5b
Case study 9
1c; 2f; 3b; 4c; 5a; 6d; 7g
Case study 10
1e; 2b; 3c; 4f; 5d; 6a
Case study 11
1d; 2c; 3b; 4e; 5a; 6g; 7f
Case study 12
1e; 2d; 3b; 4a; 5c
Case study 13
1c; 2b; 3a; 4d
Case study 14
1d; 2e; 3b; 4a; 5f; 6c
Case study 15
1e; 2b; 3c; 4d; 5a; 6f
Case study 16
1b; 2c; 3a
Case study 17
1b; 2d; 3a; 4c
Case study 18
1b; 2a; 3c
Case study 19
1e; 2b; 3a; 4d; 5c
Case study 20
1d; 2b; 3c; 4a

Unit 4
Case study 1
1e; 2g; 3d; 4f; 5b; 6c; 7a
Case study 2
1e; 2d; 3f; 4a; 5c; 6b

Case study 3
1c; 2b; 3a

Case study 4
1d; 2e; 3c; 4b; 5h; 6a; 7f; 8g

Case study 5
1e; 2a; 3d; 4b; 5c

Case study 6
1b; 2e; 3c; 4d; 5a

Case study 7
1e; 2d; 3b; 4c; 5a

Case study 8
1c; 2d; 3a; 4b

Case study 9
1f; 2c; 3b; 4a; 5e; 6d

Case study 10
1b; 2a; 3d; 4c

Case study 11
1c; 2d; 3b; 4e; 5a

Case study 12
1c; 2b; 3a

Case study 13
1a; 2b; 3c

Case study 14
1a; 2c; 3b

Case study 15
1d; 2e; 3b; 4a; 5c

Case study 16
1a; 2e; 3c; 4d; 5b

Case study 17
1b; 2d; 3a; 4c

Case study 18
1b; 2d; 3c; 4a

Case study 19
1c; 2b; 3a

Case study 20
1b; 2c; 3a; 4d

Unit 5

Case study 1
1b; 2c; 3a

Case study 2
1b; 2c; 3a

Case study 3
1b; 2c; 3a

Case study 4
1d; 2b; 3a; 4c

Case study 5
1c; 2d; 3a; 4e; 5f; 6b

Case study 6
1a; 2c; 3b; 4d

Case study 7
1a; 2c; 3b

Case study 8
1a; 2d; 3b; 4c

Case study 9
1c; 2b; 3a

Case study 10
1e; 2b; 3c; 4d; 5a

Case study 11
1a; 2b; 3d; 4c

Case study 12
1a; 2b; 3c

Case study 13
1a; 2b; 3d; 4c; 5e

Case study 14
1b; 2c; 3a

Case study 15
1d; 2b; 3a; 4c

Case study 16
1c; 2d; 3b; 4a

Case study 17
1c; 2d; 3b; 4a

Case study 18
1d; 2b; 3a; 4c

Case study 19
1c; 2a; 3b

Case study 20
1c; 2a; 3b

Unit 6

Case study 1
1a; 2c; 3b; 4d

Case study 2
1c; 2d; 3b; 4a

Case study 3
1d; 2b; 3c; 4a

Case study 4
1c; 2d; 3a; 4b

Case study 5
1a; 2d; 3b; 4c
Case study 6
1b; 2a; 3c
Case study 7
1c; 2d; 3b; 4a
Case study 8
1e; 2c; 3d; 4a; 5b
Case study 9
1c; 2b; 3a; 4d
Case study 10
1c; 2f; 3b; 4d; 5e; 6a
Case study 11
1d; 2c; 3a; 4b
Case study 12
1b; 2d; 3c; 4a; 5e
Case study 13
1b; 2c; 3a
Case study 14
1b; 2c; 3a
Case study 15
1c; 2e; 3a; 4b; 5d
Case study 16
1d; 2c; 3e; 4a; 5b
Case study 17
1c; 2a; 3b; 4d
Case study 18
1c; 2e; 3a; 4b; 5d
Case study 19
1c; 2f; 3b; 4d; 5a; 6e
Case study 20
1a; 2d; 3b; 4c

Unit 7
Case study 1
1d; 2a; 3c; 4b
Case study 2
1c; 2f; 3d; 4a; 5b
Case study 3
1d; 2c; 3b; 4a
Case study 4
1a; 2b; 3c
Case study 5
1d; 2f; 3a; 4b; 5e; 6c

Case study 6
1e; 2b; 3c; 4d; 5a
Case study 7
1d; 2e; 3c; 4a; 5b
Case study 8
1c; 2d; 3a; 4e; 5b
Case study 9
1b; 2c; 3d; 4a
Case study 10
1c; 2d; 3b; 4a
Case study 11
1b; 2c; 3a
Case study 12
1a; 2c; 3b
Case study 13
1b; 2c; 3a
Case study 14
1e; 2b; 3c; 4a; 5d
Case study 15
1c; 2e; 3b; 4a; 5d; 6f
Case study 16
1c; 2a; 3b
Case study 17
1e; 2c; 3d; 4a; 5b
Case study 18
1d; 2c; 3a; 4b
Case study 19
1a; 2d; 3c; 4b
Case study 20
1b; 2c; 3a

Unit 8
Case study 1
1c; 2a; 3d; 4b
Case study 2
1c; 2a; 3b; 4d
Case study 3
1d; 2a; 3c; 4b
Case study 4
1a; 2b; 3e; 4c; 5d
Case study 5
1b; 2c; 3a
Case study 6
1a; 2c; 3b

Case study 7
1e; 2d; 3b; 4a; 5c
Case study 8
1d; 2c; 3b; 4a
Case study 9
1e; 2c; 3b; 4d; 5a
Case study 10
1b; 2c; 3a
Case study 11
1c; 2a; 3b
Case study 12
1d; 2e; 3b; 4f; 5c; 6a
Case study 13
1d; 2a; 3b; 4e; 5c
Case study 14
1b; 2a; 3d; 4c
Case study 15
1e; 2f; 3c; 4d; 5a; 6b
Case study 16
1c; 2b; 3a
Case study 17
1c; 2b; 3a
Case study 18
1e; 2d; 3a; 4c; 5b
Case study 19
1c; 2a; 3b
Case study 20
1b; 2e; 3c; 4d; 5a

Unit 9
Case study 1
1a; 2d; 3b; 4c; 5e
Case study 2
1c; 2a; 3b
Case study 3
1c; 2b; 3d; 4a; 5f
Case study 4
1b; 2c; 3a
Case study 5
1a; 2c; 3b
Case study 6
1b; 2c; 3a
Case study 7
1c; 2a; 3b; 4d

Case study 8
1a; 2b; 3c
Case study 9
1a; 2c; 3d; 4b
Case study 10
1c; 2e; 3b; 4d; 5a
Case study 11
1a; 2e; 3b; 4c; 5f; 6d
Case study 12
1f; 2h; 3d; 4i; 5e; 6g; 7a; 8b; 9c
Case study 13
1c; 2a; 3b
Case study 14
1a; 2c; 3b
Case study 15
1d; 2c; 3b; 4a
Case study 16
1d; 2a; 3c; 4b
Case study 17
1d; 2c; 3e; 4a; 5b
Case study 18
1a; 2c; 3b
Case study 19
1b; 2a; 3c
Case study 20
1b; 2c; 3a

Unit 10
Case study 1
1c; 2a; 3d; 4b
Case study 2
1b; 2c; 3a
Case study 3
1b; 2c; 3a
Case study 4
1b; 2c; 3a
Case study 5
1g; 2l; 3a; 4c; 5h; 6j; 7i; 8k;
9d; 10e; 11b; 12m; 13f
Case study 6
1e; 2a; 3c; 4b; 5d
Case study 7
1b; 2a; 3e; 4c; 5d

Case study 8
1a; 2j; 3b; 4g; 5i; 6h; 7k;
8e; 9f; 10c; 11d
Case study 9
1d; 2c; 3a; 4e; 5b
Case study 10
1d; 2e; 3c; 4b; 5a
Case study 11
1b; 2e; 3d; 4c; 5a
Case study 12
1b; 2d; 3c; 4a; 5e
Case study 13
1a; 2b; 3c
Case study 14
1c; 2e; 3b; 4d; 5a
Case study 15
1c; 2b; 3a
Case study 16
1a; 2b; 3d; 4c
Case study 17
1c; 2b; 3a
Case study 18
1d; 2e; 3c; 4b; 5a
Case study 19
1c; 2d; 3a; 4b
Case study 20
1b; 2a; 3d; 4c

Unit 11
Case study 1
1c; 2b; 3a
Case study 2
1c; 2b; 3a
Case study 3
1c; 2b; 3a
Case study 4
1a; 2c; 3e; 4d; 5b
Case study 5
1c; 2a; 3d; 4b
Case study 6
1c; 2b; 3a
Case study 7
1c; 2b; 3a
Case study 8
1d; 2a; 3c; 4b

Case study 9
1d; 2b; 3c; 4a
Case study 10
1a; 2c; 3e; 4b; 5d; 6f
Case study 11
1i; 2d; 3h; 4g; 5b; 6f; 7a; 8e; 9j; 10c
Case study 12
1c; 2a; 3d; 4b
Case study 13
1d; 2e; 3b; 4a; 5c
Case study 14
1b; 2d; 3c; 4a
Case study 15
1d; 2a; 3b; 4c
Case study 16
1c; 2b; 3a
Case study 17
1d; 2b; 3a; 4c
Case study 18
1d; 2c; 3a; 4b
Case study 19
1c; 2d; 3b; 4a
Case study 20
1b; 2d; 3a; 4e; 5c

Unit 12
Case study 1
1b; 2a; 3c
Case study 2
1d; 2e; 3c; 4a; 5b
Case study 3
1c; 2b; 3a
Case study 4
1a; 2b; 3c; 4d
Case study 5
1d; 2c; 3f; 4a; 5b; 6e
Case study 6
1c; 2e; 3b; 4d; 5a; 6f
Case study 7
1f; 2e; 3b; 4c; 5a; 6d
Case study 8
1d; 2g; 3f; 4c; 5b; 6e; 7a
Case study 9
1a; 2b; 3c

Case study 10
1d; 2c; 3b; 4a
Case study 11
1d; 2a; 3b; 4c
Case study 12
1a; 2b; 3c
Case study 13
1e; 2a; 3b; 4d; 5c
Case study 14
1d; 2g; 3c; 4e; 5a; 6f; 7b
Case study 15
1c; 2d; 3b; 4a
Case study 16
1b; 2d; 3a; 4c
Case study 17
1b; 2d; 3e; 4a; 5c
Case study 18
1c; 2b; 3a
Case study 19
1b; 2d; 3a; 4c
Case study 20
1c; 2a; 3b

Unit 13
Case study 1
1c; 2b; 3a
Case study 2
1b; 2a; 3c
Case study 3
1c; 2b; 3a
Case study 4
1e; 2d; 3b; 4c; 5a
Case study 5
1c; 2b; 3e; 4f; 5d; 6a
Case study 6
1d; 2a; 3c; 4b
Case study 7
1b; 2c; 3a
Case study 8
1c; 2d; 3b; 4a
Case study 9
1b; 2d; 3c; 4a
Case study 10
1b; 2d; 3a; 4c; 5e

Case study 11
1c; 2d; 3b; 4a
Case study 12
1e; 2b; 3c; 4a; 5d
Case study 13
1d; 2e; 3a; 4c; 5b
Case study 14
1e; 2a; 3f; 4c; 5b; 6d
Case study 15
1d; 2c; 3e; 4a; 5b; 6f
Case study 16
1e; 2d; 3a; 4b; 5c
Case study 17
1e; 2b; 3a; 4c; 5d
Case study 18
1b; 2e; 3c; 4f; 5a; 6d; 7i; 8g
Case study 19
1a; 2e; 3c; 4d; 5g; 6b; 7f
Case study 20
1d; 2b; 3c; 4a

Unit 14
Case study 1
1c; 2b; 3a
Case study 2
1d; 2b; 3a; 4c
Case study 3
1b; 2c; 3a
Case study 4
1d; 2e; 3b; 4a; 5c
Case study 5
1a; 2c; 3b
Case study 6
1b; 2d; 3a; 4c
Case study 7
1b; 2a
Case study 8
1d; 2c; 3b; 4a
Case study 9
1b; 2c; 3a
Case study 10
1d; 2c; 3b; 4a
Case study 11
1e; 2c; 3b; 4d; 5a

Case study 12
1a; 2c; 3b
Case study 13
1b; 2d; 3a; 4c
Case study 14
1d; 2c; 3b; 4a
Case study 15
1e; 2d; 3b; 4a
Case study 16
1d; 2c; 3b; 4a
Case study 17
1d; 2c; 3b; 4a
Case study 18
1d; 2c; 3e; 4a
Case study 19
1b; 2a; 3c
Case study 20
1h; 2e; 3b; 4g; 5f; 6a; 7c; 8d

Unit 15
Case study 1
1e; 2c; 3d; 4a; 5b
Case study 2
1d; 2a; 3e; 4c; 5b
Case study 3
1d; 2b; 3a; 4c
Case study 4
1e; 2g; 3d; 4b; 5c; 6f; 7a; 8h
Case study 5
1d; 2e; 3b; 4c; 5a; 6f
Case study 6
1c; 2a; 3b
Case study 7
1d; 2b; 3c; 4a
Case study 8
1c; 2b; 3a
Case study 9
1c; 2d; 3b; 4a
Case study 10
1a; 2c; 3b
Case study 11
1c; 2b; 3d; 4a
Case study 12
1b; 2a; 3d; 4c

Case study 13
1c; 2b; 3a
Case study 14
1e; 2d; 3b; 4c; 5a
Case study 15
1d; 2b; 3c; 4e; 5a
Case study 16
1d; 2b; 3c; 4a
Case study 17
1d; 2c; 3a; 4b
Case study 18
1c; 2b; 3a
Case study 19
1d; 2b; 3a; 4c
Case study 20
1a; 2b; 3c

Unit 16
Case study 1
1c; 2b; 3a; 4d
Case study 2
1c; 2b; 3a
Case study 3
1c; 2d; 3b; 4a
Case study 4
1d; 2c; 3e; 4a; 5b
Case study 5
1c; 2b; 3a
Case study 6
1c; 2d; 3b; 4a
Case study 7
1d; 2f; 3b; 4h; 5a; 6g; 7e; 8c
Case study 8
1c; 2a; 3b
Case study 9
1d; 2c; 3f; 4g; 5e; 6a; 7b
Case study 10
1c; 2d; 3b; 4f; 5a; 6g; 7e
Case study 11
1b; 2c; 3a
Case study 12
1c; 2b; 3a
Case study 13
1f; 2b; 3d; 4a; 5c; 6e

Case study 14
1d; 2e; 3b; 4f; 5a; 6g; 7c
Case study 15
1d; 2c; 3b; 4a; 5e
Case study 16
1d; 2g; 3e; 4b; 5a; 6f; 7c
Case study 17
1c; 2a; 3d; 4e; 5b
Case study 18
1i; 2a; 3c; 4d; 5g; 6h; 7j; 8f; 9e; 10b
Case study 19
1e; 2b; 3d; 4a; 5c
Case study 20
1d; 2c; 3b; 4a

Unit 17
Case study 1
1d; 2c; 3a; 4b
Case study 2
1e; 2c; 3d; 4b; 5a
Case study 3
1c; 2d; 3e; 4b; 5a
Case study 4
1e; 2c; 3a; 4d; 5b
Case study 5
1c; 2b; 3d; 4a
Case study 6
1b; 2e; 3d; 4c; 5a
Case study 7
1e; 2d; 3a; 4c; 5b
Case study 8
1d; 2c; 3a; 4b
Case study 9
1b; 2e; 3a; 4g; 5f; 6d; 7h; 8i; 9j; 10c
Case study 10
1d; 2a; 3c; 4b
Case study 11
1c; 2e; 3b; 4a; 5d
Case study 12
1d; 2a; 3b; 4c
Case study 13
1d; 2a; 3b; 4c
Case study 14
1a; 2b; 3c; 4e; 5d

Case study 15
1d; 2a; 3b; 4c
Case study 16
1b; 2a; 3e; 4c; 5f; 6d
Case study 17
1b; 2e; 3d; 4c; 5a
Case study 18
1a; 2b; 3c
Case study 19
1b; 2a; 3c
Case study 20
1d; 2c; 3b; 4a

Unit 18
Case study 1
1d; 2b; 3e; 4a; 5c
Case study 2
1c; 2d; 3a; 4b
Case study 3
1c; 2b; 3a
Case study 4
1d; 2a; 3b; 4c; 5e
Case study 5
1a; 2e; 3c; 4b; 5d
Case study 6
1c; 2a; 3b
Case study 7
1a; 2e; 3b; 4c; 5d
Case study 8
1a; 2d; 3c; 4b
Case study 9
1e; 2g; 3a; 4b; 5h; 6c; 7f; 8k; 9i; 10l;
11m; 12n; 13o; 14p; 15j; 16d; 17r
Case study 10
1c; 2a; 3b; 4d
Case study 11
1d; 2a; 3c; 4b
Case study 12
1c; 2a; 3b; 4d
Case study 13
1c; 2a; 3b
Case study 14
1b; 2d; 3a; 4c
Case study 15
1g; 2b; 3a; 4c; 5e; 6f; 7d

Case study 16
1a; 2d; 3c
Case study 17
1a; 2c; 3b
Case study 18
1c; 2a; 3b; 4d
Case study 19
1d; 2b; 3c; 4e; 5a
Case study 20
1e; 2c; 3b; 4a; 5d

Unit 19
Case study 1
1c; 2a; 3b; 4c
Case study 2
1d; 2c; 3b; 4a
Case study 3
1b; 2a; 3d; 4c
Case study 4
1d; 2a; 3b; 4c
Case study 5
1d; 2a; 3b; 4e; 5c
Case study 6
1g; 2d; 3c; 4a; 5f; 6b; 7e
Case study 7
1c; 2b; 3d; 4a
Case study 8
1d; 2a; 3c; 4b
Case study 9
1a; 2c; 3b; 4d; 5e
Case study 10
1d; 2b; 3c; 4a
Case study 11
1c; 2b; 3d; 4a
Case study 12
1d; 2c; 3b; 4a
Case study 13
1d; 2b; 3a; 4c
Case study 14
1b; 2a; 3f; 4c; 5e; 6d
Case study 15
1d; 2b; 3a; 4c
Case study 16
1d; 2c; 3a; 4b

Case study 17
1e; 2b; 3c; 4a; 5d
Case study 18
1a; 2e; 3b; 4d; 5c
Case study 19
1b; 2f; 3c; 4a; 5e; 6d
Case study 20
1a; 2e; 3b; 4c; 5d
Case study 21
1c; 2d; 3e; 4a; 5b

Unit 20
Case study 1
1a; 2d; 3b; 4c
Case study 2
1c; 2a; 3b
Case study 3
1a; 2c; 3c; 4b
Case study 4
1a; 2f; 3c; 4b; 5d; 6e
Case study 5
1c; 2a; 3b
Case study 6
1d; 2c; 3b; 4a
Case study 7
1a; 2d; 3c; 4b
Case study 8
1b; 2d; 3c; 4a
Case study 9
1c; 2b; 3e
Case study 10
1b; 2c; 3a; 4d
Case study 11
1d; 2b; 3c; 4a
Case study 12
1d; 2c; 3a; 4b
Case study 13
1c; 2d; 3a; 4b
Case study 14
1c; 2d; 3b; 4a
Case study 15
1a; 2d; 3b; 4c; 5e; 6f
Case study 16
1d; 2b; 3a; 4c; 5e

Case study 17
1a; 2b; 3c; 4e; 5d
Case study 18
1d; 2a; 3c; 4e; 5b
Case study 19
1d; 2b; 3c; 4a; 5e
Case study 20
1a; 2d; 3b; 4c
Case study 21
1c; 2b; 3a

Unit 21
Case study 1
1c; 2a; 3d; 4b
Case study 2
1d; 2b; 3c; 4a
Case study 3
1d; 2e; 3f; 4b; 5a; 6c
Case study 4
1b; 2e; 3c; 4a; 5d
Case study 5
1b; 2c; 3d; 4a
Case study 6
1e; 2a; 3b; 4c; 5d
Case study 7
1a; 2d; 3b; 4e; 5c
Case study 8
1d; 2a; 3b; 4e; 5c
Case study 9
1d; 2c; 3e; 4b; 5a

Case study 10
1c; 2b; 3a
Case study 11
1f; 2a; 3b; 4c; 5d; 6e
Case study 12
1c; 2b; 3a
Case study 13
1e; 2a; 3b; 4d; 5c; 6f
Case study 14
1a; 2d; 3c; 4b
Case study 15
1a; 2b; 3f; 4d; 5c; 6e
Case study 16
1b; 2d; 3e; 4a; 5c

Case study 17
1a; 2b; 3c; 4d; 5e; 6f; 7g; 8h
Case study 18
1a; 2f; 3d; 4e; 5g; 6i; 7h;
8j; 9b; 10k; 11c
Case study 19
1a; 2c; 3m; 4l; 5n; 6j; 7h; 8d; 9g;
10i; 11o; 12b; 13p; 14e; 15k; 16f
Case study 20
1b; 2c; 3e; 4a; 5d
Case study 21
1c; 2b; 3a

Unit 22
Case study 1
1b; 2e; 3a; 4d; 5c
Case study 2
1c; 2d; 3a; 4b
Case study 3
1d; 2e; 3b; 4c; 5a
Case study 4
1c; 2d; 3b; 4a
Case study 5
1d; 2a; 3c; 4b
Case study 6
1a; 2d; 3b; 4c
Case study 7
1d; 2c; 3a; 4e; 5b
Case study 8
1b; 2d; 3c; 4a
Case study 9
1c; 2b; 3a
Case study 10
1c; 2d; 3a; 4b; 5e
Case study 11
1b; 2a; 3d; 4c
Case study 12
1d; 2b; 3c; 4a
Case study 13
1d; 2c; 3b; 4a
Case study 14
1c; 2a; 3b; 4d; 5e
Case study 15
1d; 2c; 3b; 4a

Case study 16
1c; 2b; 3a

Case study 17
1c; 2b; 3a

Case study 18
1d; 2c; 3a; 4b

Case study 19
1a; 2d; 3b; 4c

Case study 20
1c; 2a; 3b

Case study 21
1a; 2d; 3c; 4b

Unit 23
Case study 1
1d; 2a; 3c; 4b

Case study 2
1d; 2b; 3c; 4a

Case study 3
1b; 2e; 3a; 4d; 5f; 6c; 7g

Case study 4
1b; 2c; 3d; 4a

Case study 5
1c; 2a; 3f; 4b; 5e; 6g; 7d

Case study 6
1c; 2b; 3d; 4a; 5e

Case study 7
1d; 2e; 3b; 4a; 5c

Case study 8
1a; 2b; 3c

Case study 9
1a; 2d; 3b; 4c

Case study 10
1d; 2a; 3b; 4c

Case study 11
1d; 2c; 3a; 4b; 5e

Case study 12
1b; 2c; 3e; 4d; 5a

Case study 13
1b; 2d; 3f; 4c; 5e; 6h; 7g; 8a

Case study 14
1c; 2a; 3b

Case study 15
1b; 2c; 3a; 4d; 5e; 6f; 7g

Case study 16
1c; 2b; 3a; 4d

Case study 17
1a; 2d; 3c; 4b

Case study 18
1d; 2a; 3b; 4c; 5e

Case study 19
1g; 2i; 3j; 4f; 5e; 6h; 7d; 8a; 9b; 10c

Case study 20
1c; 2d; 3f; 4g; 5a; 6g; 7e

Case study 21
1b; 2c; 3a

Unit 24
Case study 1
1e; 2a; 3b; 4c; 5d

Case study 2
1c; 2d; 3a; 4b

Case study 3
1c; 2b; 3a

Case study 4
1c; 2b; 3d; 4a

Case study 5
1a; 2c; 3b

Case study 6
1a; 2c; 3b; 4d

Case study 7
1c; 2a; 3b

Case study 8
1c; 2a; 3b

Case study 9
1d; 2b; 3c; 4a

Case study 10
1d; 2b; 3a; 4c

Case study 11
1a; 2c; 3b

Case study 12
1c; 2b; 3e; 4a; 5d

Case study 13
1c; 2b; 3a

Case study 14
1c; 2d; 3b; 4a

Case study 15
1c; 2d; 3a; 4e; 5b

Case study 16
1c; 2d; 3b; 4e; 5a
Case study 17
1a; 2c; 3d; 4b
Case study 18
1e; 2c; 3b; 4d; 5a
Case study 19
1d; 2b; 3c; 4a
Case study 20
1a; 2e; 3f; 4b; 5c; 6d
Case study 21
1b; 2c; 3d; 4a; 5e

www.ingramcontent.com/pod-product-compliance
Lightning Source LLC
Chambersburg PA
CBHW020723180526
45163CB00001B/88